AṢṬADAḶA YOGAMĀLĀ

AṢṬADAḶA YOGAMĀLĀ

(COLLECTED WORKS)

Volume 1

ARTICLES, LECTURES, MESSAGES

B.K.S. IYENGAR

ALLIED PUBLISHERS PRIVATE LIMITED
NEW DELHI MUMBAI KOLKATA LUCKNOW CHENNAI
NAGPUR BANGALORE HYDERABAD AHMEDABAD

ALLIED PUBLISHERS PRIVATE LIMITED

Regd. Off. : 15 J.N. Heredia Marg, Ballard Estate, **Mumbai**–400001
Ph.: 022-42126969 • E-mail: mumbai.books@alliedpublishers.com

47/9 Prag Narain Road, Near Kalyan Bhawan, **Lucknow**–226001
Ph.: 0522-2209942 • E-mail: lko.books@alliedpublishers.com

F-1 Sun House (First Floor), C.G. Road, Navrangpura,
Ellisbridge P.O., **Ahmedabad**–380006
Ph.: 079-26465916 • E-mail: ahmbd.books@alliedpublishers.com

3-2-844/6 & 7 Kachiguda Station Road, **Hyderabad**–500027
Ph.: 040-24619079 • E-mail: hyd.books@alliedpublishers.com

5th Main Road, Gandhinagar, **Bangalore**–560009
Ph.: 080-22262081 • E-mail: bngl.books@alliedpublishers.com

1/13-14 Asaf Ali Road, **New Delhi**–110002
Ph.: 011-23239001 • E-mail: delhi.books@alliedpublishers.com

17 Chittaranjan Avenue, **Kolkata**–700072
Ph.: 033-22129618 • E-mail: cal.books@alliedpublishers.com

60 Shiv Sunder Apartments (Ground Floor), Central Bazar Road,
Bajaj Nagar, **Nagpur**–440010
Ph.: 0712-2234210 • E-mail: ngp.books@alliedpublishers.com

751 Anna Salai, **Chennai**–600002
Ph.: 044-28523938 • E-mail: chennai.books@alliedpublishers.com

Website: www.alliedpublishers.com

First Published 2000

Reprinted 2001 (Twice), 2004, 2006, 2007, 2010, 2012

ISBN : 81-7764-046-1

Cover design : The Author
Artwork : S.M. Waugh

Published by Sunil Sachdev and printed by Ravi Sachdev at Allied Publishers Pvt. Ltd., Printing Division, A-104 Mayapuri Phase II, New Delhi - 110064

Invocatory Prayers

ॐ

Yogena cittasya padena vācāṁ
Malaṁ śarīrasyaca vaidyakena
Yopākarottaṁ pravaraṁ munīnāṁ
Patañjaliṁ prāñjalirānato'smi
Ābāhu puruṣākāraṁ
Śaṅkha cakrāsi dhāriṇaṁ
Sahasra śirasaṁ śvetaṁ
Praṇamāmi Patañjaliṁ.

I bow before the noblest of sages Patañjali, who gave yoga for serenity and sanctity of mind, grammar for clarity and purity of speech and medicine for pure, perfect health.

I prostrate before Patañjali who is crowned with a thousand headed cobra, an incarnation of Ādiśeṣa (Añanta) whose upper body has a human form, holding the conch in one arm, disk in the second, a sword of wisdom to vanquish nescience in the third and blessing humanity from the fourth arm, while his lower body is like a coiled snake.

Yastyaktvā rūpamādyaṁ prabhavati jagato'nekadhānugrahāya
Prakṣīṇakleśarāśirviṣamaviṣadharo'nekavaktrāḥ subhogī
Sarvajñānaprasūtirbhujagaparikaraḥ prītaye yasya nityaṁ
Devohīṣaḥ savovyātsitavimalatanuryogado yogayuktaḥ

I prostrate before Lord Ādiśeṣa, who manifested himself on Earth as Patañjali to grace the human race in health and harmony,

I salute Lord Ādiśeṣa of the myriad serpent heads and mouths carrying noxious poisons, discarding which he came to Earth as a single headed Patañjali in order to eradicate ignorance and vanquish sorrow.

I pay my obeisance to him, repository of all knowledge, amidst his attendant retinue.

I pray to the Lord whose primordial form shines with peace and white effulgence, pristine in body, a master of yoga, who bestows on all his yogic light to enable mankind to rest in the house of the immortal Soul.

This first volume of *Aṣṭadaḷa Yogamālā* published by Allied Publishers, Delhi, is the first volume of the first part of the "Collected Works" of Yogācārya B.K.S. Iyengar. Each part comprises several volumes which are arranged according to the following scheme:

Articles
Interviews
Question and answer sessions
Techniques of *āsanas, prāṇāyāma, dhyāna* and *śavāsana*
Therapeutic applications of yoga
Garland of aphorisms and thoughts
General Index and analytical dictionary
Addendum

Also by the same author

Light on Yoga
Light on Prāṇāyāma
Concise Light on Yoga
Art of Yoga
Tree of Yoga
Light on the Yoga Sūtras of Patañjali
The Illustrated Light on Yoga
Yoga ek Kalpataru (Marathi)
Arogyayoga (Marathi)
Light on Aṣṭāṇga Yoga

Also on "Iyengar Yoga"

Body the Shrine Yoga thy Light
70 Glorious Years
Iyengar His Life and Work
Yogapushpanjali
Yogadhārā

ABOUT THE AUTHOR

In section one of this book the author has given a wonderful and vivid account of his life and work.

We are including here a list of Yogācārya B.K.S. Iyengar's awards and recognitions which have been compiled by his students.

AWARDS AND RECOGNITIONS

1952 *Yogi Raja*, conferred by Swami Shivananda.

1962 *Yoganga Shikshaka Chakravarti*, conferred by Yogācārya T. Krishnamacharya.

1981 *Yogi Ratna*, conferred by Vishwa Yoga Sammelan.

1987 *Light on Prāṇāyāma* wins a Rs.5,000/- prize from the Lakshmibai National College of Physical Education, Gwalior, India.

1988 The Ministry of Federal Star Registration copyrights a star, with the number Monoceras Rabh 30M49sd +1i 29', in the name of Yogācārya B.K.S Iyengar.

1989 *Yoga Padmashri* conferred by Vishwa Yoga Samaj World Wide

1990 *Vashista Award* from the All India Physical Education and Allied Teacher's Association,

1991 *Padmashri Award* by the Government of India.

Fellow Concili Scientiarum confered by the International Council of *Āyurveda*, India.

1992 Life Membership of Medicina Alternativia Institute and Doctor of Science by the Open International University, Colombo, Sri Lanka.

Pune Pride Gold Medal award.

Punya Bhushan Award given by the Tridal of Pune.

1993 Gold Medal from the Indian Board of Alternative Medicines (Calcutta).

1994 *Visva Manava*, Man of the Universe, conferred by the President of Karnataka Yoga Center, Kolar District, India.

1995 *Gem of Alternative Medicine Award* by The Open International University for Complementary Medicine, (Calcutta) India.

1996 *Doctorate of Science* conferred by the University of Mysore, Karnataka, India.

1997 *Man of the Year* awarded by the American Biographical Institute.

Entered into the *International Directory of Distinguished Leadership*.

Man of the Year and *The Twentieth Century Award for Achievement* given by the International Biographical Center, Cambridge, England.

Board of Editors of the *Dictionary of International Biography*, Cambridge, England, included *Gurujī* in a pictorial testimonial for achievement and distinction published in the twenty-sixth edition of the *Dictionary of International Biography*.

Best Citizen of India awarded by the International Publishing House, India.

Vipra Ratna conferred by the Karnataka Brahmana Mahasabha.

1998 Included in a number of National, Asian and International Who's Who, Men of Achievement, Prominent Personalities of India, Contemporary and International Authors.

Awarded *Man of the Year* 1998 *by The American Biographical Institute*

Included in the *International Directory of Distinguished Leadership 1998.*

The International Biographical Centre, Cambridge, England awarded *Gurujī International Man of the Year* 1998

Twentieth Century Award for Achievement

Included in their volumes *2000 Outstanding People of the Twentieth Century and 500 Leaders of Influence*

Arsa-Kula-Sresthah conferred by the Arsa Vidya Gurukulam

1999 *Jeevan Sadhana Gaurav* award from Pune University

Gyan Kalyan Charitable Award from Sri Murli Manohar Joshi HRD and S&T Minister, Govt. of India.

Abhinava Patanjali Maharshi by Sri Chaitanya Vaishnava Vardhini Sabha.

Rotary Excellence Award from the Rotary Club of Kothrud, Pune.

Swami Vivekanand Puruskar Award by Acharya Kishore Vyas

Best Citizen of India Award, 1999, from the International Publishing House, New Delhi.

Eminent Personalities of India from The International Biographical Research Foundation of India

Yogadron Award '99 by the World Yoga Society (Calcutta)

2000 *Priyadarshani Award* from the Priyadarshani Academy (Mumbai)

CONTENTS

SECTION III – PATAÑJALI AND HIS YOGA SYSTEM

LIST OF TABLES

LIST OF ILLUSTRATIONS

Photos courtesy of Soni Studios, plate no.15 courtesy of Annie Ciekanski.

PREFACE

This is the first volume of *AṢṬADAḶA YOGAMĀLĀ* (The Garland of the Eight Petals of Yoga), a collection of my articles, speeches, talks, interviews, question-answer sessions and teachings written and delivered at different times and on different occasions.

These "Collected Works" comprise several volumes. This first volume contains my biographical works, the definition of yoga and the exposition of Pātañjala Yoga. The whole work is inspired of Patañjali's words of wisdom woven through the eight petals *(aṣṭāṅga)* of yoga, namely, *yama, niyama, āsana, prāṇāyāma, pratyāhāra, dhāraṇā, dhyāna* and *samādhi.* They are synthesised and presented in such a manner to ignite interest in the readers and inspire them to take to the practical aspect of yoga.

This collection is the brainwave of my pupils Sricharan Faeq Biria, Ph.D., of France, Patxi Lizardi, M.A., of Spain, John Evans of London and my daughter Geeta, who have been instrumental in collecting the material from different sources spread in different countries, and compiling them over the years. Probably, this volume would never have seen the dawn, if they had not first gone through this disparate material, devoting hours and hours for months together in editing and re-editing the manuscript, and Stephanie Quirk who worked patiently on the computer day and night to bring it into a harmonious and cohesive form thus making my work of further corrections and revisions easier.

As the talks and articles are from different periods of my yogic journey, repetitions were unavoidable. Some of these have been deliberately retained for the readers to observe and study the developments that evolved in me from my continual practice since the early days.

These new thoughts are maintained with coherency in the text and in the course of time may flash new thoughts and new wisdom in your *sādhanā.* As such I request the readers to accept and investigate enthusiastically these new thoughts, which may imprint in your heart and head a lasting impression that serves and guides those who seek to undertake this yogic practice in their lives.

All my pupils, who have contributed in the preparation of this work, share with me the merit and credit of this *AṢṬADAḶA YOGAMĀLĀ*.

I express my gratitude to Dr. Biria, Mr. Lizardi and my daughter Geeta for taking on the onerous work of preparing this text. They have done a wonderful job in presenting the nuances of the science and philosophy of yoga in a clear way, making it understandable to one and all.

My grateful thanks to Harper and Collins, Publishers (77-85 Fulham Palace Road, Hammersmith, London, W6 8JB), who have published all my classical books that have been cited here in *AṢṬADAḶA YOGAMĀLĀ*. This work is incomplete without reference to those publications.

I am also grateful to Allied Publishers, for willingly accepting to publish this work and the following volumes currently under preparation, acquainting the readers with the cultural and spiritual heritage of humanity.

Ramaamani Iyengar Memorial Yoga Institute, Pune
November 2000

B.K.S. IYENGAR

SECTION I

BIOGRAPHIC WORKS

HOW YOGA TRANSFORMED ME

Destiny can affect a man in a flash and alter his shape and character. In some it may affect very fast and in others it waits for hard, persistent and patient effort to experience its fructification. In my case, it is the latter which has played its role. What is destiny? Destiny is the accumulated actions and reactions of past lives, stored together to play their role in the present life. When destiny strikes like lightning and is accepted, one has to anticipate the challenges without oscillating one's mind. It has to be remembered that destiny alone is not enough. Balanced, determined efforts are necessary to build up character for progress. When destiny and efforts play together equally, they mould and change the life of that individual. If the changes are accepted, then the gates of luck open for him to move towards success and embrace its achievement.

I consider that I am one in millions who responded to the call of that flash of destiny. The moment I plunged into it, I stuck to it with faith, though failure after failure brought me despair, dejection and distress. I thought that by accepting these failures they might act as steps towards success, and so I pursued my fate's chosen path with relentless determination. After thirty-five years of persistent struggle my efforts bore fruit and made my life worth living. Call it fate or destiny or the hidden hand of God. Both fate and untiring efforts brought me to understand and realise the purpose of my life and the utilisation of my life for the good of society and the world at large.

Though it is embarrassing to speak or write about myself, I should set aside false modesty to show how my interest in yoga gathered momentum and transformed me, and how, with the new light in my yogic practice, I attracted people towards yoga and made it popular. I hope that this narration of my early life helps the students and lovers of yoga whose destiny brought them to me, to build up courage and strength in their practices.

I was born during the world influenza epidemic of 1918, in a village called Bellur, situated in the Kolar District of Karnataka State, India. The actual date of my birth is 14.12.1918, Saturday night at 3 a.m., which becomes Sunday according to Indian Standard Time. As my mother was in the grip of influenza, there was little hope of my survival, but the hands of God spared both of us. Nevertheless, I was born sick, with thin arms and legs, a protruding stomach and a heavy head. My appearance was not prepossessing and my physical weakness caused me despair.

As sorrow and pain follow each other like a chain, my health began deteriorating from bouts of illnesses like constant malaria, typhoid and as doctors suspected, tuberculosis of the lungs. All these brought me almost close to the jaws of death. I became a burden to myself and to my parents. When I was on the threshold of turning nine years, my father breathed his last, leaving a vacuum in our family. No one in the house could guide me to gain health. My studies were affected as I was forced to spend more days on a bed than at school. This made me a backbencher in the class and I always scored below the marginal passing marks. The authorities were promoting me to the higher class hoping that I may cope along with others. Study became monotonous and laborious to me.

The turning point in my life came for the better in March 1934. My *guru*, Shri T. Krishnamacharya, was my brother-in-law. He was married to my elder sister. Before his marriage, he was staying in Varanasi studying various *darśanas*. From there he went to Nepal and learnt yoga under a great master known as Shri Ramamohana Brahmacāri. After his return from North India to his native place, Karnataka, he was running yoga seminars at various places. The Maharaja of Mysore, the late Krishna Rāja Wadiar Bahadur IV, hearing of my *gurujī*, opened a *yogaśālā* in the Jaganmohan Palace of Mysore and patronised that school. He appointed my *gurujī* to teach there. The Maharaja also sent him to various places to propagate yoga.

In 1934, the Maharaja sent my *gurujī*, with his pupils, to visit Kaivalyadhāma at Lonavla and Bombay. He broke his journey at Bangalore. As I was having summer holidays, he asked me whether I could go to Mysore and stay with my sister until his return. As I had not seen the city of Mysore and had heard of the palaces and lush gardens, I willingly said "yes," to his suggestion. He gave me money to buy the ticket to go to Mysore.

When my brother-in-law returned from Bombay I asked for his permission to join my mother and my brothers and sisters in Bangalore. Instead of allowing me to go home, he suggested that I join the school in Mysore to learn and practise a few *āsanas* to gain my health. Probably, the fate that was in store for me might have been planning to change my future life. Belonging to a poor family, and with the loss of my father, becoming even poorer, we had to live according to the then prevailing conditions. So, I consented to my brother-in-law's suggestion, stayed back and joined the school, as it did not matter to me whether it was Bangalore or Mysore.

He began teaching me *āsana*, to improve my health. Having rested on a bed for years, my body had become so stiff that I could hardly bend down and extend my arm to reach my knees. As my brother-in-law had implanted the seed of yoga in me, I began to address him as *gurujī*.

Though I was struggling hard in yoga, I was not sure that yoga would do me any good, as my body was not responding. I stayed with my *guru* for two years. In the beginning, he did not show much interest in teaching me, possibly due to my weak physical condition. After one year had passed, one day, a young but advanced student who was staying with him, left forever without intimation to *gurujī*. This made my *guru* turn his attention on me to make me practise yoga daily, both morning and evening. He also became very stern, which built a fear complex in me. So, I had to do yoga as demanded by him. The hard practice of yoga, walking everyday from house to school, from school to house, from house to *yogaśālā*, from *yogaśālā* to house, as well as doing my homework, brought about severe aches and pains, and added fatigue to my weak physique. This physical exhaustion was affecting my mind and study became so difficult that I fell asleep whenever I sat for my homework. Though I was practising yoga, *gurujī* did not explain to me any of the principles or subtleties of yoga. Circumstances forced me to do as commanded by my *guru*. I did not turn to yoga as a vocation, for I was not born in the house of yogis, saints or philosophers. Now I consider that it was a stroke of good luck that yoga pursued me even though I was indifferent towards it. Soon my *guru* asked me to run classes at the *yogaśālā* whenever he stayed home.

In 1936, the Maharaja of Mysore sent my *guru* with a few pupils, including me, on a lecture-cum-demonstration tour of Northern Karnataka, which then belonged to the Bombay Presidency. A number of people including ladies wanted to learn yoga and they requested *gurujī* to start classes for them.

In those days, women were shy of practising yoga and were not ready to stand in front of grown-ups and elderly men. As I was the youngest of the group my *gurujī* asked me to conduct classes for the ladies and they gladly accepted me as their teacher. Thus, the seed of teaching yoga that was implanted in me has now grown into a mighty gigantic tree, spreading its branches in all the six continents of the world, for yoga to stay and grow healthily for centuries to come.

People began asking me to teach yoga. I was a novice in the field. Teaching demanded experience. My immature practice and limited experiences daunted my courage. On one side I was nervous of taking the responsibility and on the other, the mind kept asking, why should I not take a chance? So, with fear in my heart, I meekly accepted to teach, being careful not to take any risks, whatsoever. This meekness forced me to practise more and more in order to gain experience faster and faster for two reasons. First, to improve my health by regular practice in order to share my practice with students; and second, the joy of remaining independent at my young age. The interest in yoga came not from the love of yoga, but for the sake of earning my livelihood.

In 1937, the Deccan Gymkhana Club of Pune, invited my *guru* to send an instructor to teach yoga for six months. *Gurujī* was very keen that someone should go and teach. Six months was a very short period, but none of my *gurujī's* senior students were willing to accept this offer. At that time all his students were from the Mysore *Sanskṛt Pāṭaśāla*. I was the only one who was going to a school where English was a compulsory subject. As I knew a bit of English, *gurujī* thought of me and ordered me to go. I accepted it as I was looking for freedom from fear. I met the Club members who asked me to teach in various colleges, schools and physical education centres. This was quite a heavy responsibility for my age. Those who were coming to the classes were elder in age, bigger in size and more cultured in their behaviour.

For me it was a great delight to enter the college premises to teach yoga, when I had not even completed school education. I was weighing about thirty-two kilos and my chest measured only twenty-two inches. It increased by half an inch only after inhalation. The first humiliation I faced was when the college students laughed sarcastically at me when looking at my figure. Ironically, their behaviour made me face them boldly and accept the challenge. The second weakness in me was the language. I was neither good in English, nor in my own mother tongue, let alone the language of the land, Marathi. The third weak point was that I had no theoretical knowledge or practical experience. I was without any qualification, but was forced to call myself a yoga teacher. I was faced with the option of acquiring second hand knowledge from books or to practise vigorously, with determination to gain first hand information through subjective experience. I opted for the latter and began practising ten hours a day to master what little I had learnt from my *guru*.

Soon, the college authorities appreciated my work and my services were extended for three years. After that I continued teaching independently. The intense effort I had put in improved my health and my teaching helped me to obtain a bare minimum to carry on, covering only my basic needs. It took years of practice to gain control over my body. I slowly achieved physical health and mental stability, and my approach to the problems of life became philosophical. I confess that in the beginning my mind could not grasp the vast background of the art and science of yoga, but with devoted effort my knowledge increased. It took years of patience and hard work to attract people from all walks of life towards yoga. But I cannot put in words the suffering I underwent.

My hard practice caused agony to my body, to my nerves, to my mind and even to my self. I was tossed from one side to the other; sometimes the body refused to co-operate and at other times the mind would not bear the pain. This way my body and my mind oscillated. My energies were sapped and mental fatigue set in. If I did not try, the self within grew restless: if I tried, failure brought on dejection. Very often exhaustion brought me to the point of collapse. I could neither eat nor drink with comfort. Sleep was almost impossible due to pain and failure causing restlessness in my body and mind. Even easing myself had become a problem. Though I continued practising yoga for years, dejection and doubt tormented me and my mind found no rest except in renewed effort. Each day was an ordeal but God's grace forced me to make one more attempt for every failure. As I had no guide, I made enormous mistakes but I learnt discrimination from observing my own errors. When circumstances forced me to live on my own, I had to go without food for days. Often I lived only on a cup of tea, but the inner flame kept on goading me to do my daily practice with zeal. Slowly, I began to feel that my body was growing in strength, my restless, agitated mind was gaining stability. Though I started with the practice of yoga in 1934 it was only in 1946 that an innate interest in yoga arose in me.

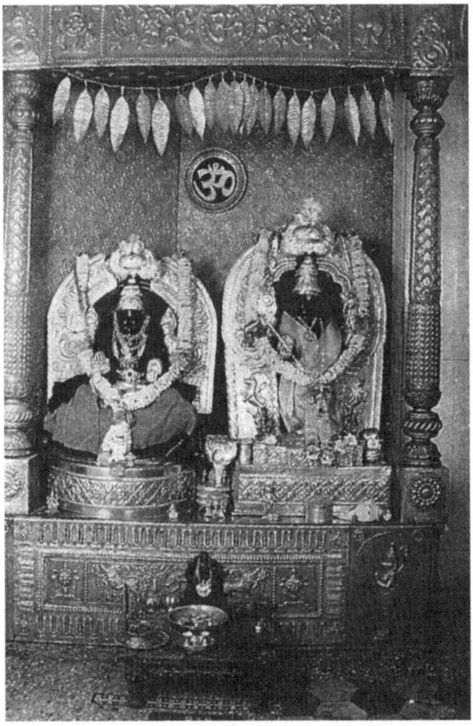

Plate n. 1 – Bālāji and Lakṣmi

I had a dream. I saw the Lord in a dream. Our family Deity Lord Venkaṭeśwara (commonly known as Bālāji) smiled at me and blessed me in a dream. I was told by the Lord, that I had no other vocation but to practise and teach yoga. The Lord blessed me with one hand and with the other hand gave me a few grains of rice. The benevolent Deity told me that from now on I should not worry about my physical survival. This dream gave me hope to continue my practices. The same night my wife too dreamt of Devi Lakṣmi, who gave her a coin, saying that She was returning the said amount She had borrowed from me long long ago.

The very next day pupils called on me for lessons and from then on, my stars have been always ascending and the grace of God continues to be upon me. My only regret now, is that I am not thanking Him as much as I was cursing Him in the days of my hard trials. From 1934 to 1946 yoga was attached to me willy-nilly. Today it is I who am attached to yoga. However it has not been all that easy since then.

In 1958, I felt that I was losing my grip on the postures. I felt dizzy, heavy and stiff. Correspondence with other yogis including my *guru* brought me no relief. I was only told that married life and age must take their toll. Even the forward bends were very painful. However, after another three years of effort I recovered and regained control, which I did not lose until 1979. In 1979, immediately after my sixtieth birthday celebrations, I had two scooter accidents. These set the clock back so much that I had to start yoga all over again as a raw beginner. All my old pains and aches re-appeared. It took me more than eight years to fight and regain control over my body and mind. This again was through my determined effort to get back into yoga, and yoga graced me to embrace it with reverence.

With all these efforts, I cannot say even today that I have completely mastered this art and science. The more I work towards refinement, the more insignificant my efforts appear to be and I feel that perfection has yet to be reached. In this way, I am learning to be content with this divine discontentment that drives me on. Practice takes my mind and intelligence closer to the core of my being. With this experience, I should like to give you all this encouragement, that even if perfection tries to elude you, do not reduce your efforts.

Yogic discipline lifted me from a sub-human level and made me a man of confidence, sincere in my efforts, hardy and honest, clear in my thinking and clean in my conscience.

If yoga had not stuck to me and I to yoga, probably this art would not have become accessible to average people nor would it have become popular. I was overlooked and branded by people as a mad cap in my early days (I may be pardoned if I say that). Now I am the proudest man on earth as I carry the message of yoga along with many of my pupils, in the form of physical health, mental poise, intellectual clarity, and spiritual solace for millions and millions of people all over the world. It is yoga guiding me in my *sādhanā* to see God in all. If yoga could do so much for me, who was not even blessed with health and good nourishment in early life, it is not difficult to imagine how much it will help those who start their practice in more fortunate circumstances.

No doubt, the art and science of yoga is vast and progress therein seems to be very very slow. As per doctors' study, due to tuberculosis, I was supposed to have only lived for twenty years or so, but the practice of yoga has not only made me live a full life of satisfaction and joy, but it has made me its messenger all over the world.

Even though age is telling upon me, I am still experiencing new feelings. I do not hesitate to share the light of my new experiences with my pupils. I live in my cells and I live in my heart. I would like to practise yoga till my last breath, as a humble service to yoga. My only wish is to prostrate before God, surrendering my last breath in a yogic posture.

MY YOGIC JOURNEY*

Though the title "My Yogic Journey" sounds very well, it is always very embarrassing to speak about oneself. When I have to speak on my yogic journey, you should know that my life is interlinked with yoga and yoga with my life. Naturally it is very, very difficult to speak of yoga and myself as different entities. Yoga being interwoven with my life, the moment I speak on yoga I am totally involved. Forget what I say about myself but take only the yogic essence to learn, adjust to conditions as circumstances demand from you, in the field of yoga.

I do not know whether destiny was there for me to do yoga or some force from childhood changed the frame of my destiny. As far as I recollect, destiny may or may not have been at all in my favour while I was in my mother's womb. She was affected by the world's epidemic disease, influenza, which consumed millions of lives. Fortunately, we both survived, but at the cost of health of the body and growth of intelligence in me. The disease tremendously retarded my physical and mental conditions. Life was a drag from birth to adolescence. My sisters and sisters-in-law used to say that my head would hang down on a repulsive body in such a way that they never touched me on account of my appearance. That was the body God gave me.

Every six months there were medical check-ups in schools. At the age of thirteen, when I was studying in the third standard of the middle school, I was suspected of having tuberculosis of the lungs and medical treatment was advised. Our economic conditions kept me away from medical treatment. As ill luck comes in chains, tuberculosis, constant malaria and a twenty-one day typhoid fever deteriorated my health further and affected not only my body but my mind also. At times I felt like committing suicide due to this parasitic life. I never played during my childhood, nor had books to read. Being weak my education moved at a snail's pace. Because of these, I could not even sit for half an hour at a stretch to read my books. Like retired people drawing their pension, I was scoring pass marks on the borderline of thirty to thirty-five percent, just enough to get through. Teachers were promoting me to the next higher class thinking that I may take pains and score better in future.

---

* Based on the talk given on the occasion of B.K.S. Iyengar's 70th Birthday at Tilak Smarak Mandir, Pune14.12.1988.

In those days there were two public examinations held throughout the state. One was the Lower Secondary School Examination, and the other was the Secondary School Leaving Certificate Examination. Unless one got through the Lower Secondary School Examination, one was not allowed to join a High School. As I failed in the Lower Secondary Examination, I had to appear again after a year to get through the examination. With great difficulty I passed in 1933 and joined the High School. Being poor, I was given 'half freeship' in 1933. In 1936, I failed in the Secondary School Leaving Certificate Examination and lost my half freeship. Thus, my education came to an end.

PLAY OF DESTINY

Destiny must have had another role for me. In 1934, when my brother-in-law was asked by the then Maharaja of Mysore to visit Bombay and Lonavla to observe the scientific progress that was going on there in the field of yoga, my brother-in-law broke his journey at Bangalore and asked my elder brother and me whether he or I could go to Mysore and stay with our sister till his return from the tour. My elder brother did not show any interest. As I was having summer holidays, I consented to join my sister, hoping to see the Maharaja and to visit the city of Mysore with its palaces and lush gardens. My brother-in-law gave me the railway fare and I took the train to Mysore. After visiting Lonavla, Bombay, Dharwar, Belgaum and other places, my brother-in-law returned to Mysore. When my holidays were coming to an end, I asked him to permit me to go to Bangalore to attend school. But he advised me to join the High School in Mysore and pursue my studies there. He tempted me when I hesitated, promising that he would teach me yoga to improve my health. As I had not experienced what health really was since my birth, I accepted this tempting offer to stay back.

After waiting for a month or so for 'D' day to arrive, and my brother-in-law would show me the way to improve my health, I was called and he taught me a few *āsanas*. When I began with my lessons, due to years of bed rest, my middle fingers could not even reach my knees when I bent forward. As he was teaching me yoga, I addressed him as *gurujī*. *Gurujī* said that if I did not make an effort, I would not gain back my health. After teaching me for a few days, he advised me to absorb his lessons before he would instruct me further. As my body was stiff like a poker, he neglected me and lost interest in teaching me. I lost my old friends in Bangalore and gained no friends in Mysore, as I was not allowed to go anywhere but to school. He would get up very early and set things for us to do every day. His temper was always running high. People call me a lion, but I don't know what you would have called my *guru* if you had seen him in his early days. My *guru* was a man of immeasurable knowledge and unpredictable moods. It was not easy to read his mind. If he said one thing at one time, he used to contradict the same at another time. We were made to accept and obey him in toto without questioning. For example, if I sat in the ordinary cross legs position, with left leg first, he would say, "Take the right first." If the right was placed first, he would say, "Take the left leg first." If I stood, he would say, "Is that the way to stand?" If I changed, he would say, "Who asked you to change?" If I took my food, using certain fingers, he would say, "Use other fingers." Subsequently, he would admonish me if I followed his earlier advice. Life became perplexing. The difference in age set fear in my heart and his presence was like a frightful nightmare.

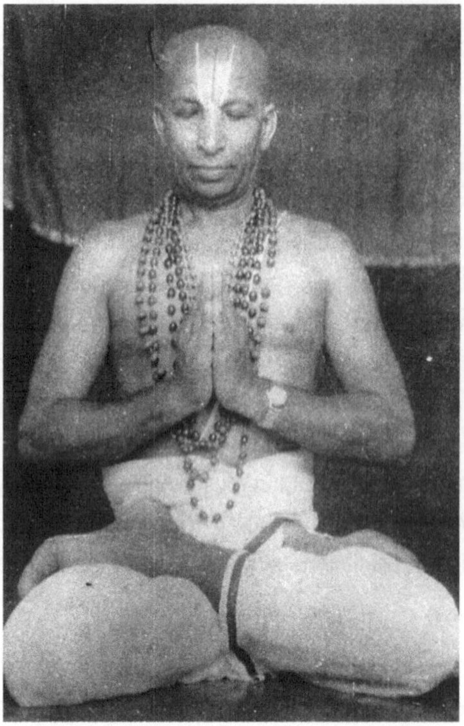

Plate n. 2 – Shri T. Krishnamacharya

Owing to my *guru's* nature, his acquaintances and friends would avoid him. I remember very well that people would walk on the left footpath, if he was on the right side.

Fear of *gurujī* created confusion in my mind, and whatever he wanted me to do, I was doing wrong. This fear and confusion in turn created an unstable mind in me. At that time, a very loveable student of *gurujī's*, by the name of Keshavamurthy, was doing yoga very well. This boy's *āsana* is recorded in the *Yogamakaranda*, a Kannada edition, written by my *gurujī* about fifty years back, and in a shorter version of it known as *Yogāsanagaḷu,* published by the University of Mysore, as part of a popular series. One fine morning this young boy, all of a sudden, left *gurujī* forever. This created a void in me, as I had no other friend except this boy. Whenever *gurujī* scolded him, me, or both together, we would console each other. In this way, we lived together for a year. His departure was a turning point in my life. *Gurujī* was a very commanding and demanding person. As I was his relative, he had more access to me than to other students. As soon as my only friend and companion left my *gurujī*, never to return, naturally *gurujī's* eyes turned on me.

In December 1935 an International YMCA convention was held in the city of Mysore. Being such a prestigious conference, the then Maharaja, Shri Krishna Rāja Wadiar Bahadur IV, a wise and benevolent king, extended an 'At Home' to the delegates and sent word to *gurujī* to give a demonstration along with a few pupils. My *gurujī* said that he would teach me a group of *āsanas* for a few days, which I should practise daily and prepare for the demonstration. Being his brother-in-law, I thought that if I failed in my presentation, the Maharaja might find a more serious fault and ridicule the whole presentation. Naturally, in order to save his honour, I said to myself, "I should do well." I struggled very hard with tears in the eyes and tremor in the body. He never asked me to rehearse before him. He only told me that I should be ready. Being weak, I was nervous to appear in public. But his words were orders. Believe me or not, I did as asked and got a coveted prize of fifty rupees from the hands of the Maharaja as a token of appreciation. Though I was in ecstasy at that moment, I was in agony with pain and tremors for months.

MY *GURU'S* UNPREDICTABLE WAYS

I will now narrate some anecdotes. One day, in 1935, V.V. Srinivas Iyengar, a well-known criminal judge of the Madras High Court, visited our *yogaśālā* in Mysore and wanted to discuss yoga with my *gurujī* and to see a demonstration. Each student was asked to do certain *āsanas* in turns. When my turn came, my *gurujī* asked me to present *Hanumānāsana*. He knew that his senior students would not do it. As I was staying with him, he knew that I would have to obey him. I went near him and whispered in his ears that I did not know *Hanumānāsana*. He at once stood up and asked me to stretch one leg straight to the front and the other back and to sit erect. That is *Hanumānāsana*. In order to avoid this very difficult *āsana*, I told him that my underwear was too tight to stretch the legs. In those days the underwear was called *Hanumān caḍḍi*. They were stitched so firmly by the tailors that even one's fingers could not pass through, between the groins and the underwear. Wrestlers used them, as the opponents could not grip the cloth. These *caḍḍis* cut the skin, leaving permanent marks and changing the colour of the skin of the leg pits. In order to escape from this torture, and knowing that I could not perform this *āsana*, I told him that the *caḍḍi* was too tight. Instead of giving me the benefit of doubt, he asked one of his senior pupils, C.M. Bhat (who later taught yoga in Bombay), to fetch a pair of scissors from the office and cut the underwear on both sides and told me to perform the *āsana*. As I didn't want to be an instrument of his wrath, I surrendered to his wishes and performed the *āsana*, but with a tear in my hamstrings which took years to heal.

In 1938, while I was in Pune, *gurujī* visited Pune. My pupils arranged a lecture on *Mīmāṁsā* and yoga at Agnihōtri Rajwade's house. While the demonstration was going on, he asked me to perform *Kaṅdāsana*. I knew the name but had never tried it as I suffered pain in my ankles, knees and groins. I expressed my innocence of the pose. He said, "Bring both feet together towards the chest, as if you were doing *namaskār* with the feet." Having tasted freedom, I had the courage to tell him that I could not do it. He flared up and in our language (Tamil), told me not to degrade him or put him to shame on the platform when so many people were watching. Well, as usual, I surrendered to his anger and did the *āsana* with great difficulty to save his honour. But my forced performance left excruciating pain in the groins. When I told him of the pains, he said I should learn to live with them. In short, when I was a student, my *gurujī's* way of teaching was that we should present any *āsana* the moment he demanded, without any comment. If we refused we were not served with food and water, we had to forgo sleep and instead we were forced to massage his legs until he said it was enough. If our fingers stopped moving, the marks of his powerful hands were on our cheeks.

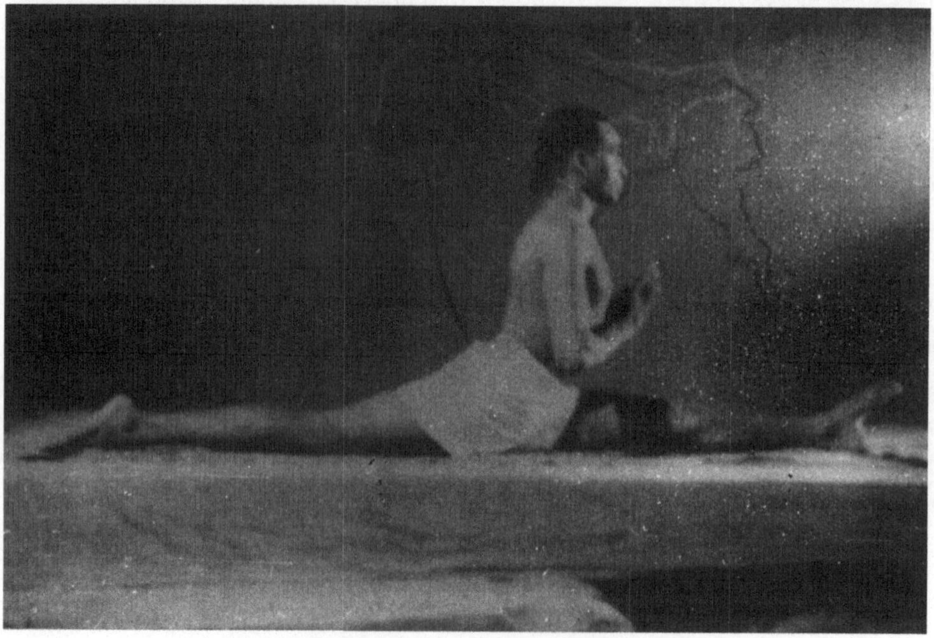

Plate n. 3 – *Hanumānāsana*

CHANGE OF CIRCUMSTANCES

I stayed for two years with my *guru* and his wife, my sister. In 1936, the Maharaja of Mysore sent *gurujī* with some of his pupils on a lecture and demonstration tour to Dharwar, Hubli, Belgaum and other places. *Gurujī* asked me to accompany him and his senior pupils. Being the most junior student, I was asked to supply water from the well for everyone's bath. The wells of Hubli and Dharwar were fifty to sixty feet deep and one had to draw water from that depth. It was a hard job to supply water for all. I did this for two or three days. The rope cut through the skin of my palms and fingers. It was beyond my physical strength to draw water for all. I told the members that I would fetch water for *gurujī* and the rest would have to get water on their own. This created friction amongst us, and complaints went to *gurujī*. *Gurujī* heard them and told me that I alone should supply water to all. This irked me and I refused to take orders and said that I was not a servant for everyone and those who wanted to have a bath, should draw water from the well for their bath. I showed my hands to *gurujī*. Instead of examining my palms, he was hurt by my curt reply and disobedience. He stopped talking to me for a few days and began calling me 'commissioner', as there was one bearing my name. I remained stubborn, which changed his attitude. He gave me the chance to demonstrate with others in public.

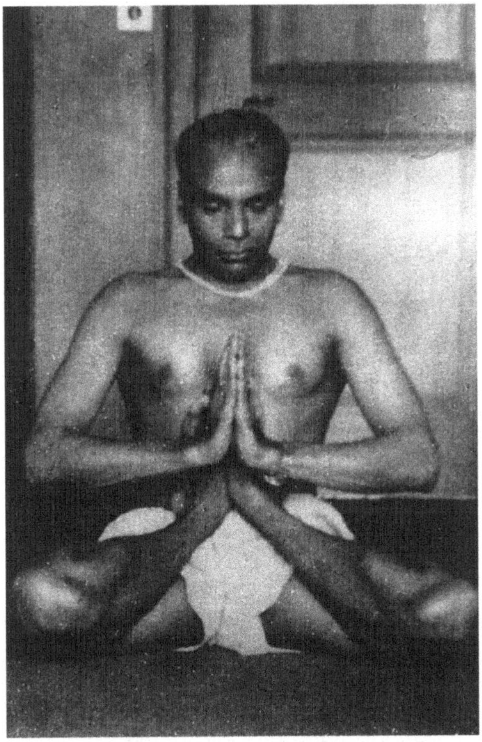

Plate n. 4 – *Kandāsana*

People became interested by our demonstrations in yoga and began asking my *gurujī* to start a yoga class for them. In the '30s, ladies did not mix with men; co-education was not yet in vogue. Girls and boys, as well as men and women were segregated. Ladies also asked *gurujī* to teach them yoga. He asked some of his senior students but the ladies being shy, preferred to learn from me, as I was the youngest in the group. This was the play of destiny. My *guru* had no other choice but to allow me to teach them. Though I knew very little, within fifteen days, the ladies who attended my class were happy with my teaching and conveyed their joy to my *gurujī*. This is how the ladies of Dharwar ignited my interest in teaching yoga.

SEED SOWN TO BECOME A YOGA TEACHER

From Dharwar, we went to Belgaum. The programmes for us were arranged in the city. There, the civil surgeon of Belgaum, Dr. V.B. Gokhale, after seeing our demonstrations, became interested in yoga and requested my *gurujī* to send some senior teachers to teach yoga for six months in schools, colleges and sports centres of Pune. *Gurujī* wanted one of his senior pupils to accept the offer, but almost all of them were reluctant to go for six months. Another reason was that they were not acquainted with the local language or with English; they only knew *Sanskṛt* and their mother tongue, Kannada. So the axe fell on me. As I was going to high school, I knew a bit of English. *Gurujī* asked me to take the responsibility of going to Pune and teaching there.

ARRIVAL AT PUNE

When I came to Pune, I was a boy of eighteen years. Dr. V.B. Gokhale told me that I should teach in schools and colleges. In those days yoga was taught individually and not collectively. I knew how to teach individually but not collectively. I thought within myself that I should face and accept this challenge. Yoga was not a popular subject then. Indiffrerent economic conditions kept people away from the pursuit of purely cultural activities, creating a void in communication. Reasons are not difficult to trace for this wanton negligence. During plunder and invasions by Timurlang, Mohammed Ghori, Mahmood Gazni and later the British and others, precious writings and materials were destroyed. People moved to remote places to save books from destruction. Hence, things became scattered and only small parts of the scriptures were retained here and there. We have to revitalise the art, science and philosophy, including yoga, to form a single chain of thought for people to clearly understand these subjects.

HEREDITY OF YOGA

You should know that many people were and still are under the impression that my method of yoga has nothing to do with the traditional art form. This is far from the truth as my *guru* had a *guru*, who also had a *guru*. My practice of yoga has a *paraṁparā* (heritage). My *guru* learnt yoga in Nepal, about two hundred and ten miles from Kathmandu, at a place called Muktinarayaṇaksetra under the able guidance of Shri Ramamohana Brahmachari. The great philosopher Ganganatha Jha (father of Amarnath Jha, the vice-chancellor of Kashi Vidya Peeth) had accepted my *guru* as his pupil. My *guru* passed *Sāṁkya, Tarka* and *Mīmāṁsa* examinations within one year, standing first in all these subjects. Ganganatha Jha advised his pupil to go to Shri Ramamohana Brahmachari, with whom he had a good relationship, and to undergo practical training in yoga with him. Soon, my *guru* went to Nepal and was accepted by Shri Ramamohana Brahmachari as his yogic pupil. He stayed there for many years and learnt this art directly from his *guru*. Hailing from Karnataka, my *guru* returned to Mysore to settle there and began teaching yoga.

Being his pupil, my method of practice is based upon his teaching. So naturally I am tradition bound.

In our community there was a great yogi by the name of Nāthamuni, the great-grandfather of Yāmunācārya. Nāthamuni wrote a treatise on yoga known as the *Yogarahasya*. Though this treatise is not available, all scholars accept that it existed and continue to quote him as the master of yoga. Hence it is not my yoga, but a purely traditional yoga. As Albert Einstein became the father of nuclear science, I consider my *guru*, and my *guru's guru* as fathers of yoga who sowed the seed to think and analyse the practical side to bring about further development in this art. The seed of the tree may be the same, but they grow in different directions, bearing fruits of different tastes. In the same way, coming from the seed, whether it is my colleagues or myself, we might have changed techniques like the branches of the tree, but all of us belong to that one tree alone. With this traditional background I carry the message of yoga when opportunities are thrown in my direction.

Here, I began teaching in schools, colleges and clubs. The college students were not only my elders, but were well educated, cultured, and civilised. I was a simpleton, not knowing how to speak or behave like them. However, I made up my mind not to get agitated or dejected but to work and prove the worthiness of yoga. By sheer will power, I began teaching and performing the *āsanas* with them without showing exhaustion. This was the turning point in winning their minds. Another reason for my inferiority complex was that I had a long tuft of hair at the back of my head, half shaved in the front. Having come from an orthodox Hindu Brahmin family, I was not allowed a hair cut. Coming out in the streets with long hair naturally was a problem. Hence, I used to hide it, using a cap. Being young, people called me a madcap, a lunatic, because when asked I proudly said that I practised yoga. I preferred to bear these hurting remarks for the sake of freedom, which permitted me to act as a freelance. I was afraid of my *gurujī's* moods more than people calling me a madcap. Freedom had come to me by chance and I did not want to lose it at any cost. If I returned, I would have to rejoin my *gurujī*. That meant living in the web of constant fear. Without hesitation, I made up my mind that I should enjoy this God given freedom, come what may. In order to maintain my freedom, I thought that I should practise more and learn to speak better English, as I was not very familiar with it. Though I read books on yoga to get the basic ideas on the subject, they did not interest me at all. I observed the positioning of the *āsana* in these books. The *Sālamba Śīrṣāsana* of one person was different from that of another. Each *āsana* was differently illustrated by the authors. I felt that these practitioners were presenting *āsana* according to their whims and fancies. Doubts and confusion led me to do all their presentations to find out by

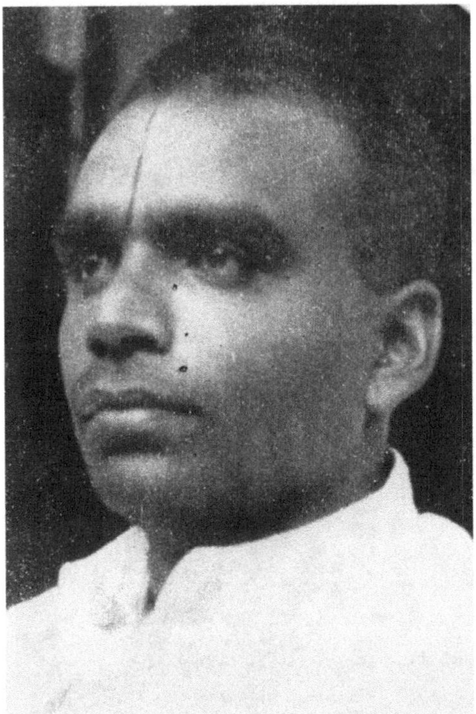

Plate n. 5 – "Long hair tuft at the back, half shaved in the front"

trial and error, to discover the correct methods and reject the wrong. I began imitating the *āsana* according to the illustrations, but they never gave me satisfaction or the right feeling. I never read or looked at books on yoga again. The moment my true journey in yoga began, trials and errors stopped daunting and taunting me.

MY FIRST SUCCESS IN A PUBLIC APPEARANCE

Pune is a main centre for wrestling, even today. Gama and his brother Imambaksh had to fight with Puransingh of Punjab in 1937. The tickets sold out like hot cakes. The wrestling match was held at the Deccan Gymkhana's Wrestling Arena *(Ākhāḍā)* where I was teaching. Though the sale of tickets was still continuing, the wrestling match ended as Imambaksh defeated Puransingh in half a second. The hands of the referee went up and the people were upset, as they had come to see the wrestling match. The crowd became restless and vandalism broke out and the police had a tough time catching the culprits. Thousands had gathered and the Deccan Gymkhana Club's honour was at stake. The members requested that I give a demonstration to attract attention and save the situation. I was more than happy to give a demonstration before world figures like Gama, Imambaksh and Puransingh, let alone the local wrestling enthusiasts. As they were all

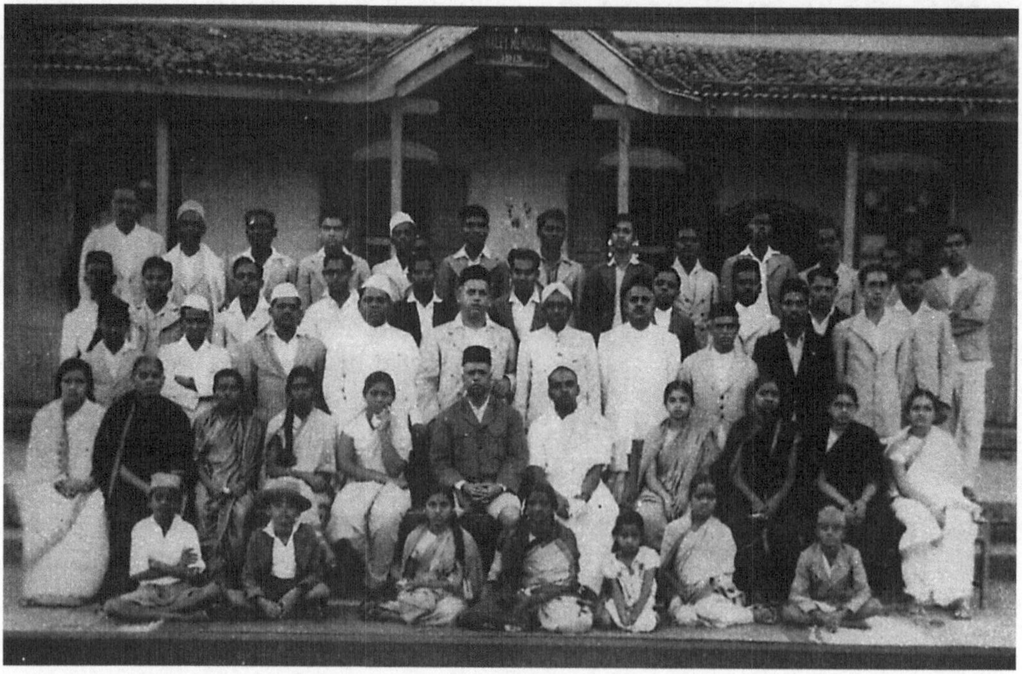

Plate n. 6 – Deccan Gymkhana – 1938

watching my demonstration, I was inspired to do well. I gave a forty minute demonstration with 'fantastic' *āsana* to start with, so that people's attention was drawn towards the demonstration. I succeeded in winning great appreciation for this art. On account of this demonstration, Gama, Imambaksh and I became very friendly.

Deccan Gymkhana owned a building next to the Post Office, where rooms were provided for guests at a nominal rent. Rooms were provided for the wrestlers adjacent to my room. Each time they went out or came in, they used to knock at my door requesting me to lock or unlock their doors. I was wonderstruck at their request and asked them why they could not lock or unlock their own doors. The locking system was above and not at the centre of the door. They could not raise their hands above their shoulders and hence, I was called to help them. Looking at their dependence upon someone, I asked them how they went to the latrine if they could not move their arms up and bend their legs? To this curious query, they said, "We cannot squat well as we cannot flex the knees fully. So we squat as far as we can bend and pass the faeces as much as we can, so we put on weight and remain uncomfortable." From the wrestlers' life of dependence, I learnt that this type of a life is also an unhealthy life. This was the foundation for an understanding of the value of yoga, where one keeps all movements of the body under control. I thought this was something in yoga to be imbibed and started accepting the challenges of school and college students, and continued to practise and teach.

PAINS

Someone asked me to speak of my body pains. As my pains and aches increased millimetre by millimetre through all parts of my body, I became an ardent student and adamant practitioner. That was the beauty of my practice. I used to bring big and heavy stones from the streets to place them on my legs, arms and head to lessen my aches and pains. Even after hours of daily practice, the *āsanas* were not coming right. Dejection as well as restlessness was writ on my face. I could not endure the strain due to the tuberculosis of my lungs. I was so rickety that one could easily count the ribs on my chest. I had no visible muscles. Naturally my body was a laughing stock for the college students. Looking at me, they used to say that yoga did not develop muscles. As I did not want them to know my medical history I gave no explanation. Unfortunately, all my students were better built than I was, so it was natural for them to make jokes about me. On account of their jokes, I became more determined within myself that this was the time to learn well. I persisted in my practices. I used to devote ten hours every day to mastering this art.

MY FIRST INNOVATION

In 1938, the ex-Principal of Ferguson College, Prof. Rajawade, who was then eighty-five years old, was suffering from dysentery. He could not even walk. At the instance of Dr. V.B. Gokhale I began teaching him. He became my *guru* for inventing methods for teaching invalids. My first inspiration to create came on account of Prof. Rajawade. Just as one lies down to do *Śavāsana*, I made him do *Supta Trikoṇāsana* in a supine position. First, I separated his legs, moved the trunk to one side and then stretched his hands sideways, as if doing standing *Utthita Trikoṇāsana*. Similarly, I began teaching him *Supta Pārśvakoṇāsana, Supta Vīrabhadrāsana, Supta Ardha Chandrāsana* and so forth. This original thinking of finding new ways continues even now, to help both healthy and unhealthy people. When I tell professors about my work with Principal Rajawade, no one believes it as he died more than five decades ago. But people forget that I have taught yoga for fifty-four years.

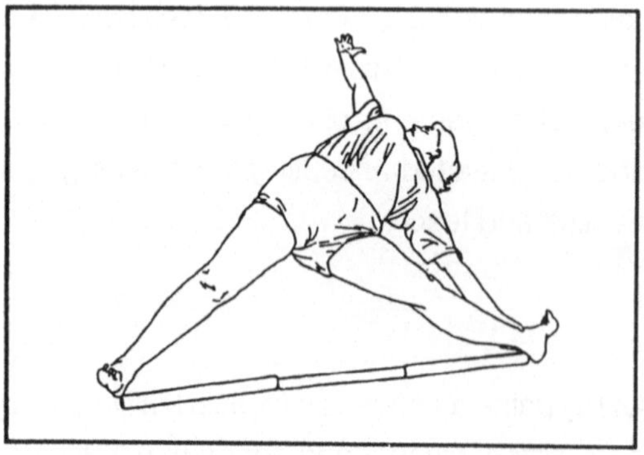

Plate n. 7 – *Supta Trikoṇāsana*

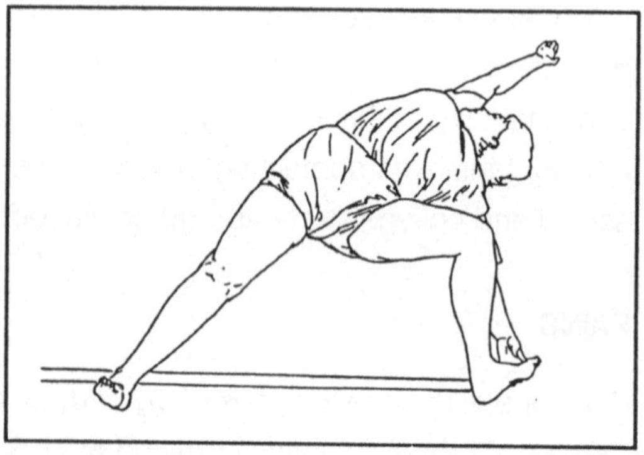

Plate n. 8 – *Supta Pārśvakoṇāsana*

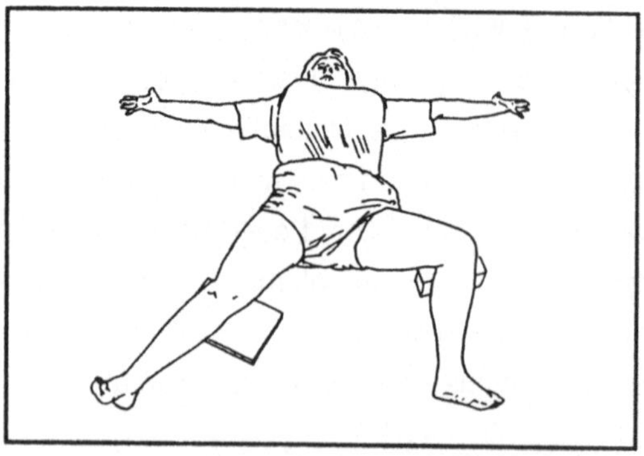

Plate n. 9 – *Supta Vīrabhadrāsana*

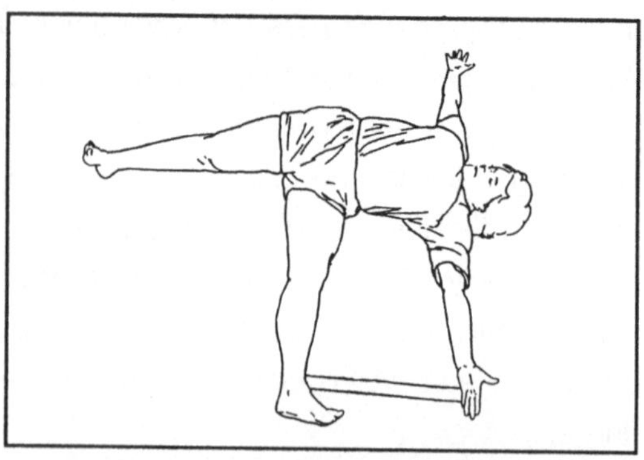

Plate n. 10 – *Supta Ardha Chandrāsana*

CHALLENGES FROM THE MEDICAL PEOPLE

Then came challenges from the doctors that yoga could not help diseased people. I accepted their patients and proved the value of yoga.

Professor D.B. Deodhar, the great "grand old man" of Indian cricket and former captain of the team of the State of Maharashtra. In 1938, he could not play cricket because of his knee injury. Prof. Deodhar being a friend of Dr. Gokhale, wanted him to operate on his knee. Instead of operating on his knee, Dr. Gokhale advised him to try yoga with me. If yoga failed, then he would operate. The Professor could not stand too long. Circumstances brought challenge upon challenge, which I accepted. With trial and error, I went on developing the intricacies of each *āsana*. Though these seemed to be a waste in the beginning, the positive results began to appear later. This increased my faith in yoga. Within a few days I flexed the professor's knees without pain. Pleased with this progress, he again started playing cricket. He began hitting century after century in first class matches, until his retirement. This inner penetration by looking into the bodies of others developed my awareness. This keen awareness taught me to focus my attention and to look and feel within myself, to penetrate the *āsana* into the inner body while doing them. In this way, I developed the awareness to penetrate the mysteries of the human body.

Though *gurujī* taught me a few *āsanas* while I was in Mysore, I depended upon my own study to find ways and means to master the subject.

HOW I BEGAN *PRĀṆĀYĀMA*

In 1941, I went to Mysore. I requested *gurujī* that he should teach me *prāṇāyāma*. Knowing the capacity of my lungs and my under-developed chest, *gurujī* said that I was not fit for *prāṇāyāma*. Whenever I approached him to teach me *prāṇāyāma* his answer was the same.

Again in 1943, I visited Mysore for a few days. As I was staying with my *gurujī* and knowing that he would not teach me *prāṇāyāma*, I thought of watching him while he practised *prāṇāyāma* in the mornings. *Gurujī* was a regular practitioner of *prāṇāyāma* always practising at a fixed time in the mornings, but he was never regular in his *āsana* practice. He was in the habit of getting up very early, but my sister was a late riser, so nobody knew that I was up to observe his practices. I wanted to see how he sat and what he did with his facial muscles. I stealthily peeped through the window and observed his movements very carefully. I wanted to learn to sit, to stretch the spinal column and relax the facial muscles. Each morning I watched his adjustments and movements, the dropping of the eyeballs, the closing of the eyes, movements of the eyelids, lift of the chest, movement of the abdominal organs, maintenance of the waist, the sound and flow of his breath. Having observed his practice minutely, I was tempted, approached him with humility and pleaded him to teach me *prāṇāyāma*. He said that it might not be possible for me to do *prāṇāyāma* in this life. His refusal to teach me was the seed for me to start the *prāṇāyāma* practices myself. Though I was determined to do it, it was not as easy as I had thought it to be. I struggled the same way to do *prāṇāyāma* as I struggled to learn the *āsana*. With failure after failure, dejection and discontent, I restlessly persisted with the practice of *prāṇāyāma* from 1944. The pains and struggles of 1934 reappeared even in the *prāṇāyāma* practices. The end of struggle, dejection and the state of restlessness came only in 1962-63 and not before, though everybody was proclaiming that yoga brought poise. I was laughing at their statements and thought it all to be nonsense. Restlessness and unhappiness prevailed over me for decades. In the beginning I could not do even one breath with any rhythm. If I took one deep inhalation, I had to open my mouth for the exhalation, as I could not release the breath through the nose. If I inhaled normally to master deep exhalation, I could not draw in the next breath due to the laboured releasing of the breath. I was under constant pressure. I was not finding the cause of this problem and my *guru's* words that I was an unfit student for *prāṇāyāma* were ringing in my ears, bringing a negative state of mind in me.

Like a religious person, each morning I would get up early for *prāṇāyāma*, and after one or two attempts I used to lie down, thinking within myself, "I cannot do it today, let me try tomorrow." This process of getting up in the early morning and not practising after one or two attempts continued for years. Then one day I made up my mind to do at least one cycle before losing heart in between. Then after an interval, I followed with a second cycle with great difficulty. I used to give up for the third cycle, as it was next to impossible. In this way, I pursued the practice daily but it was ending in failure; yet I succeeded after eight to ten years' to sit for one hour at a stretch for *prāṇāyāma*. Many may not believe that it took me such a long time.

The reason why it took me so long is on account of my spine, which could not take the load of sitting straight. As my *gurujī* was asking me always to do backbends, my spine used to go backwards in the sitting positions. I was not doing any forward bends and often avoided them for years because they were painful for me to do. This type of escape opened my eyes to re-think and re-adjust my methodologies. I realised that mobility comes with backbends, but not the strength and stability. I began the forward bends with fervour. I was determined to master each and every *āsana*, whether standing ones, sitting ones, twists, backbends, hand balances or inversions. For a few years I began practising all the *āsanas* meticulously to straighten my spine which was giving way while doing *prāṇāyāma*. When I felt strong in the spine, I again began my *prāṇāyāma* practices daily.

MY *PRĀṆĀYĀMA* PRACTICES

Do not laugh if I tell you about my efforts. I used to wake my wife up very early in the mornings to make me a cup of coffee. After preparing the coffee for me, she used to go back to sleep. The moment I sat for *prāṇāyāma*, a hooded cobra seemed to appear in front of me, hissing and ready to strike. I used to wake my wife up to see the cobra! She knew that it was just fear or hallucination. Later, while performing *Sālamba Śīrṣāsana* or any other *āsana*, this vision of the hooded cobra would return in a flash. It continued for a few years. Suprisingly, it never appeared when I was not practising yoga.

I spoke to friends and acquaintances who began to brand me as a 'mad cap'. I became nervous and wrote to Swami Shivananda of Rishikesh as well as some other yogis including my own *guru*. At that time yogis were very few, their numbers could be counted on the fingertips. No one replied. I wrote several times to my *guru*, though he regularly answered all my letters, he never touched upon my problem. I felt that they might not have undergone what it was that I was inflicted by. As no one was obliging me, I stopped writing and pestering them with my problems, but persisted in my efforts. Each time I saw the cobra I woke up my wife to sit next to me, as moral support, so I could face my nervousness with courage. This continued for nearly two to two and half years. The vision of the hooded cobra during my practices eventually disappeared on its own.

Though my *guru* never answered my queries, when he came to Pune in 1961, he asked me, "He! Sundara*, you were writing about seeing a cobra at the time of your practice. Are you still seeing it?" I replied, "No." Then he asked me "Did it touch you or bite you?" I replied, "No." Then he told me that he did not write to me because he was waiting to hear of my reaction. "As it neither touched nor struck you," he said, "you are blessed with yoga." Then he narrated the story of his colleague who had the same problem as mine. One day he went to their *guru* and requested him, "Sir, the cobra was coming to me in my practice but today it has bitten me and has made me mentally and physically sick." It seems that my *guru's guru* told that pupil, "The cobra has bitten you, you are a *yogabhraṣṭan* (fallen from grace)." My *gurujī* remembered this and said, "You have been blessed as the cobra did not touch you", and told me to fearlessly continue with yoga from then on. After this incident, the sacred syllable *Āuṁ* always flashed before me like a dazzling light. On account of this dazzling light of *Āuṁ*, I was not able to walk easily or ride a bicycle. I asked my *guru* also about this. He said that I was very fortunate to see the *ĀUṀ*. His encouragement enthused me to devote more and more of my time to yoga.

---

* My given name is Sundararāja; hence relatives used to call me Sundara.

DREAMS

There is a very famous temple called *Anañtapadmanābasvāmi* at Tiruvananthapuram. I dreamt of the temple God and, as I was prostrating before the Lord, a burning flame flew from the forehead *(Kapāla)* of the Lord, and fell on me. My *gurujī* was standing next to me. I was telling the Lord to burn me, but not to burn my *guru*. For sometime, the fire engulfed me. Though I was caught within it, it did not touch or burn me. I asked my *guru* the significance of this. He said that I was lucky to come out of the blazing fire untouched, that something was guiding me in my practice.

Similarly, once, in a dream, I got up to fix a picture of Lord Bālāji (Śrīnivāsa) as it was on my table. While nailing it to the wall, two heads of a cobra, which cover the head of the God as a crown, fell down. I was shocked and stopped nailing and looked at the picture as if to question why this was happening. The Lord appeared and said that the two heads were missing because I was using nails. I approached *gurujī* for an explanation, who told me, "You have to be re-born twice to get perfection in yoga", which I happily accepted. If I recollect this, I am happy that I can think of continuing with my yoga even after death!

THE PLAY OF DESTINY WITH MY MARRIAGE IN 1943

For years, my economic situation was very very bad. I could not earn enough to meet my daily necessities. In 1943, my *guru* wanted me to reach him in Rajamahendry (Andhra Pradesh) to give a yoga demonstration. After the demonstration, both of us returned to Bangalore. He looked at me and asked me why I was not getting married. I said, "When I can't stand on my own legs, what is the use of marrying." Instead of accepting my answer, he said, "You are teaching lots of girls. You must have fallen in love, so you are not keen to marry." My *guru* was not only a master of the scriptures but also very clever. He spoke so well that even such fanciful statements seemed true. He played with words with my mother, who was alive, as well as with my brothers and sisters saying that living alone at the age of twenty-four in Pune was bad. As I was in Bangalore, he insisted that they should get me married the same year so that I may not go astray and be a victim of bad influences. Everybody began coaxing me to get married. I wanted to settle well in life before planning for a married life. My fear was that as I couldn't look after my self, I would not be able to look after my partner. I did not want my would-be partner to suffer on account of my uncertain income. My *gurujī*, with unpalatable words, threatened me saying that I had no character and went to the extent of disowning me as his pupil.

Believe me or not, whenever I visited Bangalore, I never shaved in order to keep away offers of marriage as I knew my relatives would insist I marry. I was growing a beard and moustache (which were appearing a little here and there) so that girls would reject me. This had its effect on several occasions. Parents with their daughters would call at our house. Seeing my unshaven face, they used to discard me.

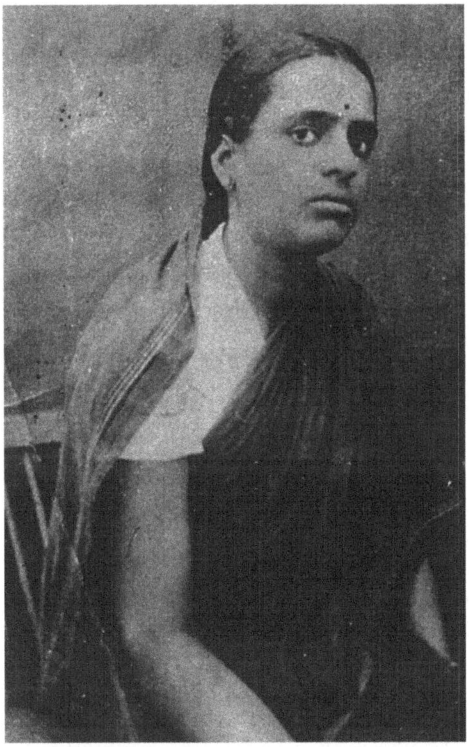

Plate n. 11 – Young Ramaamani

MY PROPOSAL WAS GOD'S DISPOSAL

One fine day it happened that destiny was waiting for my wedlock. My would-be wife Ramaa came to see me one fine morning and waited for thirteen hours, until night, because on that day I was to have come from Malur (twenty-five miles away from Bangalore). Due to some unforeseen work, I was held up and did not come until 9 p.m. This girl with her sister had waited at our house since 9 a.m. Their waiting at a strange place moved my heart. I wondered how an unmarried girl could wait so long to see me! It must be the will of God that kept her waiting. Her long embarrassing stay, at an unknown house moved me and I consented to marry her, provided she willingly accepted to marry me without any interference.

MARRIAGE

The marriage day was fixed for the 9th of July 1943. I borrowed from my pupils of Pune a sum of 1,500 rupees to meet my marriage expenses.

As I was out of touch with my pupils for three months, I immediately returned to Pune after the marriage. I contacted my pupils thereafter to renew their lessons. They shocked me. They politely stopped my lessons, saying that the amount I borrowed from them was to be treated as their wedding gifts. I blamed my stars! Fate had dragged my wife to suffer too along with me. For three months I remained without any earning. My patience paid a dividend. In November 1943, one school authority invited me to teach in their school and also some patients wanted treatment from me. This new hope made me write to my wife to come and join me. This was the first time we met after our marriage. Many of you must have read of our married life in *Body the Shrine, Yoga Thy Light*, and *Iyengar: His Life and Work*.*

OUR LIFE IN PUNE

After four months of marriage we met each other at Pune station and began our life with only the bare necessities of life. Though we could barely make ends meet, we wanted to live as a single soul, accepting both good and bad evenly with magnanimity. We spoke to each other of our wants, our drawbacks and what was close to our heart.

When Ramaa came to Pune, she knew nothing about yoga. I explained to her about yoga and my efforts in the field of yoga. All these years, I was struggling to master yoga on my own. When my wife joined me, I wanted her to help me to master my subject and I guided her to assist me in my practice. We both loved each other and got so attached that we often forgot our needs of life. She was very quick to help me in my practice. I began guiding her in the art of teaching yoga. I explained to her how to use pressure, how to hold, where to press and the way to stand and stamp and so forth. She was slightly heavier than medium size. Her weight was a blessing in disguise. Instead of carrying heavy stones on my body, I showed her ways to use her body for proper pressure, sometimes showing her how to use her knees, thighs, calf, heel, arch, sole and fingers, as the occasion needed. Many times, I used to hold her legs and arms to get my right pose. I guided her in how to place a weight on me. With the knowledge I gave her, if she were alive today, I think she would have become a top class yoga teacher for ladies.

She developed sensitivity and a gentle touch. She knew exactly where to touch to arrive at the right pose. No doubt, she sacrificed her life's interests for me, to keep me contented and able to pursue my art. She never grumbled even once and she never complained of my carelessness in looking after the family. My morning and evening practices and visiting various places in the city to teach swallowed my entire day. Often we talked to each other while I was doing inverted *āsana* for an hour! I had to cycle from one end of the city to the other, covering thirty to thirty-five miles a day. I was cycling, practising with my students as well as doing my own practices. This was sapping my energy. I began introducing her to local people and shopkeepers. Sometimes I made her teach some orthodox ladies who wanted to learn yoga. We settled between us that I should go and teach wherever I was called so that our earnings should help the children to get educated and her job was to run the family and look after the children. Not

* *Body the Shrine, Yoga Thy Light*, (Bombay, 1978, pp. 53-60), and *Iyengar: His Life and Work* (Timeless Books, USA, 1982, pp. 35-57).

once did she ask me to go for a movie or to a concert together. She never asked anything for herself. What a character she was. It was a strange coincidence that in both our families, the two of us were completely different from the other members of the families.

RAMAA'S DEATH

When fortune favoured us with a comfortable life, God snatched her away from our midst in 1973. Though she is no more with me, her life is entwined in me and yoga together. Yoga is no yoga for me without thinking of her. She has made her abode in my heart and ever lives with me as long as my conscious awareness remains in me. That is why I do not feel her loss, even after her death. Her compassion and affection towards me helped me to master this subject. If I asked for help while doing an *āsana*, she used to come at once leaving all her other work. It is on account of her that today I am what I am. I am not only grateful to her but I am sure that those who knew her are also indebted to her. But without her co-ordination and co-operation in my chosen path, you all would not have learnt what should have been learnt. You too have had the good luck to get this knowledge. The credit and merit of my work is equally shared by my wife, even though she is no more. I am indeed grateful to destiny for binding me to Ramaa in order to become both a yogi and a householder. I cannot speak more about my wife. Otherwise I will forget my journey of yoga.

SPREADING OF YOGA

To popularise yoga, I thought of working on patients recommended to me by medical professionals and showing the results of yoga on diseases. In 1945, Dr. Kini, a top class orthopaedic surgeon of Madras, had a patient struck with polio of the spinal column. She was the daughter of the late Mrs. Fatima Ismail, founder of the present famous rehabilitation centre at Mahalaxmi, Bombay. Fatima Ismail was a well-to-do lady and also a nationalist. When Shri Jayaprakash Narayaṇ went underground, he stayed at Fatima Ismail's house. The authorities came to know of this and raided her place. It seems she hid him under her cot and thus saved him from imprisonment. Dr. Kini was a friend of Dr. K.C. Gharpure, a famous surgeon in Pune. Dr. Kini wanted his patient to undergo treatment from Dr. Gharpure, as Fatima wanted to stay in Pune for its good climate. As I was teaching Dr. Gharpure and his wife (both medical practitioners), he asked me to take this case and teach yoga to improve the girl's affected spine.

The girl's mother (Fatima Ismail) was a strict disciplinarian like my *guru* and possessed a strong will power. She would stay at home and ask her children to tell me that she was not at home. Hiding herself in the house, she wanted to find out whether I taught her daughter honestly and sincerely. After a month's stay like this she came to pay my fees. At that time, she said, "Mr. Iyengar, I am really sorry, but I must confess my guilt that I was at home while you were teaching. I was watching to find out whether in my absence you really teach or if you take things casually. You are an *ustad*, a hard taskmaster. Before you, I had engaged many teachers at so many places, but not one worked with my daughter as you worked." Soon Dr. Kini examined the child and was delighted to observe that life had come in the child's spinal column and the child could take the load. Now Usha (the child) is a mother of two children. This success spread mouth to mouth, and I was approached by the proprietor of a prestigious hotel by the name of Moritore, whose daughter was affected with polio after an injection. The proprietor, Mr. Gulam Hussain Pakseema, asked me to take up his daughter's case. I agreed to try my best. She improved faster than the doctors anticipated. Now she is the mother of three children, settled in America. Her leg was affected, but I made her not only walk well but ride a bicycle too.

Like this, whenever a problematic case was presented to me, I was happy to accept the challenge to prove yoga's worth.

Let me cite another interesting case. One Mr. Pocha of Pocha Seeds had a strangulated spine, which paralysed his alimentary canal. Dr. M.S.H. Modi, a well-known physician, examined him and advised the family to shift the patient immediately to Bombay for an operation under Dr. Ginde, then a famous neuro-surgeon. He said that if the operation was delayed, the patient would be permanently paralysed. The family members took him to Bombay and admitted him to Breach Candy Hospital for an operation. After the operation, a physiotherapist was engaged for post-operative treatment. Though the treatment went on for a month, Mr. Pocha never showed signs of progress. Mr. Pocha was learning yoga from me before the accident. He had full confidence that I would help him at this juncture, for quick recovery. Dr. Ginde was reluctant to try yoga, as he was absolutely against yoga, but could not go against the wishes of his patient. I was called from Pune to meet the doctor. As soon as I met him, the first thing he said was, "No yoga, you have to work according to my directions."

Naturally, I confessed to the doctor that I knew no system other than yoga and questioned his rejection of yoga. He said that lots of yoga practitioners who learned *neti* (passing thread through the nostrils) and *dhauti* (swallowing of cloth to cleanse the alimentary canal) had developed pus formation and came to him for treatment. Observing these, he was antagonistic towards yoga. When I asked him why he did not bring it to the notice of their teachers, he said that it was the role of the patients to tell their teachers. Probably if these people had gone and informed their teachers, they would have changed their views and would have been careful to introduce these techniques. As the doctor had treated the injured yoga students, he had a dislike for yoga. So he did not want me to teach yoga to his patient. I told him that I teach only *āsana* and *prāṇāyāma* and not those techniques which he had referred to. As the patient was keen to be treated by me, the doctor was not willing to go against his patient's wishes. I made him practise simple leg movements like a therapist. He was later discharged to proceed to Pune and I began assisting him as advised by the doctor. The doctor was coming every fortnight for a check-up. Since 1954, I have been regularly conducting weekend classes in Bombay. After my classes on Sundays, we both came together to Pune by road. Twice a month, he examined the patient and said that the patient was not progressing. He was expecting recovery in three months after the spinal operation. As three months were approaching, he was worried, as he saw no signs of improvement. He gave me freedom to handle the patient but wanted progress in two weeks' time. Otherwise he would say, as the common adage goes, "The operation is successful but the patient never improved." I accepted this challenge and promised to show him progress in two weeks' time.

Mr. Pocha's bladder could not hold urine. It was dribbling all the twenty-four hours. I told Dr. Ginde that I would work first to get control over the bladder. As Mr. Pocha was my student, it was easy to teach him poses like *Supta Baddha Koṇāsana, Supta Pādānguṣṭhāsana, Ūrdhva Prasārita Pādāsana* and so forth, to strengthen the floor of the bladder. I made him sit and stand with my support. The doctor came after two weeks and was impressed with the patient's condition. Soon I made him walk with my support. Dr. Ginde laughingly said, "You labour and I get the credit. I appreciate your knowledge and will send my patients to you after I have operated." Since then, until his death, he referred his patients who needed my touch to me. Creating an interest in yoga through therapeutic means added to its popularity. I have convinced many medical practitioners that yoga is an alternative healing medicine. Even today, when they fail in their treatments, they direct their patients to me as a last resort. As I went on accepting their cases, yoga gained momentum as a science. I am always grateful to Dr. V.B. Gokhale, who in the early days inspired me to take cases and encouraged me to experiment with the value of yoga. He made me think and work with affected people.

THE WAY PEOPLE JOKE ABOUT YOGA

When I came to Pune in 1937, its population was 100,000. Very few people showed any interest in yoga and would ask me, "We are told that yoga has tremendous value and influence on the health of the individual. Can we get a child if we practice yoga?" Though I was nineteen years old, I never knew what sex was. Yet when such questions were asked, I used to say a big "Yes, provided one does yoga for three to four years." I would tell them affirmatively that yoga and God would bless them. And this happened on several occasions.

Let me narrate an interesting episode on yoga. Once on my way from Bangalore to Pune, I broke my journey at Hubli for a month to teach a few of my old pupils. It was in 1937. There was a textile mill called the Bharat Mill, now known as the Hubli Mill. An accountant of this mill had no issue at all. He asked me, whether he would be blessed with a child if he practised yoga. I said, "Yes." He asked me to teach his wife, saying that he did not need yoga, as he had no problems. According to tests, he said that his wife needed treatment and not he. Something was telling me that God would bless them if they both did yoga. He was adamant and wanted me to teach his wife only. Though I agreed to teach her, I told him that I couldn't guarantee anything, if both did not do yoga. It happened as I thought. I taught the lady for a month. Later, I was informed that the lady had conceived. I was pleased with my yoga and the innocent promise. Later, I came to know that she delivered a stillborn child. Though this news shocked me, it intensified my enthusiasm in yoga. It enhanced my faith that yoga could play wonders provided it is pursued honestly and correctly, with the right method. I felt that her husband's reluctance to do yoga was the cause of this stillborn child. God made me realise my promise only halfway because the husband had not practised and yet she, through her practice, conceived.

In 1940, I was staying in a hotel at Rasta Peth. Racegoers staying at the hotel would ask me to give them a number from one to fourteen. Innocently, I used to give them numbers, though I did not know why. Soon I came to know that they were racebirds betting on my predictions and making money out of it. They tempted their friends to contact me as an astrologer and a *brahmacārī* to make fortunes on my predictions. They began asking me to give them two figures from one to one hundred. Suspicion came on account of their daily calls. Inquiries revealed that they were betting on American Cotton opening and closing figures. If the two numbers were accurate, a rupee bet was fetching them eighty-eight rupees. When I came to know of this, I decided to refuse such requests and stopped their invasion of my time and place.

Fortunately, I was not tempted to go to the races and preferred to live an innocent life without paying much heed to my correct predictions! I attribute all these to my right practice, dedication and devotion to yoga.

I had students who had never had any children. After clinical tests, the doctors were of the opinion that they have no chances of having a child. They were blessed with many children after practising yoga.

MEETING KRISHNAJI

In 1946, J. Krishnamurti was in Pune; he had lots of followers. Somebody told me that he was the greatest thinker of the twentieth century and a world personality. As I was not reading books, or papers, I was not aware of men or events of the world. Even Yehudi Menuhin writes in his book that I talked to him as one talks to an average individual. He says, "Mr. Iyengar never knew that I was an internationally reputed violinist."

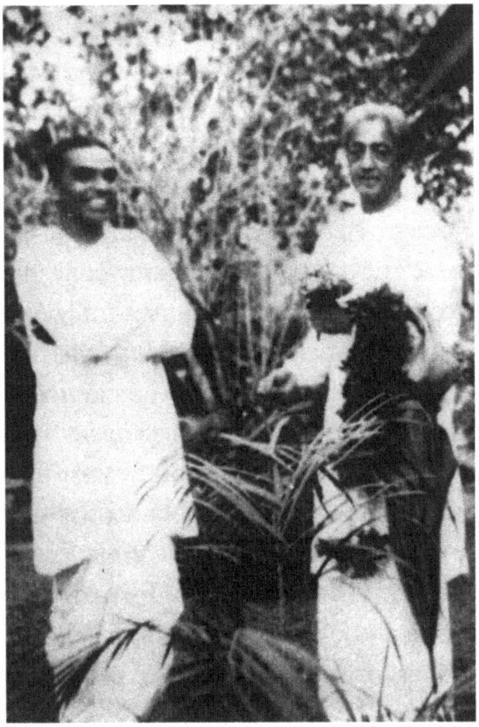

Plate n. 12 – With Krishnaji

My pupil Mr. F.P. Pocha was an old friend of Krishnaji and went to see him. My name cropped up in conversation as both were practising yoga. Mr. Pocha arranged a meeting between Krishnaji and myself and warned me that Krishnaji might ask me to teach him yoga. Krishnaji was staying at the Servants of India Society.

The day I met him, I gave a demonstration, which he watched with rapt attention. At the end of the demonstration he said, "Sir, you are a professional in yoga". I was twenty-eight years old then. I said, "Sir, I do not understand your remarks to me, nor do I know what devotion is. Sir, you are giving lectures everyday. Is not lecturing your profession? You are invited to give talks as I am invited to teach. If you call me a professional, Sir, I have every right to call you a professional speaker." He must have been shocked and surprised to hear my frank statements and moved to other topics.

After the demonstration, I asked him to show his yogic practices. He showed his reluctance to do them on the pretext that he had already done them in the morning. I left his room and was talking to his admirers who had gathered in hundreds. As I was with the group, he called me in. He was so happy that I began correcting his *āsanas*. He felt refreshed and experienced lightness and exhilaration.

Immediately, he expressed his desire to learn from me. He said that he loved to learn, but being poor himself he could not afford to pay the fees. I could not believe what he said. However, being too poor myself, I agreed to teach him on one condition, that I would come and teach him in my free time. After ascertaining the timings of discussions and talks, I said, I would come at 4 a.m. "It is too early", he said, for which I replied, "Sir, it is not possible to come at other time as I go to others to teach in order to earn my livelihood. The only free time I can spare is late noon. If you can shift your evening talks a little later, I can come and teach you." As he said that this was impossible, in the same vein, I stuck to my timings. For me, to earn and maintain my family and myself was as important as meeting people for him.

I narrated this conversation to Mr. Pocha. He told me to go and teach Krishnaji for two days instead of teaching him. I went to Krishnaji at 6 a.m. After two days I told him that I could not come at 6 a.m., as I had to go to Mr. Pocha. Krishnaji agreed to be ready at 4 a.m., and was waiting in time to open the doors. I learnt humbleness, from this great man. As I began teaching him, I made it a point to attend his talks at Tilak Smarak Mandir. The first sentence I heard was, do not criticise and do not justify. Though he repeated these words in all the talks, he used them as weapons in lectures throughout his life. He used to criticise all the religions and all the leaders of the world. But I learnt something from him, that I should not be disturbed or swayed by the opinions of others. For example, yogis all over the world criticised me, that my yoga was physical, but I was not in the habit of criticising others. You don't find me attacking or criticising others or their systems. I was and am very clear in what I am practising. I am not doing yoga for other people's comments. Let them criticise as long as they wish to. I do for the sake of doing and am keen to evolve myself in my practices. I am not keen to justify that what I do is right, nor take it for granted that my practice is perfect. I have a searching mind, hence I do not bother about others' remarks but I act to re-discover my inner body. Certainly, if occasion arises and I am attacked directly, I will reply to the criticism. I learnt another thing from him. Once, when I was explaining to him the art of stretching the legs without hurting the muscles and joints, he caught my ankle and said, "What a stupid man I am that I did not understand this much." That was his calibre as a student.

We have heard him talk of breaking one's conditioning and living unconditionally. While I was teaching him in Switzerland I used to tell his followers that Krishnaji was tied to his own conditions though he refuted it. One may say anything, but actually what is important is the way one lives. Having stayed together for five to six hours everyday, living in the same apartment, I knew his moods and way of life. One day I called his hostess to show her how Krishnaji was a conditioned personality. He always used to face the wall but not the mountains while he was balancing on his head. I just turned the carpet for him to do *Sālamba Śīrṣāsana* facing the mountains. He sat down and turned the carpet back to its original position. I just laughed and said, "Sir, why are you turning the blanket? You could have turned yourself and faced the wall instead." He laughed and said, "It did not strike me that I could do it without disturbing the blankets."

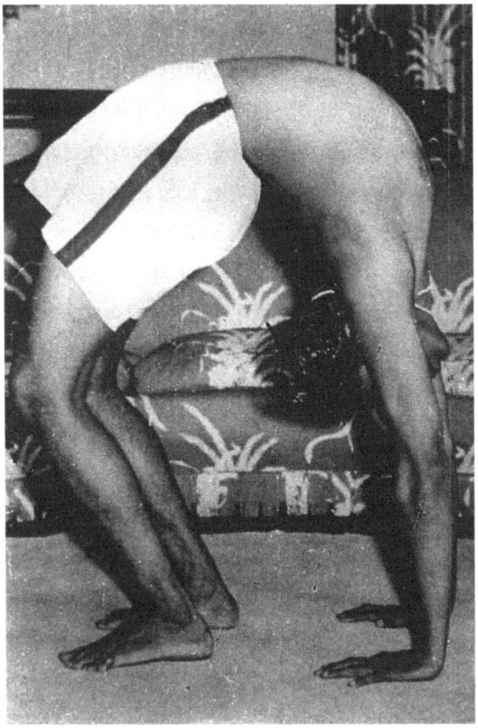

Plate n. 13 – *Ūrdhva Dhanurāsana*

Similarly, his words of challenge and response convey a negative meaning for a lay person. It may convey to one to accept all challenges without counter challenges. I say all challenges should be met equally with counter challenges. If two stones hit one another with equal force, the 'response' is light. I feel that challenge and counter challenge are meant to weigh the forces of thinking and action so that they trigger evenly for the inner intelligence to develop its own awareness in full. It means reconditioning and not unconditioning of oneself.

Once I was teaching him *Ūrdhva Dhanurāsana*. I was explaining the backbends and asked him to feel the vibration of his inner knees. He asked me to explain the vibration and how it could happen in the inner knees. I said, "Sir, don't you ask, in your talks, whether one has ever heard the sound of the trees? As the 'sound' of the tree is vibration, so too, vibrations in the knees are produced when you do backbends with firm feet. Vibrations in the tissues and fibres of the body are sure sounds to feel the right action." Like this, we used to discuss, and an intimate friendship developed.

HER MAJESTY THE QUEEN MOTHER OF BELGIUM

The Queen Mother of Belgium was eighty-four years old, when she invited me to teach her yoga. On the first day I began with simple standing poses and *Halāsana*. She was not willing to stop there. She wanted me to teach her *Sālamba Śīrṣāsana*, head-balance. I had not taught head balance to any person who was eighty-four! She was very slim with poor development of the muscles, but had very strong will power. When I looked at her, I knew she had some problems. So, I told her that before thinking of head-balance, I would like to examine her health condition. You know that in today's yogic centres, blood pressure and heart conditions are recorded before and after yogic practice. Being the Queen Mother, medical check-ups must be regular. When I asked her about her physical condition, can you guess what question she posed? She asked me, "Have you faith in yoga?" Laughingly, I said that it would be impossible for me to impart yoga

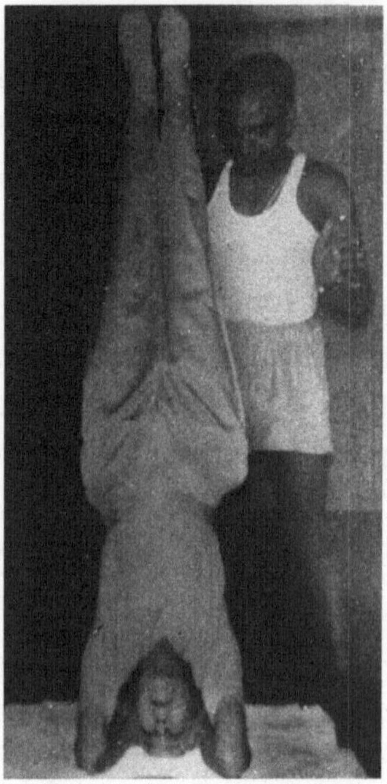

Plate n. 14 – Queen Mother in Head balance

without faith in it. I would have left the practice long ago if I had not built up faith. She asked me a simple and direct question. "Sir, if you have faith in yoga, why do you want my medical report? I may be suffering from anything. Will you teach me head-balance or not? That's all I want. If you are afraid of teaching me head-balance, then you can take the next available train to Gstaad, Switzerland, and join your esteemed friend Yehudi who recommended you to me. Please go back in case you are afraid to teach me head-balance." Observe how clear she was in her thoughts to get what she wanted. While appreciating her courage, I said to her that if she had the courage to do head-balance, I had the courage to teach her. She immediately asked me to do so. I prepared the base, by placing her head on the floor with cupped finger locks. The moment, I lifted her legs and put her on her head, she became unconscious. Her body was collapsing and her muscles and bones began sinking. I was in two minds. If I brought her down, she would say I did not take her lesson seriously. If I kept her in that pose, God alone knew what could happen. I took courage, lifted her from the ground, formed a cup shape with my feet and placed her head between the arches of my feet and waited for her to regain consciousness. After a few seconds her head moved on my feet. I thanked God as she gained consciousness and asked her whether she was on her head or not. She was pleased to know that she was on her head and asked me how she lost her consciousness. "This happened due to your high blood pressure", I said. As I had started the head-balance, I promised to teach her *Sālamba Śīrṣāsana* after taking the cooling *āsanas* that bring the pressure down.

After two weeks of yoga practice, she called her family doctor, a cardiologist, to test her heart condition. He was surprised to find the blood pressure normal with rhythmic heartbeats. He thought that his medicine had worked. She said that she did not take his medicine, but followed an Indian doctor staying as her guest and she wanted him to meet me. I was called by the Queen Mother to meet the doctor. I was introduced to the doctor who asked me what I had studied. I said, "Yoga and I gave her 'yogic pills' to bring the pressure down and it came down." With jokes like this one, we became good friends.

Similarly, Yehudi Menuhin would ask me: "My finger tips are very cold, what have I to do to warm them to play the violin?" On that spur of moment I had to think fast which adjustments would make the 'finger tips' warm. Recollecting my *āsana* practices, I used to stretch his knuckles and fingers from the back of the palms, so that the tips of the fingernails were not raised, but stretched in line with the knuckles. He at once used to feel the warmth. He was quick enough to translate my explanation of *āsana*, such as rolling of the shoulders in *Sālamba Sarvāṅgāsana*, the revolving action of the muscles of the arms and legs in *Halāsana* and to adapt them while playing. Whatever techniques I gave, he used all of them in playing his violin.

LOKANAYAK JAYAPRAKASH NARAYAN

I have met lots of saints, *sādhus*, administrators, lawyers, scientists, artists, politicians, yogis and philosophers in my life, but Shri Jayaprakash Narayan, though a politician, was one of the finest and noblest souls with a strong spiritual touch. He retained a simplicity and innocence combined with a sharp intelligence and a quick grasp of things around him. It was good fortune that took me to these people through yoga. I could never imagine that one who had grown up in such poverty ridden and difficult circumstamces would meet such glorious personalities one day. Yoga took me from that level to the present level of consciousness, which you all appreciate today. Hence, I am grateful to those with whom I came in contact, including my *gurujī*, because by observing their ways of living, their natures and habits, I learnt to weigh their ways of life with mine, not do some of what they were doing and accept some which could help me to build up my own character and develop my consciousness.

RECULTURING MY BODY

Before I conclude let me narrate my failures and how I worked to reculture my system to get back my yogic practice.

In the early days, I was fond of backbends and balancing, as they were majestic and awe-inspiring. The pride in me of these achievements made me neglect the simple forward bends, as they were not as attractive as backbends.

A SLAP ON MY PRIDE

In 1944, though I could perform all the *āsanas*, I felt no response from their actions. It was touch and go practice for two to three years. This dull response persisted, though I was doing them better. Then I began to look into each *āsana* and realised that I was performing at the cost of several cells and fibres, which remained inactive. Some parts were overacting while other parts remained dull and stupid. This observation was the turning point in my pride. I said to myself that the pride of showmanship in backbends had ruined me. I humbled myself to surrender to the *āsana* and to look within myself while doing them. This inward turning of my mind to observe my cells in action rejuvenated the cells and nerves of my body. Then I continued without loss of attention up to 1958. In that year, I began to feel dizzy and breathless in whatever *āsana* I did. This unnerved me but with determination I tried to overcome the blackouts and breathlessness by increasing the time of stay in the *āsana*, till I felt that I was going to become unconscious. I consulted my senior colleagues and *gurujī*, who told me to take yoga easy, as I was a householder and ageing. I put aside their remarks and persisted in my practice doing those very *āsanas* quite often but with intervals to break the dizziness and blackouts. It took me a year to conquer this hindrance.

I continued without interruption from 1958 to 1978. My practice was smooth and enjoyable.

In 1978, after my 60th birthday celebration, my *guru* advised me to devote time to meditation and to reduce my physical strain. I obeyed him and within three months my body lost its grace and elasticity. I realised that I ought not to respect the words of those whom I revere, but who have no experience of their own. The body was rebelling, but the will power was growing stronger to break the barriers of the body. I began practising four to five hours each day. As ill luck would have it, in June1979, I met with a very severe scooter accident injuring my left shoulder, my spine and my knees. I could not lift the shoulder up or do forward bends or twists or balances due to the injury. I began to practise yoga as if I was a raw beginner. But within three months after the first accident, I met with another accident injuring my right shoulder and right knee. As yoga means evenness, these two accidents evenly injured my body and my practice reached rock bottom. In order to come back to my 1977 standard, I practised diligently and doubly, attending to the injured parts. Though my will power and nerves were strong enough to endure hours of practice, alas, the body was revolting. But I did not surrender to my negative thoughts. With perseverance and persistence, I have re-gained seventy-five percent of my *āsana* practice with ten years of hard work. I hope I get back to my original shape. In case I fail to achieve that, I want to die with the contentment of doing the best till the last breath of my life. I am saying this in order that you build up will power and persistence to do what I did without losing heart, so that you too leave the world with joy when God calls you back.

SPREAD OF YOGA

Although Mr. Menuhin was responsible for introducing me and my art to the cream of the Western world, particularly in Europe, the credit also goes to Mrs. Beatrice Harthan, Mrs. Silva Mehta and others who helped me to take this subject to the ordinary people of Europe. Mrs. Mary Palmer became the key person to popularise my method in the United States through Ann-Arbor 'Y'. In the course of time, it spread to other parts of the world, covering all the six continents. I do not hesitate to say that my method of yoga has caught the minds of the ordinary people. Yoga has changed their lives. They have accepted yoga as their science, their art, their culture and their heritage. Now the time has come for us to think and rethink, as our ancestors were the founders of this great science. We Indians are not valuing this great art, which our *ṛṣis*, sages and yogis left for us. I want you all to ponder over this. Yoga as practised by me, has become very popular in various parts of the globe. There are about two hundred *Iyengar Yoga* centres and thirty-two *Iyengar Yoga* associations in twenty-five countries. However, nothing seems to move in our country without political influence. Even if one is not capable here, if one has political personalities in one's pocket, all facilities are extended indiscriminately.

I remember Mr. N.A. Palkhivala who said years ago that "In India, outstanding people are made only to stand out." It is true that outstanding people are kept standing out in our country.

BOOKS ON YOGA

I took six years to write *Light on Yoga* and fifteen years to write *Light on Prāṇāyāma*. Now, new books on yoga flood the market daily. If one looks at them, they are mere repetitions without originality. Though I had to struggle for years and years to learn to photograph and write on it, I am happy that *Light on Yoga* is considered as The Bible of yoga. I am grateful to my publishers, Unwin and Hyman, now Harper Collins, London, who made the book reachable to people and made it popular all over the globe. Till now, more than five hundred thousand copies of *Light on Yoga* must have been sold. This book is available in seventeen languages. *Light on Prāṇāyāma* has been translated into twelve languages. It is not a small achievement. Story books or books like *Rāmāyaṇa, Mahābhārata, Bhagavad Gītā* may exceed all sales. But the subject of yoga has absolutely no flavour, no taste and no variety. It is as dry as mathematics and yet my books and my demonstrations captured the hearts of the people. The wind of yoga is blowing in all directions. Hence, the responsibilities on you all have multiplied. There are about eight to ten thousand teachers trained by me and the Iyengar associations all over the world. In 1966, Mrs. Joyce Stewart from South Africa came all the way to London and underwent training to teach South Africans. Later, I was invited by the South Africans to teach in Mauritius, Malawi, Swaziland, Lesotho and South Africa. At Mauritius, the then Prime Minister told me, "India is our elder brother. We are acting as a bridge between South Africa and India. We are helping our elder brothers to become friends of South Africa by permitting you to teach yoga to South Africans here."

As yoga is attracting people and becoming popular as an alternative method of health and an art healing, I think this is the time for us to build ourselves up in order to carry the message of yoga directly towards a more spiritual kingdom, without forgetting the basic principles. Patañjali had such a broad outlook that suggested that one could devote and concentrate on what was most congenial. So go deep into your practices of *āsana* and *prāṇāyāma* and carry the message of yoga to people around you. Yoga is a universal religion given to us to cross over from the material world towards the spiritual kingdom.

I am really happy that the message of our heritage is carried by Western students to many parts of the globe. I request my fellow countrymen to carry the light of yoga to our own brothers and sisters in villages and to lift them up from sub-normal health to normal health and then to guide them towards spiritual health. The people in our villages have firm roots in the Indian hinterland, untouched by Western influences. Let us bring this art of yoga to fructification by revitalising our ancient thoughts and ideas. I am sure that after me, pupils, grand-pupils and great-great-grand pupils of mine will carry the message of yoga to every nook and corner of the globe so that all live as one Human Race without any geographical division or caste, colour, creed and sex.

God bless you.

MY *GURUJĪ* SHRIMAN T. KRISHNAMACHARYA

Let me first salute my direct and revered *guru,* T. Krishnamacharaya with respect and reverence, who happens to be my brother-in-law, my elder sister Naamagiri's husband. Let me also invoke Lord Patañjali through prayers before I say something of my *Gurujī,* with all the humility at my command.

Firstly, it is very embarrassing and difficult to speak of my *guru,* who was a great man, a close relative, a versatile personality and at the same time a very hard taskmaster. It was no doubt a herculean task to approach him. Secondly, my reverence for him as a great man may not allow me to do full justice. It is not an easy task for a pupil like me to talk of a master of such versatile character. Thirdly, I was hardly sixteen when I was his student. The time I lived and spent with my *Gurujī* was so short that it is not easy to sketch his life style. My mind then was raw and childish, I do not think that I had developed much of an intelligence to study and understand him, nor was I in a position to taste the wisdom of his knowledge.

As a coin has two sides, each person has two facets to their personality. It is the duty of a pupil to take the advantage of the best side of the master and overlook his shortcomings. Such a pupil will always stick to his master. It is wrong on my part to judge my master who acted as a friend, guide and philosopher and express those thoughts about him. As I am forced to speak of him today I have to say a few words about him. Yet, it is not fair to express from one's mind, the minds of others. As long as one accepts the master as a master, reverence supersedes all the other issues of the master.

Gurujī, no doubt was a gifted and talented personality. It is only possible to talk about such a person when the pupil is elevated to his master's level of intelligence.

I shall narrate some anecdotes, which may throw a light on this great personality. Many of you might have read the book on Milarepa. My *guru* was like Milarepa's *guru.* I lived with my *Gurujī* for two years and followed him similar to the way Milarepa followed his *guru,* without questioning him.

I was a boy of seven and a half years when he married my sister. He was thirty-three then and my sister was twelve. There was a difference of twenty-one years between them. My first memory of him is the day of his wedding when he came with two elephants.

Gurujī was a gifted man, with a very high intellectual calibre, powerful physical prowess and an unfaltering memory. I am sure he would have won the title of "Mr. Universe," if he had stood for such a contest. He was naturally gifted with a well-built body, proportionately muscular, expressing tremendous strength and vigour.

He was also a master of *Āyurveda*. He used to prepare *Āyurvedic* medicines and herbal oils such as *lehyams* and *tailam* at home, which were very effective when used on his patients. But he never gave any clues to how they were mixed and prepared.

Besides mastery in the fine art of music, he played Karnatak classical music on the *veeṇā*. *Gurujī* was also a wonderful cook. I don't know whether his children ever tasted the food prepared by him. He would cook only one or two dishes (during my sister's monthly periods), but they used to be so tasty that I could never decide which one was the best. I used to call his preparations *Madhupākam* – it was like honey.

He was a first-class gardener. He used to grow flowers and vegetables at his house in Mysore. He would sow any seed and by his magical touch the plant would flourish.

Coming from an orthodox Brāhmin family, he never used a charcoal fire for cooking, but would often cut wood with his own hands and used that as fuel. He used to enjoy cutting wood in the mornings from 9 o'clock to 11 or 12 o'clock. He was precise in whatever work he did; whether cooking or cutting wood; singing *vedic* hymns or playing the *veeṇā*. He would not tolerate any compromise or slackness with precision. He demanded the same from all of us. His moods and modes were very difficult to comprehend and often unpredictable. Hence, we were always alert in his presence. He was like a great Zen master in the art of teaching. He would hit us hard on our backs as if with iron rods. We were unable to forget the severity of his actions for a long time. My sister also was not spared from such blows.

You may not be knowing that after his marriage he got a job in a coffee plantation in the Hasan district of Karnataka. He used to dress differently, wearing half-pants and half-sleeved shirt, socks and shoes, a hat on his head and a stick in his hand. It was unimaginable to see a man dressed in such a manner who had studied *Ṣad-darṣanas* (the original texts of six schools of thought in Indian philosophy), with titles like *Sāṁkhyāyoga-śikhāmaṇi, Veda-kesari, Vedānta-vāgīśa, Nyāyācārya, Mīmāṁsa-ratna* and *Mīmāṁsa-tīrtha*. He was an expert in *Vāstu Ṣaśtra* – the science of scientific and aesthetic architecture, and *Jyotisya Ṣaśtra* – the science of astrology. But destiny had played its trick even on him and he had to work in a coffee plantation.

In 1931, he left the plantation job and began giving lectures on philosophy. Shri Sheshachar, a lawyer of Mysore, invited him to give a talk on the *Upaniṣads* in the town hall of Mysore. The event proved to be a turning point in his life. A hidden scholarly personality, in that garb of half-pant, half-sleeve shirt, hat, socks and shoes, was unearthed. His discourses on the *Vedas, Upaniṣads* and yoga attracted the elite of Mysore. The news of this scholar and his scholarly debate reached the ears of the then Maharaja of Mysore, His Highness Shri. Krishnaraja Wadiar IV. The Maharaja was attracted by his knowledge and personality and became his student in order to understand the scriptures and yoga. Soon he appointed him to teach *Mīmāṁsa* and yoga in the *Sanskṛt Pāṭaśālā* (school), run by the Maharaja. The Maharaja was a great patron of art, music, painting and yoga. He encouraged artists to shine in their chosen fields.

My *Gurujī* was a strict teacher. His students and even the *Pandits*, found it difficult to answer a question paper prepared by him on *Mīmāṁsa*. The students protested against him and the Maharaja soon agreed to replace him from the *Sanskṛt Pāṭaśālā* and started a *Yogaśālā* at the Jagan Mohan Palace of Mysore (now an art gallery), as he never wanted to lose such a personality. With this offer of a *Yogaśālā*, he kept the option open that *Gurujī* could go to the *Yogaśālā* whenever he wished, and gave him the recognition of *Āsthāna Vidwān* – the intelligentsia of the palace. From a plantation worker *Gurujī* had become an *Āsthāna Vidwān* and a *Yogāchārya*.

I am one of *Gurujī's* oldest pupils. Then, I was the youngest amongst the rest of his pupils. Even now, Shri Ranganath Deshikachar, a pupil of *Gurujī* who is teaching in Mysore, is above ninety years old. He is *Gurujī's* oldest and seniormost pupil, still living.

Shri Shrinivasa Rangachār, Shri Mahadeva Bhat, Shri Ranganatha Deshikachar, Shri Narayana Sharma, Shri Panduranga Rao and myself were colleagues and attended the *Yogaśālā* regularly. However, Shri Pattabhi Jois, a pupil of *Gurujī* and a student of the *Sanskṛt Pāṭaśālā*, was appointed as a yoga teacher, in place of my *guru*, to teach yoga in the *Sanskṛt Pāṭaśālā* when the *Yogaśālā* was opened. Hence, Pattabhi Jois was never a regular student at the *Yogaśālā*. *Gurujī* used to come regularly to the *Yogaśālā* in the early stages but not later. All these members were dedicated students, for whom *Gurujī* would conduct theory classes at home. Unfortunately, I was not one of them. So to some extent I missed that bus.

However, the *Yogaśālā* was meant only for the members of the Royal family. Outsiders were permitted on special requests. Therefore, it was a formidable task for an outsider to get entry into the *Yogaśālā*. *Gurujī* used to have only a selected few outsiders with him apart from the members of the Royal family, and I was fortunate to be one of them. The classes at the *Yogaśālā* were mainly devoted to teaching one to achieve perfection in *āsana*, or *āsanas* for health. The classes were held only in the evenings between 5 and 7 p.m., while the morning classes between 9 and 10:30 a.m., were meant for ailing persons.

There is a story about how I came into the picture, which may be of interest to you. *Gurujī* took my elder brother Shri Ramaswami Iyengar to Mysore in 1931 and taught him yoga. My brother could not tolerate the strict discipline and rigid rules of *Gurujī*. He could not face his anger and came to Bangalore from Mysore after a few months of study.

Then *Gurujī* took my youngest sister Jaya into yoga. She was hardly eight years old. Her practice was spasmodic, as she was young and moved with my mother. Her visits to Mysore were dependent upon my mother's visits. She got married in 1940. I think her practice of yoga dwindled after her marriage.

In 1934, *Gurujī* was sent by the Maharaja to visit the yoga centre, the Kaivalyadham of Lonavla, in order to see how the centre runs. *Gurujī*, along with his pupils had to first reach Bangalore to get to Bombay. He came to meet the family members. It was the summer vacation. He asked me to go to Mysore and help my sister, who would be alone with her young children. Here was a great chance for me. Being young, I had a great attraction towards the palace and the King. Mysore, being a capital city, was well known for its gardens and the Chamundi Hills. I had heard about it but had never seen it. It was a question of one month's stay. I consented to go.

I went to stay with my sister, helping her in household work. When *Gurujī* returned to Mysore exactly after a month, I asked his permission to return to Bangalore, as the schools were to re-open after the summer vacation. He asked me to stay on and help my sister.

My father had died in 1927 and our family was in dire poverty. My elder brothers and sisters were married and had their own families to take care of. As such, we were orphans without a father. So I thought of staying back in Mysore, so that my mother need not worry about me.

Gurujī asked me to write to my brother to get the school leaving certificate and the moment the certificate arrived I got admission to the Maharaja's High School. Three to four months passed in Mysore, with a new school, new household work for me, an entirely new atmosphere, but 'no yoga' and 'no health'.

One day, *Gurujī* called me and taught me three or four *āsanas*. He said, "Do these *āsanas*, you will regain some health." My body was like a log of wood, my middle fingers could not even reach my knee. He said, "You won't do yoga in this life. You are *anadhikārin* – not privileged. He never called me for the next lesson. I thought that was the first and the last lesson. I was caught. I could neither go back to Bangalore, nor learn yoga.

I have also talked of my companion Keshava Murthy, who was staying with *Gurujī*. He was my only companion. We shared our sorrows. One day all of a sudden, Keshava Murthy told me, "I'll just go and come," but he never returned. He just disappeared before the day dawned. *Gurujī*, being very fond of him, searched the whole of Mysore and even in the palace. But there was no trace of him. Now, I was really alone and lonely.

The big question in front of *Gurujī* was that all his pupils were married and lived away from him. He could not bind them to him. I was the only one left behind whom he could control and mould according to his wishes. The very next day, after watering the plants, he called me for a yoga lesson. Believe me! In that one day, he taught me thirty to forty *āsanas*, one after the other. He said, "You have to do it!" In a way he was helpless and so was I.

A YMCA conference was held at the Mysore Palace in 1934. *Gurujī* was totally relying upon Keshava Murthy for the demonstration. The other elderly pupils could perform only a few simple *āsanas*. Even *Gurujī* had lost the touch at that time. Being young, *Gurujī* could force me to do back bends according to his will by making me to do on his lifted legs. That is why I have written in my book *Light on Prāṇāyāma* how difficult it was for me to master *prāṇāyāma* because of overdoing back-bends at such a young age and in a short period. He taught me the advanced backbends in three days and said, "You have to perform these at the conference." He never asked me again what I do, how I do, or whether I practised or not.

When I requested him to see how I performed the postures, he said. "I will see you only on the platform." I begged him, but he was adamant in his decision. Perhaps both of us were blessed with strong will power. I did and he saw me perform on the platform. I got the first presentation of Rs. 50/-. My *Gurujī* was impressed and asked me "How did I manage?" He said, "I thought you would not do it at all, but you did it". This first demonstration of mine tied me to yoga and to *Gurujī*.

Members of the *Yogaśāla* used to hold annual gatherings where members from the Royal family and elite citizens of the city were the invited guests. Senior students were given a chance to show their skills in the demonstrations and the best ones were awarded prizes and certificates of merit. In 1935, I earned this distinction.

Gurujī had a frightful personality. His back used to be very straight even when he was aged. His eyes were so powerful that any one would be afraid to look into his eyes. Nobody could cross this intellectual giant. The pundits and scholars were afraid of him. I have attended a few of his talks in the early days. As a young and highly educated person, he was intellectually intoxicated. As nobody could come near him, surpass him, or argue with him on his level, he remained lonely. Nobody could equal him in the art of discussion. He could create a "new book" on the platform. He could create *Sanskṛt* stanzas on the spot. He was a *kavi* – a poet. The instant creation of *slokas* and stanzas *(Shīghra-kavitva)* was in his blood. This scholarly background, fiery eyes, well-built physique and a strong personality paradoxically isolated him.

To some extent, I feel that he did not get a proper channel to expose his abilities.

People were nervous of him. He was a fast walker. Nobody could keep pace with him. Nobody could match his speed. If he were walking along on one side of the pavement, the elite of Mysore would cross over to the other side.

I have already said that he was a scholar, yet he was lonely. When he was in Mylapore, Madras, a film director, Pullayya by name, was staying next door. *Gurujī* never knew of his neighbour. Once when I came to see *Gurujī* at Mylapore, I happened to see Pullayya whom I knew, standing at the doorstep. I introduced him to *Gurujī*. Being neighbours in the same place for years, they had never seen each other until I came into the picture. Since both of them were from the state of Andhra Pradesh with their common mother tongue Telugu, they became good friends later on.

Gurujī was staying at Chamundi extension. From this house the distance to the *Yogaśālā* or to the Maharaja's school was three miles. *Gurujī* tested my tolerance by not allowing me to go to the *Yogaśālā* directly from school, to attend the classes. Though it was within five minutes' walk, he wanted me to go home first and then to the *Yogaśālā*, thus walking the distance of three miles twice. Perhaps his rigidity and tests taught me a great deal in moulding my life while I settled in Pune. I learnt to bear hardships with tolerance.

The physical exertion stultefied my intelligence and I failed in my final exams. On account of this, I lost my school free-ship. Education came to a halt, but this was to be a turning point in my life. With my limited knowledge and immature experience as well as the end to my school career, the seed was sown in me to pursue yoga as my career for life. I built up courage and strength to be an independent student of yoga, becoming a stage performer, practitioner and teacher.

The Maharaja of Mysore once again asked *Gurujī* to go on a tour to promote yoga. This time, *Gurujī* asked me to tour with him. He planned to go to Chitradurga, Dharwad, Hubli and Belgaum. At Chitradurga, we met his brother Appalachar. He arranged a demonstration there.

Thereafter, we went to Dharwad where *Gurujī* entrusted me with the job of pulling water from a deep well, which I did in the beginning as an obedient pupil. I have already narrated in an earlier chapter how senior students started ill-treating me. My refusal to fetch water for them led to the first brush with my *guru*.

My early initiation into teaching at Dharwad in the year 1936 was at the instance of *Gurujī*. The women gave a good report of my teaching and that changed *Gurujī's* temperament. Then we went to Belgaum, where we met a civil surgeon, Dr V.B. Gokhle, who was impressed by *Gurujī's* talk on yoga and appreciated our demonstration. As he was Pune-based, he later asked *Gurujī* to send someone to teach in Pune. I have earlier narrated how all his senior pupils stayed away from going to Pune, citing ignorance of Marathi, as the reason. Since I knew English *Gurujī* insisted that I should go to Pune. I surrendered to his "order" as an *Āshirvād* (grace) and went to Pune which became my *Karmabhūmi*.*Gurujī* and his senior pupils went back to Mysore. I was left alone. I had to teach in Hubli and Dharwad for six months. Dr. Gokhle asked me to join him after six months. Meanwhile, I earned my fare from Dharwad to Pune and finally came to Pune in 1937.

I taught in schools and colleges. As a failed student, I never thought I would enter the premises of a college, but I did as a teacher. Not only in colleges, I also taught in universities.

My term was extended every six months for a period of three years. Then in 1940, my services were terminated, but I stayed on in Pune hoping for opportunities. I don't know what *Gurujī* saw in me. Perhaps he recognised that I while had no strength, that I had guts. He ignited the courage in me. He introduced me to my 'self' within. Or, perhaps he discovered my inner potentials.

I am basically a practitioner. Whatever little *Gurujī* taught me, I converted it into a performing art, but with a scientific base. He sowed a small seed in me and made it grow into a gigantic tree. Perhaps I am the longest practitioner of yoga, considering my age. I used to practice for hours together. Even now my practice is not less than six hours.

Direct practice gives direct knowledge. My demonstrations were not meant to show off. The yoga demonstration is *pratyakṣa pramāṇa*. *Gurujī*, in those days, stressed on yoga demonstrations. I must have given 14,000 to 15,000 demonstrations all over the world. On some occasions I have given four to five demonstrations in one day. My *guru* was very particular about yoga demonstrations. Though I have not seen him demonstrating, he insisted that we do. Whenever and whereever I gave a yoga demonstration, I used to keep him informed and he used to appreciate my ventures. Unfortunately, I did not keep those letters. We used to have very regular correspondence. He was prompt in replying.

There are several incidences where *Gurujī* not only demanded a demonstration, but also asked me to perform unknown and undone *āsanas*. In 1935 a famous criminal lawyer, Shri Shrinivasa Iyengar from Madras, and Swami Yogananda of USA, who were the guests of the Maharaja of Mysore, came to visit the *Yogaśālā*. One thing that was certain about *Gurujī* was that he would never go to see anyone, however great they might be. He commanded such a respect that these great personalities had to come to the *Yogaśālā* to see him. In an earlier chapter I have already narrated how I was forced to perform the *Hanumānāsana* in public. It may be recalled that on account of this demonstration I tore my hamstring muscles on account of which, I could not walk for two years. Still, I had to keep up my practice as I learnt that *Gurujī* could catch me unawares at any time, and ask me to do any of the *āsana*.

You will be surprised to know that almost all the difficult *āsanas* such as *Vṛśchikāsana* and *Adho Mukha Vṛkṣāsana*, the hand balancings, I learnt in public performances only. Such was the way and style of teaching of my *guru* that he would often ask his students to perform *āsana* in public, and that too, without any prior intimation or warning.

We would perform *āsanas*, while he would present *prāṇāyāma* in public. In 1935, Dr Bruce, a cardiologist and Dr Morcault, a psychology professor, visited Mysore to study the changes and stopping of the heartbeats through yogic discipline. They came to the *Yogaśālā* and wanted to test *Gurujī's* electrical heartbeats. My *guru* was very fond of castor oil. He used to drink it as though it was ghee. Until the experiment, which was going on for four to five days, he had castor oil every day. He always felt that he could do better if he took castor oil. On the sixth day of the experiment the machine stopped. It wouldn't show any beats. At first the doctors thought that there was a power failure but saw the light outside the testing room was working. Soon they realised that he had really stopped his heartbeats. They have mentioned this incident in their book.

In 1955, two doctors from the USA had come to Lonavla. They were doing research work on *prāṇāyāma*. They asked me to come to Lonavla. They wanted to test whether the blood pressure increased during *Sālamba Śīrṣāsana*. They took the readings of those who were at Lonavla. However, my blood pressure did not rise. They were surprised and asked me about *prāṇāyāma* and the stopping of heartbeats. I asked them to visit my *guru* who was an expert in *prāṇāyāma*. They came to Madras. *Gurujī* by this time had learnt a lesson. In Mysore, he did it free of charge and the researchers made money. Now, the Ford Foundation was paying two doctors, so *Gurujī* too asked for fees and he was absolutely right. For what purpose do we have to exert ourselves, when they take the credit? My *guru* permitted them to take the test when he was practising. He did not offer them a separate time. Of course they took the test and admitted that my *guru* was the first one who did something in *prāṇāyāma* where the recording showed his heartbeats had slowed down.

Gurujī came to Pune many a time. He came in 1938, '39, '40, '42, and '61. His last visit was in 1978, during my 60th birthday. Whenever he came to Pune he gave lectures and we gave demonstrations. As *guru* and *śiṣya* we were always together mentally if not physically.

Though he sometimes let me down completely, yet there was a *pāṣa,* an inner tie and an inner attachment between us. I never crossed my *guru's* words in spite of a few quarrels with him and that perhaps protected me throughout my life. Let me tell you of other encounters with my *Gurujī.* He came to Pune to stay for twenty days in 1961. His son Sribhashyam was with him too. I had arranged lectures and demonstrations at various places. He planned to go to Gaya and from there, back to Madras. But suddenly he changed his plan and came back to Pune. It was quite a surprise for me as *Gurujī* was very strict with his plans. If he had decided something, nobody could change his mind. But in 1961, he changed his plan and came to Pune, on his way back to Madras.

Fortunately, I had finished my photo session for my first book *Light on Yoga,* and I showed the photos to my *guru.* He saw the photographs and at once made a sweeping statement, "All the poses are wrong." I said, "Please, tell me where I am wrong so that I can correct them." He said, "Everything is wrong." I kept quiet. Again in 1965, before giving the book for printing, I went to him and asked him to go through the manuscript and requested him to write a "Foreword". My sister too told him, "Do write a foreword. After all, he is a young man, he has done something." But he refused. I had to accept his wish. I could not force him and came back without his foreword.

I am sure that though he let me down without writing a foreword, I had seen my book, which I presented to him after its publication, in his hand, many a time.

I told *Gurujī* I was undertaking to write a book on *prāṇāyāma,* as my publishers were insisting. He warned me, "Don't commit even a word on *prāṇāyāma* in black and white. You may speak for hours but don't write." I had to write when my pupils and publishers demanded. I finished the book and went to Madras, where one of my married daughters was staying. I went to see *Gurujī* and showed him the manuscript of the book. This time I was mum about a foreword. He took the manuscript and said, "Come tomorrow at 4 o'clock." I think he was going through the book the whole night. Next day I went, I was late by five minutes. He asked, "Why are you late? I asked you to come at 4 p.m., now it is 4.05 p.m." I said "*Gurujī,* I left early but there was a traffic jam." He said, "But you can't be late." I kept quiet. After a few moments I asked him, "*Gurujī,* did you go through the book?" He said, "Yes, I have read it. You can take it back." I asked him "How did you feel?" He said, "I have written inside." I thanked God from my heart. Without asking for a foreword, here it was.

If he had been alive, he would have definitely read my commentary on the *Yoga Sūtra.* I was a non-entity, but *Gurujī* made me a hero. I was at the nadir in this subject. I climbed the tree of yoga step by step. Perhaps *Gurujī's* eagle eyes made me think and re-think. Indirectly he taught me how to be totally aware. Today, I feel happy at heart and satisfied that I served my *guru*. There are three ways to serve the *guru;* one is to serve him physically, the second financially, and the third to impart the knowledge that was acquired from him. I served him in all the three ways.

In the early days I had to massage his legs every night. Either Keshava Murthy or I was doing it. Sometimes our nails used to touch his soft skin, I don't know how many times I used to receive blows. He would say, "Did you purposely pinch me?" I would say, "No *Gurujī*, it was not deliberate." Sometimes we used to feel sleepy and our hands would stop massaging. Again, a blow, a slap. So we learnt to be more attentive to avoid the blows. That is how my *guru* was in the '30s and '40s.

I have lived with my *guru*, I saw that he was not the same in Madras as he was in Mysore. You, who have seen him in Madras, will never know about his moods and modes. "T. Krishnamacharaya" of Mysore was not the same as "T. Krishnamacharaya" of Madras. He was as hot as fire in Mysore and as cool as water in Madras, a completely mellowed person. Probably, I have to give credit to the people of Madras (now Chennai) for having tamed and mellowed him.

Yet he was a top class teacher. In those days there were hardly any yoga teachers; we could count them on our finger tips: Swami Shivananda of Rishikesh, Kuvalayananda of Lonavla, Yogendra from Santacruz, *Gurujī* at Mysore, Iyengar from Pune, Yukteshwar from the East coast, Devananda from Lahore (this was before partition), and a few more. In the early days this subject of yoga as the greatest art of India, was ridiculed so much that only a very few select people were practising it.

People like Kuvalayananda opposed us for mass teaching. *Gurujī*, in the Mysore *Yogaśālā*, always had quite a big group in the class. He was young and energetic. I had seen him teaching in a group. That is how I could teach in schools and colleges in Pune. I could teach sportsmen and whole teams. *Gurujī's* various methods of teaching helped me to enhance and elaborate the method further.

Gurujī sowed the seed, but it took a long time to grow. Now it has spread like a gigantic tree. It has conquered the world.

Still, I emphasise, that the credit of success and popularity in yoga goes to his foremost students, including myself, who were not more than half a dozen in number. The message of yoga imparted by *Gurujī* was carried with sincerity, honesty and dedication, by these students and a note of thanks must go to them for keeping the fire of yoga alive even to this day.

The merit of the success from his pupils entirely belongs to *Gurujī* who has remained as the light to us all. Whatever we know about *Gurujī* and his work is just a bit here and there. He was like an ocean. Every one has learnt something from him. But what each one has learnt is not complete. We all have to come together, put all his words and works together. Only then can we know how big he was, how great he was.

I salute my *guru* from the bottom of my heart.

HOW I LEARNT *PRĀṆĀYĀMA**

The first thing I do every morning when I rise at 4 a.m., is to practise *prāṇāyāma*. I ask myself, if I am born today how does my first breath start? That's how I started *prāṇāyāma* each day. It may interest you all to know how my mind acted. I learned something from that approach also.

Being a sick person when I started yoga, I had no strength to stand and my lungs were not at all expansive. Naturally, breathing was a great hardship for me. I started practising *āsanas*. Then circumstances forced me to teach yoga. As I also had to teach yoga, I had to learn it. In order to learn I had to unlearn and relearn, so that the links of the chain of learning moved on and on, and it is still moving like this.

Naturally, at that time it was neither possible for me to do *prāṇāyāma*, nor was my *guru* willing to teach me. I had a narrow and collapsed chest. I did not do *prāṇāyāma* at all up to 1942. When my *guru* visited me in Pune in 1940 and I asked him about *prāṇāyāma*, he just gave an outline. My youth probably would not have taken in more than what he said anyway. He advised me to do deep breathing, which I tried, but I didn't succeed at all. I could not breathe in deeply or breathe out normally. Deep breathing was physically impossible for me. When I questioned him why I was failing to do what I tried to do, he said, "Continue. It will come." But it never came.

Each day, I would get up early in the morning with a fervour in my mind that I should sit. I had the bad habit of drinking coffee even in my early days. I used to have a cup of coffee, for clearing my bowels. Then I used to sit in *Padmāsana* to begin my *prāṇāyāma*. Within one minute, my mind would say, "No *prāṇāyāma* today." The moment I kept my fingers on my nostrils, the inner carpets of the nostrils used to rebel, and I used to gasp. So, naturally that day was a good-bye to *prāṇāyāma*.

---

* Edited from *Prāṇāyāma Symposium*. This article is excerpted from a fascinating interview with B.K.S. Iyengar by Neela Karnik, December 15, 1985. The interview was first published in its entirety in the commemorative volume, *70 Glorious Years of Yogācārya B.K.S. Iyengar*. Published by Light on Yoga Research Trust.

I went on and on like this with no solace. Even after I got married, I used to wake my dutiful wife, saying that I had to do *prāṇāyāma*, and ask for a cup of coffee. She would prepare the coffee, and until it was ready I would stay in bed. When the coffee was ready, I would clean my teeth to take coffee and my wife would go back to bed. Then, within a few minutes of sitting, my lungs could not take the deep breath and rebelled. In this way I tried and tried, but believe me, I never succeeded in my practice of *prāṇāyāma*.

Then I started doing *trāṭaka* (gazing). On a big card I used to make a black circle with rays, like the disk of the sun. I said "I can't do *prāṇāyāma*, let me do *trāṭaka*. I started gazing, without blinking the eyes. So my *prāṇāyāma* ended with *trāṭaka*. I had read in some books that *trāṭaka* would give this power or that power and so on. I used to gaze for a very long time, but nothing came to me. It so happened that *trāṭaka* brought me some discomfort in my eyes and in my brain, so I stopped doing it. I have even known yogis who developed day blindness caused by *trāṭaka*.

I was trying the *prāṇāyāma* called *ujjāyi* – deep inhalation, deep exhalation. If I failed, I used to try to do *nāḍi śodhana*, which everybody said was a very good *prāṇāyāma*. In 1944 I had an opportunity to go to Mysore with my wife. As she was pregnant with our first child, I went to take my *guru's* blessings. He was a master in *prāṇāyāma* in those days.

He never did *prāṇāyāma* in the presence of anyone. He used to do it in his own room, so there was no chance to see his practices. It so happened that one day he was sitting in a hall and doing *prāṇāyāma*. I saw how he placed his fingers on his nose, and that was the only indirect lesson I had from him.

I returned to Pune and again started trying. I could not sit straight like him at all, because of all the backbends in my early days. My spine used to curve backwards if I sat straight. I had no power to resist. Naturally, without resistance I could not sit straight and *prāṇāyāma* never came. Up to 1960 my *prāṇāyāma* was a thorough failure. It was a long process, but you have to appreciate my patience and impatience balancing together. Others would have given up, but I never did.

Each morning, I used to get up religiously at four, to sit for *prāṇāyāma*. I would sit for two or three minutes, and then I used to open my mouth to take in air. Or, if I did two breaths, I had to wait for a few minutes to take another deep breath. Throughout I was restless. As I could not do *prāṇāyāma* in *Padmāsana*, I tried lying down. After two or three breaths, I used to feel heavy in my head. This way I tried relentlessly to do *prāṇāyāma*, oscillating between sitting *āsanas* and *Śavāsana*.

All yoga masters say that when you are not in mood, you do *prāṇāyāma* and you regain your humour. I'm the only man who says that if you are moody, or at times have an upset mind, you cannot do *prāṇāyāma*. Through my failures, I learnt some good points also.

Sometimes I used to feel very fresh with two or three breaths, and at other times moody, with heaviness in the lungs and tension in the brain.

Somebody gave me a book written by a gentleman in the 1800s, which said, "If you keep a cotton on the chest when you exhale, it should not shake." Reading this, I started exhaling and I couldn't inhale at all. Books explained the quality of exhalation, but no mention of the quality of inhalation could be found.

I was teaching Krishnamurthi in Pune in 1946, and his theory of passive alertness was for me like maintaining a loose cotton in front of the chest and exhaling without disturbing the fibres of the cotton. He coined new words, but the action was old. I started doing inhalation with that passive alertness. When I inhaled with passive alertness without feeling the touch of the breath in my nostrils, my heart would start beating loudly. So I was caught in between, not knowing how to go on. So I began with 'soft' inhalation bringing a gentle touch to the inner carpet of the nose. I felt a sensation of exhilaration and quietness. This, I thought, must be the right method and I began manipulating the intercostal muscles of the chest, the fingers on the nose and so forth.

From this exhilarating fragrance, I started learning to gently place the fingers on my nose as I had seen my *gurujī* doing the digital placement of the fingers on the nose in 1944. My own student, Yehudi Menuhin, to some extent was an indirect *guru* from whom I learnt the placing of the fingers very accurately on the nostril passages, though he never knew that I learned from him. I observed his fingering work, the mobility of the knuckles on the violin strings and the placement of the tip of the thumb on the bow and fingers on the strings. This gave me the clue of placing the thumb and fingers on the nose to control the inner carpet of the membranes and to trace the exact air passage for my *prāṇāyāma*.

In 1962, I was in Gstaad, Switzerland. The weather was very good that year. As usual, I used to get up at 4 a.m., prepare my own coffee, and practise *prāṇāyāma*. One day, I was delighted to feel the fragrance of that inhalation, which was not too cold, nor too warm. Some sensations came and those sensations gave me the key to enjoy the act of inhaling and exhaling. That's the first feeling I got out of my practice of *prāṇāyāma*.

As I said, I was doing too many backbends, I could even stay in *Kapotāsana* for fifteen minutes; one day I made up my mind to do forward bends like *Jānu Śīrṣāsana* – I could not stay in it even for a few minutes. My spine and back muscles became sore and I couldn't bear the soreness when I used to do forward bends. It was as if somebody was using a sledgehammer on my back.

Then I determined that if I could do backbends, I should learn to do in forward bends too. Since then, I keep a day for forward bends and my pupils follow the same routine. In that learning of forward bends, my spine started resisting in such a manner that I felt soreness with unbearable pain. Similarly, while sitting in *prāṇāyāma*, my spine started shrinking and sinking, due to soreness, which made me realise the importance of forward bends. I understood then that forward bending was as important and essential as the backbends.

SECTION II

YOGA EXPLAINED

YOGA DEFINED*

Is yoga a physical discipline, a mental discipline or both?

It is hard for a common man to grasp the intricacies of the traditional definition that "yoga is the process of stilling the consciousness and then merging the individual soul *(jīvātmā)* with the Universal Soul *(Paramātmā)*". Following the pedagogical adage of leading the pupil "from the concrete to the abstract", the average intellect can be made to understand what yoga is by exploring the concrete in him, the body. Communication, communion and proper understanding exist between body and nerves, nerves and mind, mind and intelligence, intelligence and will, will and consciousness, consciousness and conscience and conscience and self. It is hard to begin directly with the abstract, the soul,** until these vehicles of *ātmā* operate at their highest level of efficiency

MISLEADERS GALORE

Though yoga is one, it is at the same time fascinating and baffling. Unfortunately owing to various interpretations it lends itself easily to be abused by both intellectuals and ignoramuses. Books and articles on yoga are often written by persons with mere theoretical knowledge; and those who practise tend to be fanatical about their own set of practices but are not keen on expanding its knowledge. Hence, interest in yoga does not get ignited. Some masters either declare the beginner unfit from the start or praise someone sky-high as if he had been born for it

Even today we tend to quarrel over the meaning and modes of yoga at conferences or in the course of a speech or in articles. It reminds one of the story of the description of an elephant given by six blind men. The first one touching the tail cried aloud that the elephant was like a flywhisk. The second one grasped the leg and for him the elephant was like a pillar. The third felt the flank and remarked that the animal was like a flat wall. The fourth one held on to the

---

* From *Bhavan's Journal*, September, 1977.

** See the author's commentaries on *Y.S.*, II.27, *Light on the Yoga Sūtras of Patañjali*, Harper Collins, London, 1993.

ear, and rejecting the opinions of the other, took the view that the beast was like a winnowing fan. The fifth and sixth respectively described the elephant as a spear and a hissing serpent, since the former had placed his hand on the tusk and the latter on the trunk. The interpretations of the six blind men varied according to the limited 'light' of each one. Perhaps the blind men might have had doubts that their descriptions did not fit into the whole reality of the elephant.

YOGA UNITES

While I am not posing myself as a 'seer', I feel that the interpretation of yoga according to one's own frame of mind is very much in vogue. Unlike the blind men however, whose assertions are stated categorically, as though any other exposition was completely untenable, one could assert with authority that yoga was merely physical, another, with equal authority, could assert that it was more mental and spiritual. A third person could label it as science or call it an art, education, religion, philosophy or even hocus pocus, without giving a thought to the development of man's total being.

Yoga covers all these and more. It transforms the sincere practitioner into an integrated personality. It helps the harmonious development of body,* consciousness and self. It develops a feeling of oneness between man and nature, man and man, and man and his Maker and thus aids one to experience the feeling of identification with the Self.

THE FOUR AND THE EIGHT

Our sages enumerated four paths for the evolution of man: *jñāna* (knowledge), *bhakti* (love or devotion), *karma* (action) and *yoga* (control of the consciousness). The trouble and confusion arose with these names when each path began to be called 'yoga', *jñāna yoga, bhakti yoga* and *karma yoga*. As the last path could not be called *yoga yoga*, the subject was sub-divided, bearing different names. Thus, we have *mantra yoga* (the yoga of thoughtful prayer), *laya yoga* (the yoga of love and dissolution in the object of devotion), *haṭha yoga* (the yoga of firmness and determined discipline) and *rāja yoga* (the royal path of yoga). If one carefully examines these so-called divisions of yoga, one finds that those ways explained are almost identical, with emphasis on one or the other facet of the subject, depending upon the favourite field chosen by the author.

---

* Here the author means the physical, physiological, organic, cellular, psychological body, and not merely the flesh and bones.

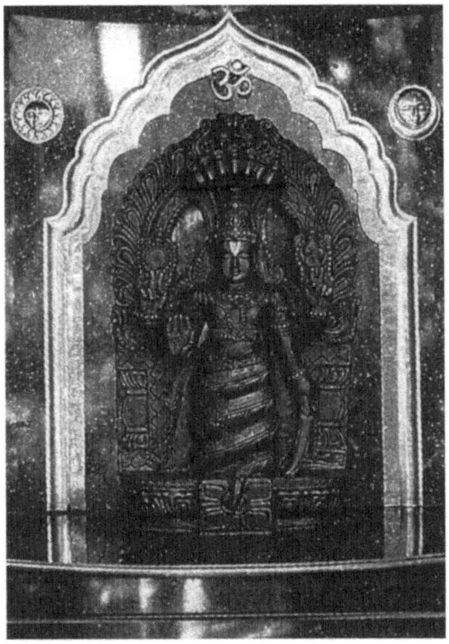

Plate n. 15 – Patañjali

Man is a product of intellect *(vidyā)*, intelligence *(buddhi)*, emotion, action and determined will. While the seat of the intellect is the head, the seat of the emotion is the mind. The hands and feet are meant to be the limbs for action. If one is to be pure in action, in love (lust free emotional life) or in intellectual pursuits, the foundation is the path of yoga. Patañjali, the codifier of yoga, has not called his treatise *'rāja yoga'*, but has enumerated it as *aṣṭāṅga yoga* (eight petalled yoga). The first of these petals is *yama* (social discipline) – the great commandments, transcending creed, geographical origin, age and time, namely, *ahiṁsā* (non-violence), *satya* (truth), *asteya* (non-stealing), *brahmacarya* (continence) and *aparigraha* (non-coveting). The second petal is *niyama* (individual discipline) encompassing *śauca* (purity), *santoṣa* (contentment), *tapas* (ardour or austerity), *svādhyāya* (study of the Self) and *Īśvara praṇidhāna* (devotion to the Lord). The third petal is *āsana* (posture) which brings physical health as well as mental steadiness and lightness. The fourth petal is *prāṇāyāma* (control on breathing), which makes the body and mind fit instruments for the purpose of concentration. The senses are brought under control directly by the mind in the fifth petal, *pratyāhāra*. Then comes the sixth petal, *dhāraṇā* (complete attention of the consciousness on a single point or task). The seventh petal, *dhyāna* or meditation, is an uninterrupted flow of concentration. *Samādhi* is the eighth petal, where the body and senses are at rest as if in sleep, but the mind and reason are alert as if one is awake, beyond the pale of consciousness.

Svātmārāma, author of *Haṭhayoga Pradīpikā*, speaks of six petals or aspects of yoga *(ṣaḍāṅga yoga)*. He says that "one cannot obtain perfection in *rāja yoga* without *haṭha yoga*, nor perfection in *haṭha yoga* without *rāja yoga* and that both should be practised till perfection is attained." *(H.Y.P.,* I.1, II.76).

He explains the various terms for the pinnacle of yoga as one and the same: namely *rāja yoga*, *samādhi*, *unmanī* (radiant Self), *manonmanī* (extinction of mind), *amaratva* (immortality), *laya* (absorption), *manolaya* (pensive mind), *tattva* (truth), *śūnya* (the void), *aśūnya* (the non-void), *śūnyāśūnya* (void and yet non-void), *paramapada* (the supreme state), *amanaskatva* (supreme, positive, still and silent state that is beyond the mind), *advaita* (monism), *nirālamba* (supportless), *nirañjana* (pure), *jīvanmukti* (free), *sahajāvasthā* (natural intuitive state), and *turīyā* (trance) (*H.Y.P.*, IV, 3-4). When the text is so clear, it is beyond my comprehension why we are quarrelling about words. Practitioners – not discerning their own hidden ego – assert with a superior air that they practice *rāja yoga* or *jñāna yoga* and thus show their contempt for other practices. When one has reached the state mentioned above, the *sādhanā* or effort is at an end. As long as the effort has not ceased, as long as the duality between the dweller (the soul) and the dwelling (the body) exists, it does not really matter by which name the *sādhanā* is called. But the most important point is how the soul uses the body to express itself so that the body loses instantaneously the feeling of its existence but the existence of the self alone is felt.

DISCOVER THE 'EMPEROR'

Yoga is the knowledge of the Self. Knowledge of the Self does not impart negligence or carelessness about the body or the mind. Knowledge of the Self encompasses the knowledge relating to the gross and subtle sheaths of the Self.

The absolute pre-requisites to reach the highest state in yoga are peace in body and poise in the consciousness. Peace in the body is acquired only through the practice of *āsanas* and *prāṇāyāma*. If these practices are done with *prajñā* (penetrating discernment) it is ethics in practice. Watching each and every part of the body and observing whether the *buddhi* is penetrating its depth or not, leads the practitioner towards *prajñāna yoga*. Merely practising as a routine without deep penetration, may be coined as *ajñāna yoga* (yoga of ignorance).

Instead of quarrelling about various types of yoga, my advice to the *sādhaka* is to devote time on the path one has taken to practise in order to develop a sense of perfection not only in *sādhanā* but also acquire mental and spiritual transformation in oneself. I assure those who are afraid of *haṭha yoga* practice, that it does not make one excessively body-conscious, but makes one energetic, intelligent and sensitive. It takes the *sādhaka* from *ajñāna sādhanā* to *jñāna sādhanā*. This is the way that the various yogas teach the *sādhaka* to move from *ajñāna yoga* towards *prajñāna yoga*. Instead of quarrelling about the types of yoga, it would be more to the point to observe one's own practice and improve its quality. When yoga is practised with the intelligence penetrating each and every corner of this empire the body, then its emperor, the Self, is discovered.

I think this is enough to let us conclude that yoga is neither physical nor mental or spiritual, but all these three disciplines are yoked and unified together and integrated in order to make man a whole man.

YOGA DESCRIBED*

Actually, yoga is based on principles of morality *(yama* and *niyama),* physical discipline *(āsana* and *prāṇāyāma),* mental alertness *(pratyāhāra* and *dhāraṇā)* and spiritual awakening *(dhyāna* and *samādhi).* We have been endowed with a body so that the self can express itself and it is the bounden duty of each of us to treat the body with that respect which is its due. Hence, it begins with the ethical discipline and ends with the sight of the self.

Nowhere have the yogis of yore said that the body is to be treated as something untouchable. On the contrary, they advised that it's the body's intelligence be sublimated and transformed to the level of the intelligence of the self. Showing negligence towards the body is as good as contempt of the Self, because the Self dwells in the body. Therefore, it is in our hands to find a means in the *sādhanā* to sublimate and transform the body to the level of the Self. Hence, maintenance of the *sādhanā* (which should be yogic) is morality and negligence and disrespect to the body is immorality.

DISCOVER THE TRUE PERSONALITY

No single facet can be practised without reference to the other facets of yoga. Only in the beginning are some external and internal divisions demarcated in order to learn well. For thoroughness in the yogic *sādhanā,* each movement of the body, mind and intelligence is made a tool in the quest of the Self. Whether one practises *āsana, prāṇāyāma* or meditation, a certain qualitative morality is demanded by each posture, each movement of inspiration or expiration, as well as adjustments required for the intelligence in the art of meditation. Each movement has to be observed and the adjustments made immediately and precisely.

In the practice of *āsana,* the mind is kept alert and the brain as a witnessing instrument, so the *sādhaka* realises that yoga is not simply a physical discipline but a great mental discipline.

---

* From *Yuva Bhārati,* February, 1978.

Accurate performance of *āsana* heightens one's total awareness, reaching out to each and every pore of the skin, as it were. This way, the intellectual energy of the body is gradually raised to the level of the spiritual intelligence.

CONTACT THE UNIVERSAL SOUL

Let us consider the aspect of *prāṇāyāma*. Normally inhalation is known as the intake of energy, exhalation – the output of energy and retention – the distribution of energy. In the philosophical language inhalation means drawing in of cosmic energy, whereby the cosmic force comes in contact with the individual soul *(jīvātmā)*. In exhalation the individual soul *(jīvātmā)* goes out in the form of breath to come in contact with its Maker, the Universal Soul *(Paramātmā)*. Inhalation-retention *(antara kuṁbhaka)* is the process through which the cosmic consciousness (that has been taken in from the cosmic force), is accepted and held together to mingle and merge in the body. In this process the intelligence is not attached to one focal point, but all-pervasive points. The exhalation-retention *(bāhya kuṁbhaka)* is nothing but the purging of the brain and complete surrender of one's intelligence and ego to the Universal Soul that is within us all. Thus, this *prāṇāyāmic* process makes the body, the brain and mind fit vehicles for meditation.

In meditation, the body should be as firm as a diamond, alert and sharp as a razor. The brain, which is situated inside the skull, has to be kept passive, gentle and sensitive like the thin end of a leaf, which moves to the gentlest touch of the breeze. The passivity of the brain helps us to study and quieten every movement of the ears, tongue, nose, skin, mind, intelligence and consciousness. In this passive and alert state of the brain, the super mind *(manas cakra)*, situated in the centre of the heart, reveals itself by uncovering layer after layer, intelligence, consciousness and conscience to reach the Self. The conscious intelligent power tosses between the head and the heart - not physical but spiritual. By conscious effort the *sādhaka* purges the load of the brain and makes it become silent, so that poise is cultivated within himself. This state of impersonal being is the true personality of man.

YOGA – A SPIRITUAL DISCIPLINE

In the state of attention the sense of *(asmitā)* 'I' functions in the brain, while in deep sleep the energy of the brain and the sense of 'I' descend to the seat of the spiritual heart. Here the energy of the heart and consciousness keeps up its function. In meditation, the spine has to be held straight, the body firm, like a pillar and the intelligent power, released from the cells of the brain, descends towards the seat of the consciousness. At the same time, the energy of the body consciousness is raised up to receive the descending energy of the brain. This simultaneous action stops the thinking processes and brooding thoughts and makes the intelligence dissolve in the seat of the conscience *(antaḥkaraṇa)*, leading the *sādhaka* to a composed, peaceful, calm, motiveless and motionless state so that his self dissolves in the Self. This is how the *sādhaka* discovers his true personality - the *ātman*, through the discipline of yoga.

YOGA – AN ANCIENT CULTURE*

India is a land enriched by its ancient but ever fresh and flourishing culture. Although the country was ruled or misruled by foreigners for centuries, our people did not lose heart in their heritage. They had a firm conviction in their inner selves and a strong faith in their way of life, which protected them from cultural poverty. Facing calamities, they understood the meaning of life and passed on this heritage to posterity.

Yoga, an ancient but perfect science, deals with the evolution of humanity. This evolution includes all aspects of one's being, from bodily health to Self-realisation. Yoga means union – the union of body with consciousness and consciousness with the soul. Yoga cultivates the ways of maintaining a balanced attitude in day-to-day life and endows skill in the performance of one's actions.

Yoga is not tied to any religion. It is appropriate for all people in all locations. As yoga is concerned with the betterment of the life of each human being, it can be viewed as a universal religion and culture. Yoga alone is able to reach the richest and the poorest, the cities and the remotest countryside. No special place or paraphernalia are needed. Yoga requires only a will to practise, and an available space, in your own house, in which this can be done.

YOGA COMES TO THE WEST

In 1954, Mr. Yehudi Menuhin (the world-famous violinist) invited me to Switzerland and Great Britain. Since then, I have been working to convey the message of yoga to the general public in the Western world. At the time of my first visit, the popular impression of yoga was quite different from what it is today.

Over the last thirty years, many individuals and organisations have played significant roles in bringing yoga to the West and in helping to make its benefits more widely known.

---

* Based on an article in *The Daily*, December 14, 1987.

Realising that happiness, peace and genuine freedom have been eluding them, more people in the West began searching for something that gives them those qualities and many have turned to the East for solace and inspiration. However, the search for peace cannot come from outside. It must begin from within, otherwise peace eludes the searcher forever. It is from yogic practice that one learns to distinguish the essentials from the non-essentials, and to live a simple, straightforward and peaceful life. As the aim of mankind is to know the Self, yoga helps in culturing mankind irrespective of place, class, caste and religion.

SELF ANALYSIS AND YOGA*

Friends, I offer my respects to my revered *guru* in Madras, aged about ninety-six, who introduced me to this art about fifty years ago, and to sage Patañjali, who is for us the father of yoga, medicine and grammar. Whatever I present and whatever words I say, the credit and merit of that goes to my *guru* and to the sage Patañjali, and whatever mistakes you find are mine.

To pronounce the word "yoga" is easy; to penetrate the depth of its meaning is very difficult. Like the rays of the sun, which emanate in various directions, similarly, wherever yoga touches us, it conveys the essence of life. It is one of the noblest of all the arts of our civilisation.

According to Patañjali, yoga is *citta vṛtti nirodha. Citta* is the consciousness, which vibrates, whether our thoughts move or not. Yoga is a method of stilling the vibration of consciousness entirely to reach a state of silence within. Another meaning of yoga is to bring the individual soul in contact with the Universal Soul. According to the *Bhagavad Gītā*, a skilful action, a talented presentation of anything, is yoga. In other words, it is a creation of balance and harmony between the various regions and frontiers of the body, mind and consciousness, with the very core of being. Think of water in a lake, which on its surface is even, though there may be dents and bumps at the bottom. Similarly, in this lake of the human body, there are such irregularities, yet it is possible to spread the flow of consciousness evenly. Patañjali expresses this same idea in these words: *citta prasādanaṁ.* He says that yoga diffuses the consciousness, intelligence and awareness, and spreads them in the system without any interruptions.

Patañjali discusses the theory of five afflictions as the philosophy of sorrow in the second chapter of his aphorisms on yoga. They are physical sorrows, mental sorrows and spiritual sorrows. *Avidyā* and *asmitā* refer to want of spiritual wisdom, seeing through the senses of perception, thinking with the mind and intelligence as if one is seeing through the soul. These two are known as the intellectual defects of a human being. In *rāga* and *dveṣa* he explains the

---

* An excerpt from B.K.S. Iyengar's September 1, 1984 lecture/demonstration at Davies Symphony Hall, San Francisco.

sorrows as emotional imbalances: pleasures attract desires and they multiply, bringing unhappiness though they appear pleasurable for the time being. If pleasures are not satisfied, they lead to sorrows. Then there is the instinctive fear of death, *abhiniveśa*, which has to be learned through understanding. Observing the mind, the brain, the self, and the defects of intelligence of the head, of the heart and instinct, he shows the ways to transform them into intuitive knowledge. This intuitive knowledge is the essence of yoga. Through these afflictions, the consciousness moves in various directions bringing disturbances in health and happiness in the form of diseases, sluggishness, heaviness of the breath, tremor of the body, and so on. After analysing the reasons for the sorrows, he analyses how man can reach a state of unalloyed blissful happiness and maintain it eternally. He says that the inner being coming in contact with external observations is the cause of unhappiness. A wise man learns not only the art of renunciation, but to see things as a witness. He uses the same vehicles of the soul: the organs of action, senses of perception, the mind, the intelligence, the consciousness, to serve the core of the being; whereas for average men it is the other way round: the core of the being is made the servant of these organs. The former leads one to experience the river of tranquillity, the essence of being flowing through each and every cell, so that the joy is not tainted by pain, or pleasure. Having experienced the essence of the unalloyed bliss flowing in each cell, he feels life and death as two sides of the same coin, loses the fear of death, and lives in the eternal being. This is what yoga teaches us: to reach the zenith of growth to experience absolute freedom, absolute beatitude, without any divisions, or polarities between body, consciousness and soul. When all these three are mingled together, then the entire man appears as a universal entity. There is no other art, no other science, except yoga, that can give perfect health, perfect happiness and universality of life in this world.

Yoga has eight aspects, but I call it eight petals*. All these eight aspects are nothing but petals on the path of action, path of knowledge and path of love. If one petal dries out, the others too slowly fade. The practices of the eight-petalled yoga help to increase the calibre of the intelligence by destroying the impurities of the body and consciousness, so that the crown of wisdom radiates in each individual, making him friendly and compassionate to himself, to his neighbours and to his society.

I know that many of you are keen to see what I do, more than listening to me. As an artist on the platform, as a performer, I have to curtail words and present my practice through direct perception, so that you can receive how the self can radiate through its vehicle, the body. This human machine has hundreds of muscles, hundreds of joints, miles and miles of blood gushing

---

* cf. Pathway to Salvation, p. 95., and Table n. 15.

through the entire system, moment to moment. The two ventilators, the respiratory and circulatory systems, keep all the other systems functioning harmoniously, understanding each other without words, communicating between themselves and with each part of the body, making each cell appear as a true self for the practitioner. That is how the yoga has to be practised. *Sādhanā* is like an ocean *(sāgar)*. My presentation is just a drop of that ocean.

YOGA – A UNIVERSAL CULTURE*

The birthplace of yoga might be in India, but it belongs to the whole universe. It embraces all the religions. Religion is auspicious. Religion is realisation. Religion is that which upholds, sustains and supports the one who is falling or fallen or about to fall physically, morally, mentally, intellectually or spiritually. Yoga supports and sustains by using the vehicles of the Self – the body, the organs of action, the senses of perception and the consciousness (mind, intelligence and ego) – to do right and virtuous actions. In this sense yoga is a religion. Self has no religion, but its vehicles have religion. Their religion is realisation of the Self. This religion of the vehicles of the Self is not created by human beings. Its religion is not set by man, but by God. The realisation of the Self is a divine religion, where a human being goes beyond religions that are created by human beings.

Yoga is a vast subject. It is as immeasurable as its subject matter – the Self. One can make a beginning, though one may not know the end. There can be an end to ignorance, but there is no end to knowledge. Yoga is as deep as the ocean. When it is hard enough to touch the surface, then gauge how much more difficult it must be to know its depth.

Yoga is communion. Unfortunately we observe that the human mind is in a disintegrated state. We hardly feel the communion between the body and mind, mind and intelligence, and intelligence and the self. This disparity causes *viyoga*. *Viyoga* means disintegration whereas yoga means integration. The individual consciousness coming in contact with the universal consciousness, is yoga.

Yoga is a complete subject, since it is an art, a science and a philosophy.

Yoga is to still the ruffles or the ramblings of consciousness. The consciousness exists and expresses itself with multiple facets. As the sun shoots millions and millions of rays in all directions in the form of energy to illumine and provide warmth to the Universe, the consciousness also throws up millions and millions of rays in the form of thoughts. But these rays are so disintegrated that one cannot perceive or conceive the consciousness. It is through yoga alone that one can bring these disintegrated and scattered ramblings of energy to re-integrate in the

* USA 1979.

consciousness. Yoga is meant to keep the conscious centre in a state of alertness without any oscillation, so that the power of the Self abides in its own grandeur.

Yoga is a discipline. The word *anuśāsanam* means law. It is the law that disciplines the human being. It is the discipline, which brings all one's hidden energies and powers together for integration. Yogic discipline is not merely external ethics, but it is the ethics of consciousness, which consists of the mind, intelligence and ego. Hence, yoga cultivates ethics in the mind, intelligence and ego, so that none of these behave unethically or immorally.

Yoga is the means and it is the end too. All the antagonistic tendencies arise from consciousness within and without, as well as from society. Whenever we try to associate ourselves with yoga, these interferences dissociate us. Our body, organs of action, senses of perception, mind, intelligence and ego, distract us from yoga through disarrayed actions, thoughts, approaches and behaviour. This is done constantly, bringing unwanted interference in our lives.

We are our own enemies. Antisocial elements create further problems that strengthen our own antagonistic tendencies. Therefore, we need a constructive approach to transform ourselves. This is possible through a yogic approach, which totally changes each cell of our organic body and mind as well as intelligence, so that all the sheaths of the self have the capacity to face the transformation; whereas in dissociation, they turn their back on the self.

The complicated job of correcting these antagonistic tendencies is entrusted to *aṣṭāṅga yoga:* This eight-petalled yogic approach is multifaceted with *yama, niyama, āsana, prāṇāyāma, pratyāhāra, dhāraṇā, dhyāna* and *samādhi.* These are not steps of yoga, but weapons of yoga to fight our own enemies that are hidden inside us. These enemies are ignorance, ego, attachment, aversion, fear, desire, anger. greed, pride, delusion or infatuation and malice. We have to learn to use these eight aspects of yoga as weapons to subdue all the physical, mental and emotional impediments.

Though the parts of a tree have separate identities, the tree as a whole is unique. In yoga too, *yama* as the root and *niyama* as the trunk support, unite and interconnect the tree of yoga. Various aspects of yoga eradicate the gross, the subtle and hidden antagonistic tendencies that are stored within us in the form of subliminal impressions *(saṁskāra).* When *yama* and *niyama* are followed, they make the path of yoga easy to tread upon. Unfortunately, now many of us have forgotten the fundamentals of a moral foundation. Our minds nurture motives. Therefore, we cannot trace our real consciousness. We observe the mind only at the level of motivation, but we do not examine whether the motivations are based on morality or not. Even spiritual endeavour is impossible without motivation. Any good action is impossible without right motivation. Motivation must be based on the kindness of the heart. Without incorporating the principles of *yama* and *niyama* the practices of yoga are like a dry and diseased tree which can fall at any moment. This is the reason why the root of yoga should remain firm in order to feel the Self.

Learn to approach yoga without prejudices in the mind. Do not demarcate yoga as physical, moral, mental and spiritual, or as *haṭha yoga* and *rāja yoga*. Neither Lord Patañjali, the saviour of yoga or Svātmārāma, the author of *Haṭhayoga Pradīpikā*, demarcated or separated yoga as physical, mental or spiritual. It is you and anti-yogis who coloured and gave names and forms to this pure subject with ideas, prejudices and thoughts. As a businessman sells his goods under attractive names, labels and packaging, yogic science and art too are sold under different labels.

Rāja means a king. The Self is the king. *Ha* is the Self (sun) and *ṭha* is the consciousness (moon). The pure consciousness meeting the Self is *haṭha yoga*.

As the moon borrows energy from the sun, the consciousness draws energy from the Self. If one realises this and works with that in the heart, then illumination shines forth. The physical energy and the mental energy meet the Self. This is what *haṭha yoga* conveys. Without using the body and consciousness, it is hard to reach the Self. Yoga is accomplished by utilising and channelling properly the energies of body and consciousness.

We all have two types of intelligence. One is factual intelligence and the other is analytical intelligence. One is the basic and original intelligence while the other is a cultivated intelligence. Factual intelligence is single faceted and has an unshakeable determination to reach the goal, whereas analytical intelligence is multifaceted with multiple goals and therefore is infirm. The logical, analytical brain calculates and demarcates; the factual brain unites. Logical brain argues. It is like having plenty of smoke but no fire. Factual brain, being an experiencing brain, eradicates confusion without demarcation.

In *Sanskṛt* this factual intelligence is called *vyavasāyātmika buddhi*. The factual intelligence gives subjective knowledge and the analytical intelligence gives objective knowledge. When you think of yoga, it is analytical intelligence, when you experience yoga, it is factual intelligence. Thinking differentiates the subject and there comes the division between the body, consciousness and the individual self. When the analysing intelligence is put to the test through practice, for synthesis, it becomes factual. A view of the subject is known through the analytical intelligence and converting the views into ways to reach the goal becomes factual intelligence.

For example, you like to perform *Padmāsana* (the lotus pose). The brain begins to work objectively. You begin to work with knees, ankles, hip joints and ligaments of the knees. All these parts become objects for trial. If these parts of the body trigger themselves and perform, you are joyous of the accomplishment.

Now, the intelligence wants to perform *Padmāsana* but the different parts of the legs do not co-operate. Due to stiffness they refuse to obey the dictates of the mind to achieve the pose. Then the analytical view has to be changed in order to learn the way of doing the pose and to find the movements that bring elasticity in the joints, as well as co-ordination. This is *vicāra* – insight.

If you cross your legs in *Padmāsana*, it becomes factual knowledge. As you get used to the *āsana*, the intelligence interacts with it totally to check whether the flow of energy is even or uneven on both the sides. This kind of approach in thinking, acting, observing and adjusting generates a synthesis in understanding the action. This is *jñāna*. It is *jñāna mārga* in the performance of *Padmāsana*. *Karma mārga* is the linking of the thread between the analytical knowledge and factual knowledge through action. This judicial work of the intelligence is the bridge between the acting factor and the thinking factor. The correct posture results from this kind of intelligence. If you work for the accomplishment of the *āsana*, with love, devotion and dedication, *jñāna*, *karma* and *bhakti* get involved and interwoven in the performance of the *āsana*.

As people go to church for worship, the yogis say why not make your own bodies a temple or a church and worship the Lord – the Self within. Jesus Christ has said, "The body is the temple of soul." The yogis say, "Make the body holy as it is the temple of soul". Hence, the yogic discipline commences from the body.

Many people often discard yoga saying that it is a sectarian religion. These days everyone wants to be free from religion. You may discard the concept of religion, but can you discard your own existence? You cannot discard your body, mind and intelligence. It is your duty to clean and purify them. Is it not a righteous duty to make them pure? Recognise this duty as religion. Yoga asks you to go towards realisation of the Self, that is religion.

Yoga commences with the purification of the gross body, refines it and then moves to clean the mind and intelligence. It transforms the body, mind and intelligence to the level of the Self. This is the goal of yoga that each practitioner has to realise. It is the analytical brain that demarcates *jñāna*, *bhakti*, *karma* and *yoga* but not the experiential intelligence. You may analyse for the sake of simplicity, but not for the sake of convenience. Analysis is simple, synthesis is difficult. Disintegration is simple, integration is difficult. Diversity of attention does not need any effort but unity in attention needs effort. Explanations become easier if I say that each yoga is different from the other. If I say that they are one and the same, it is hard for you to grasp, because brainwashing has been going on for ages.

Nothing can be achieved without knowledge, action, devotion and will. Without them you cannot reach perfection. Each person may integrate the subject in their own style of thinking, but one should not lead others towards a complex state of confusion. The truth is a fact. Yoga is the science which leads to the knowledge of truth. Unfortunately, innocents who are ignorant of the subject, get misguided by certain self-motivated writings.

Do not accept the truth with blind faith, but at the same time do not reject the truth blindly. The moment confusion is eradicated, faith sets in for further discovery and re-discovery.

Anatomy speaks of muscles, bones, joints, vessels and nerves. Yogic anatomy goes beyond this. The clarity that the yogis had about involuntary muscles and organs was incredible. The yogis knew how to contract, elongate and revolve the organic body. They knew the place, the originating point and terminus of the *nāḍis*, as well as their functions. Besides these, they were aware of the energy centres and their metaphysical as well as spiritual significance.

In the third chapter of the *Yoga Sūtra*, Patañjali speaks about the accomplishments, including the full control of physical, mental and spiritual bodies, while in the *Haṭhayoga Pradīpikā*, Svātmārāma speaks about the method to bring control over involuntary organs. They had the subjective living anatomy of man at the tips of their fingers.

Modern scientists have a very good knowledge of theoretical aspect, but very little is known about the practical aspect. We have to blend both, the objective knowledge of the occident with the subjective experience of the orient, to leap forward in knowing man's unknown organic body, mental body and metaphysical body.

Prāṇāyāma is one of the most important techniques of yoga. Let us see how the above concepts can be applied in the practice of *prāṇāyāma*. You all know that the intake of energy is inhalation. The output of energy is exhalation. Inhalation-retention is the distribution of energy whereas exhalation-retention is emptying the load of the neurons of the brain.

Our energy is dissipated in various directions at the physical, physiological, mental, intellectual and spiritual levels. *Prāṇāyāma* teaches us the method to stop this dissipation.

Even if you limit your attention to this body, it has about 700 muscles, 300 joints, 100,000 km of blood vessels, 16,000 km of nerve current and 15,000 millions of nerve cells. People ask me why one has to do so many *āsanas*. I hope you understand now why yogis have so extensively presented the *yogāsanas* for this complex human system. The varieties of *āsana* and methods to approach them help the energy to flow in their channels properly and uninterruptedly without waste. The words *ghaṭa śuddhi* (purification of body) and *nāḍī śuddhi* (purification of *nāḍīs*) indicate this meaning. *Ghaṭa* is body, which includes muscles, bones, organs and circulation, whereas *nāḍī* means nervous system, including the zones in which the vital energy flows. *Prāṇāyāma* plays the role of carrying energy to the remotest parts of our body.

Does *prāṇāyāma* end there? No. It has a philosophy of its own. The inhalation is the intake of cosmic breath; exhalation is individual energy coming out to unite with the cosmic breath. In inhalation-retention the cosmic energy communes with the individual energy and in exhalation-retention, the individual energy reaches out to commune with the Cosmic Force.

Some people doubt whether the breath and *prāṇa* are the same. For yogis the breath is energy. The breath not only carries the gross atmospheric energy but also nuclear energies. The steady, slow, regulated and subtle breath is the one that connects and establishes the relationship between the individual *(pinḍāṇda)* and the universal *(brahmāṇda)*.

Breathing is normally done by the brain. As the brain needs a lot of oxygen, it draws the energy, causing the air to be sucked in. Thus, one feels the stress in the brain from its need for oxygen. Similarly, to release the carbon dioxide, the brain cells create exhalation. Because the brain acts as the main instrument, in normal breathing, the stress is felt, whereas in *prāṇāyāmic* breathing, thanks to the use of *bhandas* this stress is not felt in the brain; hence, it becomes a passive witness.

The breath is gross and the energy hidden in that gross breath is subtle and fine. It is called *prāṇa*. The breath nourishes the system and produces energy. The energy within us is atomic as it comes in contact with cosmic energy, which is then converted into divine energy. As one can use nuclear energy for destructive as well as constructive purposes, so too the energy, which is vitalised with cosmic energy, can be utilised by man either for destructive or for constructive use. *Prāṇāyāma* is the method that makes this union of vital and cosmic energy divine. Hence, it is a positively constructive technique.

The change that occurs at the energy level leads one towards meditation. Meditation gives a positive divine silence. When one proceeds towards meditation without the practice of *prāṇāyāma*, it leads one towards negative silence. Negative silence gives sensual silence. The sensual silence may give tranquillity but not the unalloyed poise.

In *prāṇāyāma*, the breath charges the nerves with its energy. This energy charges the individual's mind with the sharpness of attention, tranquillity and silence as well. This state of consciousness leads one to experience the self, which is in the state of poise. The nerves are the links between the mind and the consciousness, consciousness and self and from the self *(asmitā)* to the Self *(nirāsmitā)*. Yogic practice gives a formidable strength to the nervous system, which can hold any amount of stress, wield any amount of strength and speed. If the nerves are shaky, the mind is shaky. Here, one ends up as a mental patient. When the breath leads the nerves, mind and consciousness to be on par with each other, it is true *prāṇāyāma.*

When you are engaged with thought or work you normally breathe from the abdomen. When you are emotionally involved, the breath moves in the upper portion of the chest. In a deep alert state, the middle chest breathes and the sleepy or dull state, the breathing is done with the lower lungs.

As far as a yogi is concerned, he touches all these parts in each breath. He does a total deep inhalation, as well as a total deep exhalation. All the compartments of the torso are opened for him. He achieves harmony, rhythm, depth, as well as total fullness.

Avoid strain, during inhalation, exhalation or retention. The normal inhalation contracts the cells of the brain and exhalation dilates them. Yogic *prāṇāyāma* neither contracts nor dilates the brain. It doesn't create any strain on the brain, but keeps it in a restful state. In *prāṇāyāma* practice, the brain is kept in a meditative state, while the body is held in an active state.

How does one know what is correct *prāṇāyāma* and what is false *prāṇāyāma?*

When one breathes by puffing the intercostal muscles, it is the muscle expansion and not the expansion and diffusion of the breath. In this case, the muscles are puffed and the lungs remain empty. In *prāṇāyāma*, the physical expansion or muscular expansion is not expected. If they are used, it is false *prāṇāyāma*. In correct *prāṇāyāma*, not only is physical freedom essential but also the elasticity of the lungs. The lungs have to be mobile, soft and sensitive to receive the energy that is expected to respond. The moment you see food, saliva oozes from the mouth; likewise the alveoli (the air sacs) have to receive the nectar of the breath with the feeling of exhilaration. While doing the *prāṇāyāma*, one should not get carried away with motion. Rather, one has to watch the receptivity of lungs, passivity of the brain, fullness in oneself and recession of nerves. All these have to go together.

You might have heard about Dilip Kumar Roy, who has an *āśram* called Hari Krishna Mandir, in Pune. Yesterday I received a letter saying that he had an attack of paralysis and dilation of the heart. When he asked me, before my departure to the USA, to help him, I met him in Mumbai and told him to do certain things, but unfortunately his doctors had asked him to do *bhastrikā prāṇāyāma* and he said that he had called me to teach him that *prāṇāyāma*. Tell me, how does this breathing help such a patient? Will it give any rest to the patient? Harsh breathing at this stage leads towards further haemorrhage. Some say that this type of breathing awakens *kuṇḍalini* and innocent people follow it. Is it not violence to the brain? Why put wrong ideas in the heads of innocent people? The pure and holy *kuṇḍalinī* is awakened only in those who are pure in body and holy in their heart. One may invite serious problems by doing wrong *prāṇāyāma* and bring a bad name to yoga. Scrutinise and analyse this great science before coming to any conclusion.

As *prāṇāyāma* is misinterpreted as harsh breathing, so also is the retention of breath *(kuṁbhaka)* misunderstood.

People take it for granted that by holding the breath, the brain remains under control as thoughts are arrested and desires get vanquished. With a competitive mind, they test how long the breath can be held. If you see them, their eyes get red and their ears get blocked, creating great tension in the throat and brain. Here, they hold the brain and not the breath. The stress is felt while breathing, the nerves become restless and restlessness makes one depressed. They may even hate to live in this world. They mistake this to be desirelessness. They think that their restlessness is a sign of hate against the visible world. These wrong practices deceive the practitioners. Such renunciation is not genuine renunciation. As *prāṇāyāma* is a stepping stone to spiritual life, one has to practise it carefully and watchfully. The practice of *prāṇāyāma* is considered by all yogis to be the highest penance *(tapas).*

Prāṇāyāma is meant to store energy. That is why it is done with *mudrās* and *bandhas* like *Jālandhara, Mūla* and *Uḍḍīyāṇa.* The flow of breath is controlled at the nostrils with the fingers. This controlled action is called *prāṇāyāma mudrā.* You build a dam to store water; the *mudrās* and *bandhas* are like dams that store energy so that it is not allowed to dissipate.

In *prāṇāyāma,* the flow of the breath must be kept slow, smooth and soft. The depth cannot be penetrated with harsh breathing. The distribution of energy is done horizontally, vertically and circumferentially and the consciousness also is expanded and controlled.

Prāṇāyāma leads essentially towards calmness and quietness so that the senses of perception and mind are not made to wander. They turn automatically towards the Self.

Prāṇāyāma is a foundation for *pratyāhāra, dhāraṇā, dhyāna* and *samādhi,* where the inward journey begins. Therefore, I stress these two limbs – the *āsana* and *prāṇāyāma,* as they lead one towards the inner journey.

(A demonstration and a question and answer session followed this lecture).

IS YOGA ART, SCIENCE, RELIGION OR PHILOSOPHY?*

Very often, people ask me to explain what exactly yoga means. Is it art, science, religion or philosophy? It is natural that such doubts excite the curiosity of those who are interested in yoga.

My answer to all of them is that yoga is not any one of these and at the same time all of the above combined together. It is independent and it is a consummation of all these faculties, transcending the realm of one's thoughts. It is the silver cloud that takes man from the plane of the body towards the realisation of the Self. One has to analyse, experiment and experience yoga in all the above categories and expel notions of doubt one by one to understand the significance of yoga. First let me explain the preceding expressions.

Art means skill. It is skilfulness in doing anything that is a result of knowledge, practice and its display. Science is systematised knowledge of any kind: it is a study of facts with experimentation. Art is experiential knowledge. Religion is a set of beliefs, practices and a moral code of conduct for human affairs. Philosophy stands for rational investigation and critical study of truths and principles of a state of being.

Yoga is the art of education to attain the realisation of the Self. We all live in nature's bounty consisting of the flora and fauna, which, if exploited with moderation, are there for our right enjoyment. The practice of yoga with skill, executed by repeated efforts and guided by principles from which springs creative beauty with the expression of true happiness within oneself, becomes subjective knowledge. Yoga, as subjective knowledge, is art. When yoga is learnt well, it is as nourishing and tasteful as wholesome food. It expresses the inner being of the practitioner as it refines his body, consciousness and self. He lives in it as if the earth is heaven.

As a science, yoga helps us to know ourselves through tests, experiments, experiences and observations. It makes us know what we are and how yoga is to be applied. But to taste that knowledge, we have to practise, like any artist who devotes and dedicates his time for his quest.

---

* From B.K.S. Iyengar's 60th birthday celebrations souvenir book, Puṇe, 1978.

As a religion, yoga has universal moral codes: non-violence (in action, word and thought) *(ahiṁsā)*, truthfulness *(satya)*, non-covetousness *(asteya)*, celibacy *(brahmacarya)* and non-possession beyond needs *(aparigraha)*. It has disciplines like cleanliness within and without *(śauca)*, contentment with the situation in which one is placed without malice or hatred *(santoṣa)*, burning desire to realise the truth *(tapas)*, study of the Self *(svādhyāya)*, and surrender of all actions to the Lord *(Īśvara praṇidhāna)*. It is a divine religion as it leads towards the realisation of the Self, a path leading to the realisation of God.

Philosophy deals mostly with the views of righteous life. *Vedānta* shows the ways of reaching the highest state of one's state of life. *Vedānta (veda* = knowledge and *anta* = end) is the consummation of all knowledge. Thus, *vedānta* means wisdom. It lives in the two expressions 'sustain' and 'abstain'. Fortunately, yoga guides in both philosophy and *vedānta*. As a philosophy, it leads to the art of living. The true art of living lies in understanding how to live with nature without disturbing the order of things as well as ourselves. Yoga helps us to distinguish the true and everlasting happiness and peace *(śreya)* from false and ephemeral pleasures, which are coupled with pain *(preya)*. To sustain what is good involves practice *(abhyāsa)*. To abstain from what retards evolution is renunciation *(vairāgya)*. Abstinence involves giving up pleasures which are not only congenial for living in peace and harmony, but also those that bring conflict, pain, sorrow and unhappiness. Observance of discipline and control of the senses and mind leads to the realisation of lasting unbiased happiness. This is yogic culture. Only a realised soul, through the light of his divine culture, free from bias, can illumine mankind. He shines like a lamp in darkness and illumines the consciousness of those who come to him for light. This is how a true culture participates in the creation of a civilisation, or gives birth to the true 'religion' of man.

Before ending, I quote from the *Śvetāśvatara Upaniṣad:* "God is one and all pervading, but people call Him according to their understanding, by different names". In the same way, yoga is one. As the trunk is one, but branches are many, yoga is one, but it embraces all its branches at the same time.

YOGA – A SCIENCE THAT LEADS ONE TO GOD

Yoga as a science deals with the health of the body and harmony of the mind and consciousness. It is this training of body and consciousness which leads to the experience of eternal tranquillity of the Self. In this way, yoga engulfs the whole of man for his evolution from the base – the body – to the extreme end – that of the Self.

In spite of the development of various branches of medicine for physical and emotional diseases, the administration of drugs alone does not free man from the host of ailments that human flesh is heir to. Health is a perfect state of equilibrium of the entire human system. It has to be earned by sheer discriminative hard work along with ethical observances.

The body is the dwelling place of the Self, and yet it is the most abused instrument of man. This body has an amazing power to recover. Knowing this, let us direct our intelligence and hasten to change our outlook and habits in order to re-educate ourselves completely by adopting the right food, proper *yogāsanas* and *prāṇāyāma* and train the consciousness to keep it free from envy and negative thoughts for a healthy condition. This way of re-education goes a long way in saving the life force for one to realise the source of being.

The body is the shrine where the Divine Spark dwells. Whether it is for enjoyment in life *(bhoga)* or for freedom from suffering *(mokṣa)* the body has to be taken care of.

According to the *Vedas*, there is no peace or happiness without health. These sacred scriptures proclaim that *ātmā* is unattainable by those who are weak. Lord Buddha had said that the greatest gift is health. When such are the words of the immortals, is it not our bounden duty to endeavour constantly to maintain this body, the God-given gift? Lord Patañjali emphasises that persistent, long and uninterrupted efforts, done with advertence (attention, heedfulness) alone, can lead us to that unalloyed perfection of body and consciousness where all divisions of body, consciousness and individual self vanish. This is the essence of a sound self and a sound mind, in a sound body.

Patañjali analyses in detail the causes which create disharmony in body and mind and lead man to misery and unhappiness. The nine forms of obstacles are said to be: disease *(vyādhi)*, mental laziness *(styāna)*, doubt *(saṁśaya)*, negligence *(pramāda)*, physical laziness *(ālasya)*, indiscipline of the senses *(avirati)*, erroneous views *(bhrāntidarśana)*, lack of perseverance *(alabdhabhūmikatva)* and backsliding *(anavasthitatva)*. The symptoms are pain *(duḥkha)*, despair *(daurmanasya)*, unsteadiness of the body *(angamejayatva)* and unrhythmic breathing *(śvāsapraśvāsa)*. (*Y.S.*, I.30-31).

Everyone has one or the other of the above mentioned impediments. One has to think and work to overcome these causes of unhappiness in order to obtain undisturbed peace. Patañjali points out the ways and means showing three types of discipline: moral, physical and mental. Moral discipline is of two types: individual and social ethics.

The moral, physical and mental disciplines consist of the physical practice of postures *(āsana)* and rhythmic breathing *(prāṇāyāma)*. *Prāṇa* means breath and *āyāma* means lengthening out. These two disciplines tone and help to cultivate the individual along with the social ethics, physical and mental health, in order to live and let live.

According to the *yoga śāstra* (yogic texts), there are as many *āsanas* as there are living species. Their names always have significance; they range from insects and reptiles to sages and incarnations of God. They point out the essential unity of life, expressing the same Divine Essence that pervades all. The practice of *āsanas* and *prāṇāyāma* helps to circulate oxygenated blood to every part of the body and eliminate toxins from the system*.

After undergoing the moral and physical disciplines, one becomes fit to practice the mental disciplines. They are withdrawal of the senses and emancipation from the domination of the exterior tempting objects. Here begin the subtle aspects of yoga *(dhāraṇā, dhyāna* and *samādhi)*, for the realisation of the Divine Essence *(paramātman)* in us.

If the body is not taken care of, then the hosts of sorrow and unhappiness enters in the form of disease and desecrates this temple of God. If we are vigilant, diseases and other evils shall not touch us. Hence, yoga is taught to attain perfect health and good life leading one towards God with an enduring and everlasting joy.

---

* For more information on this subject, see my books, *Light on Yoga* and *Light on Prāṇāyāma*, Harper Collins Ltd., London, UK. See also *Body the Shrine, Yoga thy Light*, Bombay, 1978, pp. 53-60, and *Iyengar, His Life and Work*, Timeless Books, USA, 1987, pp. 35-57

PATHWAY TO SALVATION*

The culmination of yoga is samādhi.
After attaining this, the yogi shines like the sun
and illumines those who take refuge in him.

In Europe, America or India the questions I am posed as a practitioner of yoga are usually as follows: Can you swallow acid, chew glass and walk on fire and water? Can you read the future? Are you a clairvoyant? Could you make yourself invisible? What happens after death? Do you practise *haṭha yoga* or *rāja yoga?*

Such questions imply a misunderstanding of yoga. They are only looking for certain sensational powers acquired perhaps through the practice of yoga, which however are certainly not to be taken as the goal to be achieved in yogic practice. Yoga is for the search of the Self and this search is not meant for public attraction or attention.

According to Patañjali, the aim of yoga is to bring stillness in mental impulses and thought-waves. Shri Svātmārāma, another authority, tells us that all our movements are caused by positive and negative currents, termed as *piṅgalā* and *iḍā*, sun and moon, *prāṇa* and *apāna*. According to him, the harmonious union of these positive and negative currents is yoga. Shri Krishna in the *Bhagavad Gītā* describes the true yogi as one who keeps tranquillity of mind in heat and cold, success and failure, pain and pleasure, and evil and good; so he remains calm and composed through the ups and downs of life. Yoga is putting body and mind to the divine purpose of service and sacrifice. Shri Krishna further states that all actions performed gracefully and with joy are to be considered yogic actions.

Yoga is the art of bringing together the *jīvātmā* (individual self) with the *paramātmā* (the All-Pervading Soul or the Universal Self). Hence, yoga is the re-discovery of experiencing the eternal *puruṣa*, or the Self.

---

* From *Bhavan's Journal*, December 9, 1973.

MĀRGA OR *PATH*

The *ātmā* or the soul is free, but the influence of intelligence and mind taints it; hence the search for reality becomes essential. However due to ignorance of the true nature of the soul, we dwell in the senses. In order to discard this ignorance the *ṛṣis* of old pointed out various paths for Self-realisation:

a) *Jñāna mārga:* the path of knowledge in which the seeker learns to discriminate between the real and the unreal.

b) *Karma mārga:* the path of selfless service without looking for the benefits accruing from such service.

c) *Bhakti mārga:* the path of love and devotion.

d) *Yoga mārga:* the path that studies the activities of the consciousness and brings them under control.

All impulses such as desire, passion and possessiveness originate from the mind, which is also the source of thinking and understanding. All these four paths guide the consciousness to withdraw from these impulses and then direct it to develop stability first and afterwards, to go towards the realisation of the Self.

While the paths may differ at their starting point, they all have the same goal: Self-realisation. According to one's destiny created by the subliminal impressions *(saṁskāra)*, the path may be long or short, devious or straight; but each one is expected to work to the fullest extent, according to his capacity, to realise the inner light.

Man is blessed with head, heart and hands, which correspond to *jñāna*, *bhakti* and *karma*. They complement each other, for *karma* cannot be perfect without knowledge and love; *bhakti* cannot be understood without action and knowledge, and *jñāna* (knowledge) cannot be gained without love and action.

It is very interesting to note how the path of yoga is connected to these three paths and embraces all of them in their approach to the spiritual quest of mankind. Knowledge, love and action constitute man. These three – knowledge, love and action – are inter-woven. Yoga helps to acquire true knowledge, true love and true action. Unless the body and consciousness are purified, knowledge cannot be complete, love cannot be full, or action unselfish. To neglect the body and the consciousness is to betray the Self. No culture is worthy of its name if it does not seek the harmony of the human trinity – body, consciousness and Self.

MEANS OF YOGA

Consciousness is in constant movement. As consciousness is the king of the senses and mind, the stilling of consciousness is called *rāja yoga*. All are not endowed to be able to still the consciousness at once; hence, Svātmārāma stresses that body and breath (the source of life) must be first brought under control.

Body, consciousness and Self have been given by God to be utilised for right living. Yoga embraces the body, the consciousness and the Self of all and as such it is a 'Universal Culture', and also a 'Universal Religion'.

Patañjali has given us the eight yogic means in the form of *yama, niyama, āsana, prāṇāyāma, pratyāhāra, dhāraṇā, dhyāna* and *samādhi*, to purify the consciousness and then lead that purified consciousness towards the light of the Self.

YAMA is a collective name comprising non-violence, truthfulness, non-covetousness, continence and the rejection of acquiring superfluous wealth. As these ethics apply to everybody, they naturally become the Universal Principles. Class, time and place play no part in following them.

Ahiṁsā (non-violence): Is to draw back from infliction of any type of injury whether physical or mental, done knowingly or unknowingly, by thought or deed. When hatred and animosity are abandoned, an all-embracing cosmic love settles in one.

Satya (truth): Is to be ruthlessly truthful and honest with oneself. One's speech becomes infallible and whatever one thinks and says turns out to be true.

Asteya (non-covetousness, non-stealing and non-misappropriation): By this, the *sādhaka's* desires are controlled and his wants reduced; then things come to him without asking.

Brahmacarya (continence): This is enjoined in all matters of sex, whether it is mere desire or actual. This purity opens the gates of knowledge towards perfection.

Aparigraha (non-possessiveness, greedlessness): This is not to desire things that are unnecessary for the maintenance of life: for desire is followed by attachment, attachment leads one towards aversion and avarice towards jealousy and hatred. It is very difficult to know where need ends and when greed begins. But the practice of yoga guides the *sādhaka* with discriminative faculty and distinguishes the need and greed and protects the *sādhaka*. If desire stretches forth in an unending chain, it leads finally to the destruction of right conduct. Hence the principles of *yama* are advised.

NIYAMA is composed of five principles: purity, contentment, austerity, study of the scriptures, and surrender of all actions to the Lord.

Śauca (means purity): It is of two kinds, internal and external. Both must be cultivated. External purity means cleanliness i.e., being untainted by our environmental surroundings in body and mental behaviour. Internal purity is the rooting out of selfishness, egoism, passion, anger, possessiveness, attachment and aversion.

Santoṣa (contentment): Contentment reduces desire and makes one cheerful.

Tapas (penance): Enables one to endure hardship and adversity, by discipline of the body and senses so that the consciousness moves closer to the Self.

Svādhyāya (self-study): The education of oneself to deal with the search for truth and Self-knowledge.

Īśvara praṇidhāna (surrender to God): Is the surrender of all of one's actions to the Lord and confiding oneself entirely to His Will.

Yama and *niyama* calm the disturbed mind and bring contentment. They are great universal principles to be cultivated by every human being in order to realise the four aims of life *(puruṣārtha)*. These are *dharma, artha, kāma* and *mokṣa.*

a) *Dharma* is to live in accordance with ethical laws, as spiritual realisation is impossible without observation of morality.

b) *Artha* is to work for the means of livelihood and the necessities of food and shelter. One must be able to live without the fear of constant want. Wealth alone cannot give lasting joy and its enjoyment requires a sound body and mind. It is equally true that a poorly nourished body and the haunting fear of survival are the fertile ground for the seeds of disease and worry.

c) *Kāma* is the enjoyment of life. Neither lasting peace nor enjoyment of life is possible without a sound body.

d) *Mokṣa*, the last, is emancipation. The enlightened man realises that power, pleasure, wealth and knowledge do not bring emancipation and freedom. He tries to rise above his *tāmasic, rājasic* and *sāttvic* qualities by gaining freedom from his emotions.

The body plays a vital part in attaining the fourfold aims of life. The sages knew very well that though the body wears out, it is nevertheless an instrument to attain realisation and as such has to be kept in good condition.

Traditionally the body has five layers or sheaths – the physical, the vital, the mental, the intellectual and the blissful. To penetrate these layers, constant discipline, sustained practice and tireless efforts are required. The aim of yoga is to experience the state of unalloyed bliss.

ĀSANA together with *PRĀṆĀYĀMA* purify the body and mind. These techniques are unrivalled both in their preventive as well as in their curative effects. The *āsanas* are innumerable, catering to the various needs of the muscular, digestive, glandular, nervous and other systems of the body. Just as a goldsmith heats gold to burn out the impurities, *āsana* too helps in supplying well-oxygenated blood to the body to burn the toxins and purge them out.

Āsana influences not only physical, physiological and biological changes but also neuro-psychological ones. The aspirant does not take up the practice of *āsana* for the sake of sensual pleasure or showmanship, but directs his practice towards the betterment of his life and the realisation of the Self. It is fallacious to believe that maintaining a sitting posture with comfort alone will eradicate the scores of evils and infirmities man is heir to. Nor is health to be mistaken for mere existence. Health is the delicate balance and harmony in body, mind, intelligence, consciousness and self, where physical disabilities and mental distractions vanish and the gates of the Self open.

The type of food taken is important for *āsana*. It should be neither too hot nor too cold. It must not be excessively pungent, sour, salty or bitter. Our outlook on life is determined to a large extent by what and how we eat. If each morsel is taken to enable one to serve the divine, then one is on the right path. It is true that character is influenced by the food we eat and it is equally true to say that the practice of yoga changes the food and eating habits of the aspirant. The sages tell us that yoga is not for him who sleeps too much or keeps awake too much. Moderation in one's living habits is the rule.

Āsana and *prāṇāyāma* should be done in a clean and airy place. Fold a blanket or two and spread it on a carpet, that is sufficient for the practice of *āsana* and *prāṇāyāma*, provided the floor underneath is even. There is no age limit and no geographical restriction. Differences of sex and health too are no drawback. All that is required for success in yoga is cheerfulness, perseverance, courage, correct knowledge of the techniques to be followed, moderation in one's habits and faith in the practice of yoga. Then the effects of yogic practice as enumerated by the sages follow. These are beauty and strength, clarity of speech and expression, calmness of the nerves, an increase of one's digestive power and a happy disposition that is revealed in a face full of smiles.

The mastery of *āsana* also leads to freedom from dualities. The duality between the body and the consciousness, and the consciousness and the Self vanishes, resulting in tranquillity. To live in the Infinite is the result of yoga. This happens only when the aspirant's attempts become effortless *(sahajāvasthā)*. He gains health, strength, firmness and lightness. He becomes sharper and learns humility. Thus the essence of the practice of *āsana* is to light the path to the spiritual awakening of the practitioner. His senses withdraw inwards, vanity gradually begins to fade out and divinity pervades.

Yama, niyama and *āsana* are known as *bahiraṅga sādhanā*.

Prāṇāyāma is part of *bahiraṅga sādhanā*, and *pratyāhāra* is considered as a transitory state between *bahiraṅga* and *antaraṅga sādhanā*.*

Prāṇāyāma or breath control consists of three basic movements: inspiration, retention and expiration. Inspiration is the intake of energy. Retention is the interval of time or restraint of breath after full inhalation or after full exhalation. It is the cultivation of the art of silence in a motionless state, or cradling the divine energy within. Expiration is the emptying of the mind and brain of all thoughts and the surrendering of the self to the Universal Self.

The practice of *prāṇāyāma* brings illumination as it purges the all-powerful brain and forces it to surrender to the seat of the consciousness. Thus the impurity and the arrogance of the 'I', which covers the core, is destroyed. The regular practice of *prāṇāyāma* rids one of fear, develops strong will power, clarity and correctness in thinking. Consciousness becomes stable and fickleness is eradicated. Then the imposition of discipline is no longer forced and an urge for natural discipline begins in *sādhanā*.

If a man born blind were graced and granted by God to see for a moment a glimpse of the beauty and grandeur of the world, who would be able to measure his ecstasy? Similarly, if yoga bestows a glimpse of the Divine to the *sādhaka*, is it not worth all the pain and hard work implied in the practice of yoga?

DHĀRAṆĀ, is to focus all one's attention to bring the subject (Self) and the object (consciousness) together; while in *DHYĀNA*, the Self and consciousness become a single unit. This is similar to *tailadhāra* (pouring oil from one vessel to another), where the oil flows steadily without any splashes. It cannot be explained but only experienced. It is a state of complete

---

* See Table "The evolutionary stages in *sādhanā*, according to the three main texts on yoga". Page n. 145, Table n. 7.

peace and oneness with the Universe and the creator. One exists without the awareness of 'I'. There is no sensation of consciousness, breath, nor any type of movement or anything else existing, except infinite peace and joy *(ānanda)*. This joy cannot be perceived by the senses, the mind or the consciousness.

SAMĀDHI is the experience of unalloyed bliss, the last facet of yoga. This unalloyed bliss of the *puruṣa* becomes the real instrument for God realisation. In all fields, creativity means transcending consciousness of the "I". The musician can bring forth delicate and subtle divine sounds only by forgetting himself. The poet distils the quintessence of language and the artist presents the wondrous world of line and colour only by transcending the self. The yogi too is creative within himself and the experience of this new creation within himself touches a state where neither time, nor cause and effect affect him. His forgetfulness of the self *(asmitā)* is the awareness of an integrated personality. Body, consciousness and self are integrated and united with the Self *(puruṣa)*. In this state of purity and wisdom, the yogi shines forth with humility and simplicity. Such a yogi radiates like the sun with no barriers or limitations. Not only is he illumined but he also illumines all who come into his orbit.

YOGA – A PATH TO *ĀTMA DARŚANA* *

Caught as we are in a web of words, it is rather difficult to define 'yoga' so as to satisfy everybody. God is one, yet He is named and described in different ways. Yoga too is one, but each interpreter qualifies it according to his own whims and fancy. Yoga has been defined as 'yoking' or 'uniting'.

Yoking the body, the senses, the mind, the intelligence and consciousness together, in order to unite the self with the Universal Soul is yoga. This yoking is achieved by firm discipline, whereby the right character is developed. This yoking, union and integration results in consciousness of perfect purity.

Yoga leads to that state in which neither the physical, mental, intellectual or spiritual fluctuations, nor the dualities like the consciousness of the body, mind and self take place. All movements in the seat of consciousness are silenced as if life and death have no difference.

The body should be neither neglected nor pampered. It is the only instrument and the only resource we are provided with to meet our Creator, the Lord. It is to be understood that the body, the temple of the soul, is not for mere muscle building, but for spiritual practice and experience. It may be fashionable to despise the body as something non-spiritual. Yet, none can afford to neglect it. The moment we neglect or pamper it, aversion or attachment to it increases and the right royal road to *ātma darśana* is lost.

Great saints like Shri Ramakrishna Paramahamsa, Swami Vivekananda and Bhagawan Ramana Maharshi were not free from the onslaught of diseases. But they had the inner strength to bear with tolerance the afflictions of the body and did not allow the stability of their emotional and intellectual centres to get disturbed.

---

* Published in *Bhavan's Journal*, November 12, 1972. It is difficult to give an exact translation of the term *ātma darśana*. *Ātmā* means Self and *darśana* means insight or enlightenment. So, *ātma darśana* means Self-enlightenment.

Can ordinary people like us endure suffering as they did? We may boast about our capacity to put up with pain, but when we are faced with reality, the bitter truth surfaces, that we cannot really bear pain. Pain and suffering therefore force us to take cognisance of our body.

It is not only the pain that makes us realise that we are bound to the body. Pleasure very quickly tends to enmesh us in its snares. The senses of perception and the organs of action, with their strong outward tendencies draw the consciousness to the pleasures of the world making a permanent impact on man.

Attracted to the pleasures of life, the individual begins to believe that such pleasures are eternal, whereas in fact they are transitory. Caught in the giddy whirl of pleasures, he is blinded and fails to realise this fact.

A discriminating person however, sees through the ephemeral veil of sensory pleasures and learns to channel the outgoing energy of the senses inwards. He turns that energy back to the shrine of the Divinity, the Soul.

The *Kaṭha Upaniṣad* reminds us that the body is important in the spiritual quest. It compares the body to a chariot, the senses to the horses, the mind to the reins, the intelligence to the charioteer and the *jīvātmā* (soul) to the master of the chariot. If something goes wrong with the chariot, or the horses, or the reins, or the charioteer, not only the chariot and the charioteer, but also the master, comes to grief.

Similarly, if something goes wrong with the body, God-realisation through Self-realisation cannot be reached.

The body like a boat carries the in-dweller, the Self, from the shores of bondage to the shores of emancipation. Emancipation is after all freedom from the entanglement and allurement of the senses and mind.

A number of qualities are pre-requisites for experiencing the state of freedom. Freedom demands purity in body, senses, mind and intelligence as well as humility and tenacity.

Besides these, faith, courage and uninterrupted intelligent awareness are to be present whether one is wide awake, half asleep, or in deep slumber. The *sādhaka* has to live with a mind free from selfishness in his daily chores and practices. This is poise in action. This poise leads to that serenity that one hankers for. Yoga assures and offers complete stability to integrate the body, mind, intelligence and consciousness.

To realise this integration, yoga outlines codes of moral conduct, physical and vital disciplines, and disciplines the senses and the intelligence in order to reach the state of oneness, where dualities vanish and the seeker becomes the seer.

On the effects of yoga, Patañjali very beautifully says, *"Yogāṅgānuṣṭhānāt aśuddhikṣaye jñānadīptiḥ āvivekakhyāteḥ".* (*Y.S.*, II.28). This means that by adherence to the practice of yoga, impurities of body and consciousness are destroyed and the pure light of knowledge and wisdom is kindled. This quote from Patañjali is more than enough to illustrate the importance of yoga as a path for refinement and spiritual enlightenment or *ātma darśana.*

YOGA – FREEDOM THROUGH DISCIPLINE*

Thank you for inviting me to Oxford. Oxford is one of the most enlightened educational centres of the world. I come from a place where there was not even a primary school. Perhaps you all know that some years ago, I succeeded in building a primary school in my village so that the coming generation may be fortunate enough to have the benefits of education. I have never stepped into a college. Having no formal education, I feel somewhat embarrassed and humbled to address educated people like you in this temple of education?

With my shortcomings, I feel the joy in myself to be speaking to enlightened people like you. I feel this is a great honour and I am proud of this occasion.

PURPOSE OF EDUCATION

Real education is that which develops the conscious mind to a greater receptivity. Many of you might have read my book *Light on Yoga,* and may have practised yoga under the guidance of my pupils who are teaching here. The book conveys objectively the facets of what I experienced. Though the book does not reveal everything in totality, one should be content with it, as it provides a firm foundation to go from part to part to know the whole. It is commonly understood that one has to begin with different parts in order to know and absorb the whole through self-education.

Education is that which teaches us first to know thoroughly the parts, so that one moves on to know the whole. In the art of learning one begins compartmentally, working clearly, in order to experience the whole one day. Education is complete when it makes one realise one's ignorance and light the lamp of inquiry for progress. Education brings about the realisation of what one does not know and how much has been left out of the known.

---

* Talk at Oxford, 20th June 1976.

BHOGA, ROGA AND *YOGA*

Indian philosophy has six main streams of thought: *Nyāya, Vaiśeṣika, Sāṁkhya, Yoga, Pūrva Mīmāṁsā* and *Uttara Mīmāṁsā* (now known as *Vedānta*). My subject is yoga and I am only eligible to say a few words on yoga.

Yoga is as old as civilisation. It begins with the discipline and cultivation of character and it culminates in emancipation and freedom. Between 500 and 200 BC, the sage Patañjali codified this yogic journey, explaining it as great art, science and philosophy and at the same time showed ways to evolve, step by step, from the periphery of the body towards the core of being, to reach the zenith of evolution.

Yoga co-ordinates activities of the body, the consciousness and the individual self harmoniously. These three entities act heterogeneously. The body goes against the consciousness and the consciousness goes against the self. Similarly the self goes against the current of consciousness or the body goes against the thoughts of consciousness and the self. Sometimes, the body and consciousness may act in co-ordination, but the self does not go along. The body and mind may say, "Smoke!", but the self may not agree. The self guides but the smoker does not listen to the call. Yoga makes these heterogeneous actions blend homogeneously as one listens to the call of the inner voice.

Heterogeneity is *bhoga* and homogeneity is yoga. Complete co-ordination is yoga and noncoordination is *bhoga*. *Bhoga* means the joy of worldly and sensual pleasure. Sensual pleasure does not lead one towards pure tranquillity but towards *roga* or disease. Yoga helps one's intelligence to get acquainted with the Self. *Bhoga* or worldly pleasures, associates one with the senses and the mind. Yoga associates and unites the body with the consciousness (mind, intelligence and ego) and then both to the Self.

The aim of yoga is Self-realisation. The goal of *bhoga* is sensual pleasure leading gradually towards suffering. Yoga leads one towards emancipation, but *bhoga* leads to *roga* or diseases. As pleasures incite one to overindulge, they make one suffer with pain and affliction, whereas yoga makes one enjoy the pleasures of the world without inviting disease. *Bhoga* binds one, leading to discomfort and disease, which may end up in early death.

Nowadays, drinking, smoking, sensual enjoyments and meditation go together. How can *roga*, *bhoga* and yoga go together? Moderation in *bhoga* and intense attention in yoga is the path of physical, mental, intellectual and spiritual health. Let us not live a lifeless life, but adopt a dynamic, positive and natural way of life through the yogic process. Yoga teaches one to lead a natural life and to experience the divinity within one's self.

FROM COMPLEXITY TO SIMPLICITY

Patañjali, in the very first aphorism uses the word *anuśāsanam* (codes of discipline) and comes later to *pratiprasava*, (*Y.S.*, II.10), that is, going back towards the core of being, the culmination of seeking or search.

According to yoga, mind is a gross sense while intelligence, ego and consciousness are considered as subtle senses. The mind, being more peripheral than intelligence, it is the outermost sheath of consciousness.

Patañjali teaches one how to peel the layer of the mind and to educate the *citta*, so that it experiences simplicity through yoga. Through this experience, the clashes of thoughts within man come to an end. *Citta* as consciousness acts as the first great principle in man. It comprises the mind *(manas)*, intelligence *(buddhi)* and ego *(ahaṁkāra)*; hence, it is a complex entity.

However this journey from complexity to simplicity, will not be an easy one. It is a journey from a difficult and complex state of being towards a simple, innocent state without any ignorance or arrogance. The complex state of *citta* is known today as stress and strain. If one can face life without stress and strain, it becomes easy. This complex *citta* acts as a springboard to think and act in order to reach the serene state of simplicity and rhythm in life. The effect of yoga is like that of the fragrance of roses covered with thorns. One has to hold the rose with great care to enjoy its fragrance. Similarly, millions of thorns prick the body, mind, intelligence, ego and consciousness with unbearable pain. Yet these have to be endured patiently. Yoga teaches the art of overcoming pain and affliction as well as methods to avoid them. When man faces the ups and downs in life, he learns through trial and error. In the beginning one is bound to commit mistakes and suffer. From these mistakes one realises what is right and what is wrong and learns to build up strength of character, avoiding the thorns of desire, which are not congenial to life. This, for me, is education, where the gates of study and understanding open for emancipation.

We have all experienced the simplicity of consciousness in childhood. As we grow, it becomes hard to be as simple and as innocent as we were in childhood. We lose that innocence because our behaviour gets complicated as we grow. The more the modes become complicated, the more difficult yoga seems. For a doctor the body is a complex object, for a psychologist the mind is a complex object. Having known the complexity of the consciousness and the body, a yogi tries to simplify their modes and behaviour. He cleanses the body and removes the taints from the consciousness so that the consciousness experiences the Self with crystal clarity that is ever pure and colourless (untainted).

In order to understand this simplicity of the consciousness and purity of the Self, one needs a matured knowledge *(paripakva jñāna)*. We go to educational institutions to acquire knowledge. But to learn yoga, the institution is not outside. You have to step into your own university within the body, the mind and the intelligence. The body is an educational centre. The intelligence is its chancellor and volition is its vice-chancellor. Here the intelligence cannot work unless it is ignited by volition. Volition is will power. In yoga terminology, it is called *icchā śakti* or *preraṇā śakti*. Will power has the strength to take a decision. Intelligence, without volition is impotent. Intelligence and will power, both being dynamic in their own ways, approach each other and get ignited and electrified. When the mind and intelligence come closer to each other, intelligence becomes meek, because the mind – being tricky – makes the intelligence oscillate. Yoga creates a state of equilibrium by training the mind and will power so that the will power is sharpened and the mind is tamed. Then the intelligence shines out with clarity and purity and steps out of the shadow of either the will or the mind.

The will, consciousness (mind, intelligence and ego), senses of perception, organs of action and body are the vehicles of the Self. Patañjali offers methods to discipline these vehicles and to train them towards purity, cleanliness and clarity. This quality is a simplicity and humility where arrogance loses its presence. The path of yoga is such that both discipline and freedom are found in it. If discipline is the root, then freedom is the fruit. In yoga, discipline and freedom, freedom and discipline go hand in hand.

OBJECTIVE KNOWLEDGE AND SUBJECTIVE EXPERIENCE

Knowledge has two facets. One is objective and the other subjective. Objective knowledge is based on speculation, thinking and analysis, whereas subjective knowledge is to verify the objective knowledge with experience. Subjective knowledge comes through practical experience and objective knowledge is earned through theoretical study. Yoga is both a practical as well as a theoretical subject, but it is neither blind practice nor a discursive one. Any practice needs some objective knowledge. One puts this objective knowledge or the acquired knowledge into practice, so that one experiences the reality of the objective knowledge. This experienced knowledge again leads towards the act of rethinking, reanalysing and reprocessing to set oneself for a new avenue in knowledge. Due to this renewal of knowledge, practice takes a new shape, leading each objective knowledge into subjective experience and at the same time that subjective experience guides one to express accurately the objective knowledge. This cycle of knowledge from the objective to the subjective and from the subjective to the objective produces a certain reaction in one and develops a memory tasting like a ripe fruit.

This memory is not merely remembrance of imprints but it is like the butter that is churned out of knowledge and experience. This accumulated memory is cleansed and clarified by our re-thinking and re-experiencing process. Wrong and unwanted memories are discarded and ripe memories retained. It is actually the ripe memory that stops the fluctuations of the inquiring and acquiring mind. When this cycle comes to an end, then the mind, intelligence and consciousness remain like an ocean without waves.

Thus the yogic method combines and blends the theoretical and practical approaches, offering stability for the *sādhaka* to experience the real.

FROM *ADHYĀTMAVIDYĀ* TO *ĀTMAVIDYĀ*

Vidyā means knowledge. *Adhyātmavidyā* means knowledge concerning the Self, with its various sheaths and functions. Knowing and coming in direct contact with the Self is *ātmavidyā*. Discipline begins with *adhyātmavidyā* and freedom comes with *ātmavidyā*.

As a flower has several petals, the flower of yoga has eight petals or eight disciplines. These are *yama, niyama, āsana, prāṇāyāma, pratyāhāra, dhāraṇā, dhyāna* and *samādhi*. These petals or disciplines take one towards clarity of consciousness and conscience and blossom into *adhyātmavidyā* (the knowledge that liberates, B.G. X, 32) and *ātmavidyā* (the knowledge of the Self).

YAMA AND *NIYAMA*

We are well acquainted with the principles of *yama*. If one watches carefully, one realises that one often breaks the principles of *yama* because of undisciplined thought-force and actions. One becomes the slave of the senses of perception and organs of action. The senses of perception entice and cause the organs of action to act. Practice of the principles of *yama* tames the organs of action and *niyama* educates and disciplines the senses of perception not to entice the organs of action.

ĀSANA AND *PRĀṆĀYĀMA*

Desires are never ending. The thirst of desire cannot be quenched soon. One does not become desireless at once. Desires cannot be discarded easily and they do not vanish on their own. The yogic method gradually checks and controls them. The journey of right education begins with *yama*. The known desires, which are recognisable, are checked by the disciplines of *yama* and *niyama*, while the deep rooted desires, which may not surface soon are worked out by the other *aṅga* of yoga. The taming of the physiological and psychological body begins with *āsana* and *prāṇāyāma*, a starting point to remove the darkness of ignorance. The mind, which is very near the outer body, gets attracted easily, even when there is slight indisposition. Diseases of the body, like flatulence, cold, fever, uneasiness and so forth are recognised immediately but mental diseases are not recognised so easily. It should be known that the practice of *āsana* is not meant just for physical health, but for a healthy, balanced and calm mind. Through the organic body, *āsana* makes the consciousness to penetrate deep within. Both psyche (mind) and soma (body) are treated through *āsana*. It helps one to know the known mind, while *prāṇāyāma* takes one to bring to the surface the unknown inner mind.

Practice of *āsana* produces a lot of energy, while *prāṇāyāma* takes this produced vital energy to the remotest parts of the body for physiological and energetic nourishment and for the development of sensitivity and dynamic awareness in intelligence. This flow of energy makes the intelligence aware and attentive to feel each part of the body from the periphery to the core or from the skin to the Self. If this penetration is not there, insensitivity develops and becomes a breeding ground for disease. Therefore, *āsana* and *prāṇāyāma* are a preventive as well as curative system. Though medical science has enriched us with its understanding of the functioning of the anatomical and physiological bodies, it has not shown the changes that take place in the body with the fusion of energy and consciousness. *Āsana* and *prāṇāyāma* do that beautifully, enriching the functions of the vehicles of man as a whole. Yet credit has to be given to modern science which has provided artificial limbs, transplantation of organs and so forth.

PRATYĀHĀRA

Āsana produces energy and *prāṇāyāma* distributes energy: when the intelligence reaches each fibre and cell of the body, the old and stale energy is brought out and new energy is circulated. *Prāṇāyāma* deflates this energy and *pratyāhāra* reabsorbs it from all corners of the body. In *prāṇāyāma*, the brain is made to remain quiet, while in *pratyāhāra*, the seat of the mind is cultivated to remain silent. In this way the brawn, the brain and the mind are made to remain stable, quiet and silent.

Cream is present in milk. One churns the milk to separate cream from milk. Similarly, the various aspects of yoga help the energy to get saturated like cream in the form of clear intelligence, and allow the energy to flow uninterruptedly as *dhāraṇā* and *dhyāna* from the core of the being to the skin and from the skin to the core. This is the essence of yoga.

NO *DHYĀNA* WITHOUT *JÑĀNA*

Nowadays it has become very common for everybody to talk about *dhyāna* or meditation. Without *jñāna* (knowledge), there is no *dhyāna* and without *dhyāna* there is no *jñāna*. A ripe knowledge *(paripakva jñāna)* leads one towards *dhyāna*. From *yama* to *pratyāhāra*, the 'gross knowable' is known, but the subtle has yet to be known. These subtle senses are the intelligence, ego and consciousness. In *dhāraṇā* the intelligence surfaces clearly and becomes known.

In *dhyāna* the 'I' and the 'I - ness' are humbled and the practitioner transforms himself from the individual self towards the Universal Self. Thus, these seven petals of yoga take the practitioner to breathe in the spiritual fragrance by integrating the body to the mind; the mind to the intelligence; the intelligence to the self; and the self to the Self. In this state, the intelligence gets matured, quietened, placid and serene. Now there is nothing for the intelligence to 'know'. This is the absolute state of consciousness, one without a second.

Up to the state of *dhāraṇā* there is a method, a technique, but for *dhyāna* and *samādhi* there is no technique. A teacher is necessary to guide the student up to *dhāraṇā*, whereas in *dhyāna* the student becomes the master and the same master residing within, guides him as his pupil.

Dhyāna leads towards *Īśvara praṇidhāna*. *Japa* and *bhajan* make the consciousness move towards the seer. They are considered as preparatory steps for *dhyāna*.

a) *Japa*

Often one is advised to repeat the *japa āuṁ*. Repetition of *āuṁ* is considered as meditation. But *japa* and *dhyāna* are not the same. *Japa sādhanā* may lead one towards *dhyāna* but *japa* cannot be *dhyāna*. In *dhyāna* there is no word, there is no verbal expression.

Āuṁ is a word. It is symbolic, but it has *śabda* or sound. It is composed of three letters: *ā*, *u* and *ṁ*. These letters are not picked up out of the blue. When you open your mouth, the first syllable that is produced is in the form of the sound *ā*. The very opening of the mouth is a pronouncement of *ā*. The middle syllable is *u* which is neither opening nor closing the mouth but a movement. When the mouth completely closes it is *ṁ*. The syllable *āuṁ* is the base for all words. The creation of words is called *śabda brahma*. Words have resonant sounds. Sound has a rhythm. This rhythmic sound is called *nāda brahma*. No *śabda* can be uttered without these three syllables, Hence, it is considered Divine.

The Supreme Soul has no name or form. Names and forms belong to objects, but the subject has no name or form. God cannot be expressed. We name a baby and call it by that name. By which name can we call the Supreme? In spite of knowing that the Supreme has no name, there is an urge to call Him by name. So the Supreme or God is called by various names.

Āuṁ is the root of verbal expression. *Āuṁ* begins from the navel and ends in the mouth and the sound merges back into the navel. Even a dumb or mute person has his own expression of sound. The moment he tries to express his efforts, the resonance is *āuṁ*. It might not be clear to us but the sound that comes has *ā, u, ṁ*. As we cannot live without food, air and water, similarly we cannot live without words. Speech is a gross expression of words. Even in our thinking process, the words are present and sound exists in all our movements.

In order to bring the wandering mind to a state of stability, *japa* is taught. Then one is advised to know the meaning of the word and then to feel the word with its meaning. Word and meaning may be objective but the experience of the word and its meaning is subjective. One should not allow one's experiences to become mechanical and static. One should develop freshness in word, thought and deed so that experience too, is fresh.

ĀUṀ is called *praṇava*. That word reveals a new meaning each time it is pronounced. A new challenge sets in and sets the mind to search the depths of one's consciousness.

Patañjali gives several methods for the single-pointedness of the consciousness *(citta)* in *Samādhi Pāda*. The *japa āuṁ* is one of these methods. The *mantra āuṁ* is given to one and all as *dhyāna*, but it is a *japa*, a prayer. This is not *dhyāna*. *Japa* is not *dhyāna*. *Japa* is a means towards *dhyāna*. In *dhyāna*, *japa* disappears.

b) *Bhajan* and *bhakti*

Bhajans are musical compositions on the Lord, with the purpose of bringing back the wandering mind to contemplate on the quality and praise of the Lord. The singing of *bhajans*, going to temples and churches, gazing at the idol of the Lord, are externally expressed forms of devotion; whereas total surrender of the Self to the Supreme Lord is the subtlest of devotion, known as *bhakti*, i.e. devotion and dedication. *Bhajan* and *japa* are a kind of preparation to gravitate the mind towards the Supreme. *Bhajan* and *nāma japa* (repetition of the name of the Lord) is meant to distract the mind from sensual objects and to bring the mind into a state of controlled discipline. The attachment and love for the Lord is far superior to the attachment of mundane thoughts. *Bhajans (nāma smaraṇa)* and *japa* prepare one physically and mentally for devotion, but real devotion has to come from within.

DHYĀNA – A PATH TO MATURED INTELLIGENCE AND INNOCENCE

Meditation is the continuous process of keeping the consciousness in a thoughtfully thoughtless state.

Consciousness is like a magnet. Thoughts are like iron. As the magnet pulls the iron towards itself, the consciousness pulls the thoughts towards itself. Therefore, keeping the consciousness thoughtfully thoughtless or thoughtlessly thoughtful is meditation.

One should differentiate between sensual tranquillity and spiritual poise. Sensual tranquillity is tainted whereas spiritual tranquillity is unalloyed bliss.

A man sleeping for ten hours realises chronological time only as he wakes up. In deep sleep he is not aware of the time. He does not know whether he slept for one hour or ten hours. His body and consciousness *(citta)* remain in an objectless or thoughtless state. The moment he is awake the *citta* fills with many thoughts. Meditation is a state wherein one simulates consciously that quality of thoughtlessness, which requires tremendous pensive action without any tension and emotional upheaval.

Meditation is not a negative state but a positive and pure state of living. As one cannot express the actual experience of sleep, similarly, one cannot express meditation, but lives in it. The moment it is expressed, know that it is not meditation but an expression, which may not be proper to the experiences. In sleep one is thoughtless and the moment one wakes up one is full of thoughts. In meditation one remains thoughtfully thoughtless or thoughtlessly thoughtful. If sleep is a negative state of consciousness, meditation is a positive state of consciousness. It is living in moments without being caught in the actual movements of moments. In this state of meditation, cause and effect vanishes, timeless time is experienced and one witnesses the timeless space.

Psychological time has a beginning and an end, whereas chronological time *(kāla)* has no beginning and no end. That is timeless space. In meditation both the thoughtful state and the thoughtless state are evenly balanced.

A matured intellectual person can never remain in the state of innocence, because his ego does not allow him to remain innocent; while in the highest state of meditation, the ego is silenced and intelligence becomes innocent. This state of innocence in matured intelligence is meditation. Though we are born as simple beings we create complications as we grow, while yoga helps us to return to the original state of simplicity.

PURE, SIMPLE AND SACRED EXISTENCE

Real evolution is the evolution of inner awareness, which expands and penetrates deep within and without. Though it is easy to feel the purity and divinity within, it is hard to maintain this uninterruptedly. One has to question oneself and analyse how this divine purity fades very often and gets unknowingly interrupted. So both purity and simplicity should not be lost in our *sādhanā*. One has to recharge the filtered memory to ripen again so that it guides one in the right path of yogic practices and saves one from the fall from purified life. The *yogāgni* (fire of yoga) should be burning throughout one's yogic practices with this ripened memory until one reaches the goal. Memory is dropped only when the goal is reached. The goal is the soul. Nothing remains at this state except the pure being which is *sat*. *Sat* is a pure and sacred existence, free from bondage, free from everything. This ultimate freedom comes through dedicated and devoted practices of yogic discipline in daily life.

YOGA – A FOUNT FOR ALL SPIRITUAL PATHS*

Before beginning my talk, I wish to express my gratitude to the members of the Central Salt & Marine Chemicals Research Institute, Bhāvnagar, for inviting me to the Third Seminar or Science of Human Development sponsored by the Research Institute.

Though most of the invitees gave talks, I have preferred to give a lecture-cum-demonstration, so that one can see directly how the different aspects of yoga develop and culture the physical, physiological, psychological, mental, intellectual and causal sheaths of man and evolve him towards unalloyed peace, emancipation and freedom.

Before proceeding with my demonstration, let me explain to you what yoga means. According to the *Upaniṣads*, yoga is the union of the individual soul with the Universal Soul or God. In simple terms, yoga is the art and science of removing the polarities between body and consciousness and consciousness and Self. It cultures the mind of the *sādhaka* in order that they experience the state of Universality within themselves. Mind, with its thoughts, moves fast like mercury. Yoga begins with the work of stilling the waves of thought so that the very consciousness is diffused to experience the state of silence, equilibrium and oneness.

Though consciousness moves in each of us like quavering and withering leaves in various directions, a thought arises in each of us to aim at something that may bring real peace and poise in life. It may be music, dance, sports, painting, sculpture, yoga or philosophy. But the final aim of all is to live a life free from misery. In philosophical terminology, this is *mukti mārga* or the path of absolute freedom.

In order to experience the presence of the Self in one's daily life, one has to study to have the knowledge and understanding of the core of being or *ātman*.

A vessel is needed to store water. Even the vessel that contains water should have a support in the form of a perfect base to place it on the ground. Then the ground becomes the

---

* Lecture-demonstration delivered at the Third Seminar on Science of Human Development, Bhavnagar (26-28 February 1989), organised by the Forum for Advancement of Science of Human Development.

support for the vessel as the vessel becomes the container of water. We search for hangers to hang clothes on. To rest, we go in for mats. Similarly, in order to understand the knowledge of the Self and to experience its presence, we must accept the need for support. This support is the body. Hence, the body as support, becomes the shrine of the Self. This way one needs the support of the other. Even to experience absolute freedom *(mokṣa* or *kaivalya)* a support is essential. This support may be in the form of the path of action, path of knowledge, path of devotion or path of yoga. The path of yoga shows the ways of stopping the waves of consciousness so that the consciousness experiences poise and peace from the state of stillness and evolves further to feel the inner being.

Whatever path one chooses for practice, one needs the supports of confidence or faith *(śraddhā)*, zeal *(utsāha)* and forbearance *(kṣmā)*. Effort with confidence *(śraddhā)* is the key to unlock the doors of absolute freedom through knowledge, action and devotion. The path of yoga braids *karma*, *jñāna* and *bhakti* into one.

The reasons for the fluctuations and wanderings of the consciousness are want of understanding *(avidyā)*, pride *(asmitā – tāmasic* by nature), attachment *(rāga)*, aversion *(dveṣa)* and attachment to life or fear of death *(abhiniveśa)*. These cause distress and invite waves of thoughts *(citta vṛtti)* in one's consciousness. Besides these intellectual, emotional and instinctive wants, Sage Patañjali enumerates many more supporting impediments that affect peace of mind. (*Y.S.*, I.30 and I.31). They are physical ailments, doubt, carelessness, laziness, sense gratifications, sorrows, despair, tremors of the body and heavy or unrhythmic breathing.

Patañjali then explains the means in the form of eight petals of yoga* for facing and conquering these distractions and developing a composed consciousness. He braids these eight petals of yoga together in the form of *tapas*, *svādhyāya* and *Īśvara praṇidhāna* as *kriyā yoga*.

Tapas is a blazing practice with a religious fervour, wherein the impurities of the body, the senses and the mind are burnt off. *Tapas* can be easily termed as the path of action. Here, a man is made to accept his inevitable destiny with composure. Actually, the fruits of action accrue from action. This is known as destiny or fate. *Svādhyāya* is to study and understand, through the spiritual scriptures, the true knowledge. *Svādhyāya (Sva* = Self; *adhyāya* = study; i.e. Self-study) helps us to experience the never changing eternal truth, which is ever the same in all circumstances. This study to know and experience the eternal truth is the path of knowledge. By this knowledge, the aspirant develops equipoise and diffuses his consciousness with equanimity, like the light of the sun, which shines evenly on the earth when the sky is clear.

* c.f. Author's *Light on the Yoga Sūtras of Patañjali*, Table n. 6, page n. 104.

Practice of *svādhyāya* guides man to realise that the support of the consciousness is a non-differentiating clean entity. It is unchangeable, eternal and exists anywhere and everywhere. It has no beginning, no middle and no end. It is without want. Understanding the non-differentiating clean entity, i.e., the core of the being and then to work on it to reach the goal of spiritual endeavour, is *vedānta*.

Nature *(prakṛti)* has three qualities: *sattva*, *rajas* and *tamas*. Knowledge (*jñāna*) also has three facets: acquired knowledge *(śāstrika jñāna)*, knowledge of memory *(smṛti jñāna)* and experienced knowledge *(ānubhavika jñāna)*. Knowledge earned through scriptures *(śāstra)* is *rājasic jñāna*. It has just a scholarly or academic value. The knowledge of memory *(smṛti jñāna)* gained through desires *(vāsanā)* is *tāmasic jñāna*. It mostly deals with perverse knowledge, where the transient is mistaken for the permanent, the impure for the pure, pain for pleasure and non-self for self. (*Y.S.* II.5). Subjective experience through right understanding and action is pure knowledge *(ānubhavika jñāna)*. It is also called *vyavasāyātmikā buddhi* (experienced subjective knowledge), *rasātmaka jñāna* (essence of experienced knowledge that is filtered repeatedly) and becomes *sāttvic jñāna (sāttvic* knowledge).

Normally food *(āhāra)*, sleep *(nidrā)*, enticement *(moha)* and fear *(bhaya)* eat away a person's energy. Besides these, one is caught in lust, greed, anger, ignorance, pride and competition. These engage one to be busy at other times. So one has no time to devote to the knowledge combined with practice, which gives power to renounce the temporal joys and experience unalloyed bliss. If one gives a thought to this sensual knowledge *(vāsanā jñāna)* and realises that it is the root of all desire, attachment and pain which are obstacles in the path of acquiring true knowledge and bliss, one begins to act to control them.

If one is caught up in improper thoughts, emotions and actions, they result in endless pain and ignorance in mild, medium and intense degrees. They are caused through greed, anger and delusion. This is *vāsanā jñāna*. (*Y.S.*, II.34).

Patañjali, in *Y.S.*, II.17, relates that the conjunction between the seer *(puruṣa)*, and the seen *(prakṛti)* is the cause of pain and says that the avoidance of union between them is a remedy to become free from pain and sorrow. This is an academic or *śāstric jñāna* or knowledge earned through the scriptures.

Patañjali, as an experienced person in all aspects of knowledge, comes out with *ānubhavika* and *rasātmaka jñāna*. He says that the process of the conjunction of the seer *(svāmi)* with the seen *(sva)* is for unfolding the inherent powers of nature and Self or the seer so that the seer discovers his own true nature. (*Y.S.*, II.23).

It is very interesting to note that Patañjali enumerates the *āgama* (the traditional sacred texts, the scriptural references and the scriptural authorities) along with *pratyakṣa* (direct perception) and *anumāna* (inference), as one of the three means of *pramāṇa* or right knowledge. (*Y.S.*, I.7). But later he declares that the knowledge and wisdom of the one who has been bestowed with the truth-bearing state of direct spiritual perception (*ṛtambharā prajñā* or seasoned intelligence) is distinct from and beyond the knowledge gleaned from books, testimony or inference. (*Y.S.*, I.48-49). Though Patañjali in the beginning advises book knowledge as a support, later he says that they are not necessary as the purpose is served by *rasātmaka jñāna* and *ṛtambhara jñāna*.

The senses, mind and intelligence are the abode of lust and lust is the eternal enemy (*nityavairi*) of knowledge. Hence, knowledge or *jñāna* has to be earned through *tapas* and *svādhyāya*.

Tapas, as *karma*, covers *yama*, *niyama*, *āsana* and *prāṇāyāma*. *Svādhyāya* as *jñāna* embraces *pratyāhāra* and *dhāraṇā* while *dhyāna* and *samādhi* act as the gateway towards the path of taking refuge at the feet of the Universal Soul or God. This is *bhakti* or *śaraṇāgati mārga* (the path of surrender of oneself to God), or *Īśvara praṇidhāna* (*Īśvara* = God; *praṇidhāna* = directing one's eyes and thought towards).

The aspirant (*sādhaka*) should practice for the sake of practice (*sādhanā*). Let the effects of practice come and go. But, the *sādhaka* must remain steadfast with his *sādhanā* harmoniously blending the intelligence of the head and the heart, so that his practice remains true and pure. In this way, the shrine of the Self as well as the Self, remain wedded to each other. The supporter and the supported are made to appear as one. Experiencing this unique state of oneness is yoga.

As two eyes are required to see the beauty of creation, *tapas* and *svādhyāya* develop *jñāna* and *vijñāna*, which function as two eyes to observe and feel the spiritual growth in the *sādhaka*. *Jñāna* is the way of understanding the scriptural texts on the soul (*ātmā*) and *vijñāna* is the understanding of the relationship between soul and God. Through study, the practitioner knows that he is made up of five elements besides mind, intelligence and ego and realises that they are all part and parcel of God.

Īśvara praṇidhāna is the surrender of one's Self to the Almighty. His grace and blessings are essential for *jñāna*. To earn this grace, *bhakti* acts as the seed. Practice of yoga ploughs the supporter of the Self – the body – by keeping it clean and clear of all impediments in order to bring out the best of the fervent, spiritual knowledge. This is *prajñāna*.

A potter cannot make anything without clay. A goldsmith cannot make ornaments without gold or silver. Similarly, man cannot move without the grace of God who is an indestructible seed *(avināśi bīja)*. Practice of yoga ploughs the body to bring out the best of the harvest.

When yogic *sādhanā* is ripe, knowledge grows. As knowledge grows, the actions become mature and perfect and with this perfection, the *sādhaka* becomes divine and lives in contact with the divinity.

As sesame seeds have to be pressed to extract oil, the practitioner of yoga extracts and squeezes out spiritual knowledge by bringing the intelligence of his head and heart to work in harmony. This is yogic *svādhyāya* so that he dedicates his life to serve humanity as a command from the Lord and at the same time surrender himself to the Lord.

In *prāṇāyāma*, energy is not only distributed to all parts of the body, but also stored in the storehouse of the lungs to use when necessary. *Prāṇāyāma* fuses the two antagonistic elements water and fire, for the production of a new energy as bio-energy or *prāṇa*, to take one towards meditation.

Meditation is the fruit of consistent practice of ethical, physical, vital and intellectual disciplines of yoga. Meditation is the act of bringing the complex *citta* to a state of simplicity without any sign of arrogance.

As the rivers Gangā, Yamunā and Sarasvati have their confluence at *Triveṇi* (the modern *Prayāg)*, so also in yoga the *bahiraṅga sādhanā*, of *āsana* and *prāṇāyāma*, and the *antaraṅga sādhanā* of *dhāraṇā* and *dhyāna* interweave the body, mind, intelligence and consciousness to reach their confluence at the seat of the Self *(antarātmā)*. Thus, yoga braids *karma*, *jñāna* and *bhakti* together and becomes the fount of all spiritual paths and the nectar of life.

WHY DO WE DO YOGA?

Manuṣyāṇāṁ sahasreṣu
kaścid yatati siddhaye /
Yatatām api siddhānāṁ
kaścin māṁ vetti tattvataḥ //
(*B.G.*, VII.3)

(Hardly one among thousands of men strives
for perfection, and of those yogis who strive
and succeed, scarcely one knows Me in truth).

This *śloka* is a great encouragement for yoga students. We do not know whether we reach spiritual enlightenment or not, but Patañjali too wants us to continue the *sādhanā* without giving a thought to success or failure.

Caturvidhā bhajante mām
janāḥ sukṛtino'rjuna /
ārto jijñāsu arthārthī
jñānī ca bharatarṣabha //
(*B.G.*, VII.16)

Here, Lord Krishna encourages the *sādhaka* to pursue the path with this advice, "There are four types of devotees who worship Me, Arjuna, among them some pray to have worldly possessions, some pray to be free from afflictions and sorrows, others pray for knowledge, while the man of wisdom prays for the sake of prayer without any motive, O best of Bharatas!".

Similarly, Patañjali explains four types of devotees in yoga who act with different motivations. Some may do it to get rid of ailments, some out of curiosity, some to gain name and fame and some for the sake of emancipation.

This way each one begins yoga in order to have good health, or to make a career out of it or for enjoyment of worldly pleasures, or for spiritual enlightenment.

Patañjali explains at the very beginning of the *Yoga Sūtra,* that consciousness (mind, intelligence and ego) gets involved with the thought waves and forgets its true element in nature.

This conjunction of the three components of consciousness with the thoughts perceived or conceived creates desires. Desires act at once without letting the man use his discriminative faculty. So, man becomes a victim of his own thoughts and deeds.

The spokes of the wheel of desires, fulfilments and frustrations get cycled and recycled as subliminal impressions *(saṁskāra),* life after life.

The cycles of subliminal impressions remain unmanifest before birth, get manifested during the life span and dissolve into the unmanifest after death by addition or subtraction.

WHAT ARE THESE SUBLIMINAL IMPRESSIONS *(SAṀSKĀRA)?*

The subliminal impressions are formed on account of our accumulated merits and demerits in many past lives. They become the cause of pleasure and pain in this life. The cultivation of modes and moods of this life becomes a springboard for the next life. Hence, Patañjali's yoga expositions come in handy to minimise the impressions so that the practitioner can build up a free will and make his own destiny. He accepts the fruits of past actions and faces them courageously without being caught in that web.

As nature is eternal, so too, is life eternal. As nature revolves as past, present and future, life too revolves between birth, death and rebirth.

HOW YOGA FREES ONE FROM MOTIVATION

Uninterrupted practice of yoga done with devotion keeps the practitioner free from motivation, desire or reward and develops his discriminative intelligence. With this discriminative intelligence, he keeps his mind free from the contact of tempting objects and yokes it to the Self. The Self is unmoving, unrotating and always remains in the state of the present.

Yoking the mind, intelligence and consciousness to the Self is possible only through the yogic disciplines which make the body firm and pure, mind stable, intelligence clear and consciousness sanctified in order to be one with the Self.

This is precisely what the practice of yoga does. Patañjali emphatically says, "Through reverential practice of yoga, the fire which emanates from practice burns out the impurities of body, mind and intelligence and bestows the consciousness with the crown of wisdom for it to rest on the lap of the Self" (*Y.S.,* II.28). From then on the never-changing intuitive light of the Self radiates and frees the practitioner from the actions that are filled with afflictions.

Thus, the practice of yoga not only eradicates such afflictive actions, but also leads one towards emancipation.

In the zodiac, the nine planets, as servants of God, maintain a rhythmic universal order. We have nine gates in our body. They are: two eyes, two ears, two nostrils, mouth, the organs of excretion and organs of generation *(Śvetāśvatara Upaniṣad,** III.18). The lack of control over these nine gates generate nine distractions which are: disease, sluggishness, doubt, carelessness, idleness, sensual gratification, living in the world of illusion, not being able to hold on to what is undertaken and inability to maintain the progress achieved.

By regular practice of yoga, these nine gates are controlled and the energy, which was going to waste, is constructively channelled and used for the realisation of the Self.

"The embodied soul, having controlled his nature and having relegated all actions to the mansion of nine gates, the body, dwells happily in God, neither working nor causing work to be done." (*B.G.,* V.13).

As one installs a device in the form of a metallic rod on the top of a house to divert lightning and prevent it from striking the building, the practice of yoga protects the practitioner by minimising the effects of the zodiac and frees him from bondage. As the yoga *sādhaka* becomes clean, he becomes the son of God. Being the son of God, the servants of God (the nine planets) cannot taunt him.

Thus, the main purpose of yoga is to free oneself from fluctuations of the consciousness and afflictions of the body by obstructing the recurrence of mixed sorrows and pleasures and then guarding that they do not take place any more.

This is why I continue doing my daily practice uninterruptedly and I wish all those who are practising regularly with intensity reach that state of emancipation which is free from afflictions of sorrows.

That is why yoga is practised.

---

* *Kathopaniṣad* (V.1) enumerates eleven gates. See: *Yoga and Peace*, p. 134.

YOGA SAṀPAT – THE WEALTH OF YOGA*

Today is a very auspicious day for all the *yoga sādhakas*. Its importance is three-fold. Today is *Dhanvañtarī Jayañtī***, *Patañjali Jayañtī* and *Dhanatrayodaśī*.

Lord Dhanvañtarī, the physician of Gods, and an incarnation of Lord Vishnu, appeared on this earth with a pot of nectar during the *samudra mañthana* (the churning of the ocean)***. The Gods and demons churned the ocean in order to get nectar. They received many other things before the nectar. They were given liberty to choose whatever they wanted and they did. Last came the nectar and both opted for the same. The Lord, in the form of Mohinī, enticed the demons with her beauty and distributed the nectar amongst the Gods. However, man inherited both divine and demonic qualities. He has to combat his demonic nature and nurture his strength towards divinity.

Today is *Patañjali Jayañtī* also. As Lord Vishnu appeared to the Gods and demons with a pot of nectar, the couch of Lord Vishnu appeared on this earth as Patañjali, to offer the nectar of yoga for man's emancipation.

Today is *Dhanatrayodaśī* day, the second day of *Diwālī* – the festival of lights. *Dhana* is wealth, treasure. This is a day on which wealth is worshipped in order to become prosperous.

This is a unique day since man was gifted with both yoga and *bhoga* – nectar and intoxicating things, with divine and demonic qualities – for him to choose.

A human being is a creation of God. It is God who generates life within us, organises our life and diminishes us through death. The child inherits certain qualities from his parents and also acquires certain qualities on his own. Similarly, we inherit qualities of God from the Creator and acquire certain demonic qualities on our own. If yoga is an inherited quality, then *bhoga* is

---

* Lecture delivered by *Gurujī* on 11.11.1993.

** Jayañtī = Birthday.

*** See the author's *Tree of Yoga*, part four, chapter on *prāṇāyāma*, first edition pp. 124-126. Harper Collins, London

not only an inherited quality but also an acquired quality. We want emancipation as well as enjoyment. The spiritual and worldly tendencies are both inherent in us. Therefore, we have to begin yoga to minimise the intoxicating effects of worldly pleasures, so that one day we progress towards emancipation.

Knowing very well these two sides of us, Patañjali, with his great compassion, presented a well-balanced path of yoga so that we get pleasure (accomplishments) as well as freedom (emancipation).

All of us are blessed with the spiritual wealth, which is like immovable property. This spiritual wealth is nothing but spiritual tendencies that we own. It is known as *ṣaḍ saṁpat* (the six spiritual properties). These qualities are found in each individual. They are:

Table n. 1 – *Śaḍ-saṁpat* (six spiritual properties)

1. *Śama*	tranquillity, calmness, absence of passion
2. *Dama*	power of training, self-restraint, restraint of the senses
3. *Titikṣā*	power of endurance, patience, forbearance
4. *Uparati*	cessation of tendency towards pleasures, desisting from sensual enjoyments
5. *Śraddhā*	reverential faith, trust, confidence
6. *Samādhāna*	the tendency to set right mental energies and attitudes, satisfaction, steadfastness

Wealth is such that if it is used properly or invested in a right direction, it can be redoubled and increased. The *ṣaḍ saṁpat* can also be multiplied if we invest it properly.

Patañjali offers us the eightfold path of yoga to invest these six kinds of spiritual wealth in order to multiply the spiritual tendencies within us.

In order to follow the path of yoga each individual has been gifted with the first and the primary wealth – *prakṛti* (basic or primary resources).

Prakṛti is a wealth. It can be used as a means, directing its flow either for enjoyment *(bhoga)* or enlightenment *(apavarga).* Here the wealth of yoga is spiritual materialism *(siddhi* or accomplishment), *apavarga* is pure spiritual enlightenment. As practitioners of yoga, we have to be very careful to use this wealth essentially towards emancipation. Let us see the *prākṛtic* wealth: *Prakṛti* has three inherent components or qualities, namely: a) *Sattva* – luminosity, bringing clarity and brightness. b) *Rajas* – vibrancy, or bringing volition to do something. c) *Tamas* – inertia, dormancy, leading one towards steadiness or firmness.

From these three-fold resources *prakṛti* evolves and offers man, consciousness (the mind, the intelligence, the ego), the senses of perception, the organs of action and the body, made up of five gross and five subtle elements.

Table n. 2 - The disciplines of *aṣṭāṅga yoga* and the development of *ṣaḍ saṁpat*

Aṣṭāṅga Yoga	**Kind of discipline**	**Enhancing *Prākṛtic Saṁpat***	**Developing *Ṣaḍ Saṁpad***	**Achieving *Puruṣārtha***
1. Yama	Social	A disciplined conduct to channel the moral energy and the behaviour of the organs of actions *(karmendriya)*, practice of ethics outside ourselves	*Dama*	*Dharma*
2. Niyama	Individual	An individual effort to develop the capacity to bear the spiritual emotion (disciplining the *jñānendriya)*, ethics to be practiced and followed within us	*Śama*	*Dharma*
3. Āsana	Wholistic postures	Postures to generate energy in order to develop physical, psychological, organic, ethical and mental endurance	*Titīkṣā*	*Artha*
4. Prāṇāyāma	Disciplining vital energy	Channeling the earned, stored and endured vital energy, spreading the vital energy and sharpening the consciousness	*Titīksā*	*Artha*
5. Pratyāhāra	Sensual and mental *(manaṣ)*	Channeling and disciplining the energy of the mind, controlling the fluctuating mind, organs of action and senses of perception after earning *prajñā*	*Uparati*	*Kāma*
6. Dhāraṇā	Concentration, discipline of *buddhi*	Channeling and disciplining the energy of the intelligence with *jñāna* and *prajñā*	*Śraddhā*	*Kāma*
7. Dhyāna	Meditation, controlling ego	Disciplining the intelligence in order to get *jñāna* and *prajñā* to develop humbleness and then decentralise the intelligence resulting in consciousness, devoid of ego *(ahaṁkāra)*. That is the purification of consciousness.	*Śraddhā*	threshold for *mokṣa*
8. Samādhi	Absorption Self-realisation	Merging the consciousness *(citta)* and conscience in the Self or *ātman*	*Samadhāna*	***Mokṣa***

The eight-fold path has a unique importance since it helps to enhance the material and the spiritual wealth and then it takes us to conquer the real and eternal wealth, i.e. knowing and identifying the Self. (See Table n. 2)

Yama and *niyama*, explained by Patañjali and Svātmārāma (see Table n. 3), have a vast scope to discipline our life with moral and ethical values. They are meant to train, channel and purify the energy of the organs of action and senses of perception. They improve our behaviour and self-control, so that we overcome bad and evil attitudes.

Yama and *niyama* teach the way of life. The principles of *yama* tame the organs of action. *Yama* strengthens *dama* – the restraint of senses; whereas the principles of *niyama* bring *śama* – calmness and quietness in mind due to simplicity in life.

Table n. 3 - *Yama* in the texts on yoga

***Yama* according to Patañjali**	**Divine qualities according to *Bhagavad Gītā***
1. *Ahiṁsā* (non-violence, fearlessness, tolerance)	1. *Abhayam* (fearlessness) *Ahiṁsā* (harmlessness) *Akrodha* (devoid of anger)
2. *Satya* (truthfulness, honesty)	2. *Satyam* (truthfulness)
3. *Asteya* (non-stealing, non-covetousness, dispassion, desirelessness)	3. *Adroha* (non-treacherousness)
4. *Brahmacarya* (celibacy, continence)	4. *Teja* (sharpness)
5. *Aparigraha* (non-acquisition, non-receiving of gifts, non-possession)	5. *Alolupatvam* (non-indulgence)
Additional *yama* according to Svātmārāma	
6. *Kṣamā* (forgiveness)	6. *Kṣamā* (forgiveness)
7. *Dhṛti* (steady intelligence, firmness, surety, certainty of intellect)	7. *Dhṛti* (steadfastness)
8. *Dayā* (compassion)	8. *Dayā* (compassion) *Mārdava* (softness)
9. *Ārjava* (simplicity, straightforwardness, uprightness)	9. *Ārjava* (uprightness)
10. *Mitāhāra* (moderation in diet; balanced, suitable, pure and palatable diet)	10. *Śauca* (cleanliness)

Table n. 4 - *Niyama* in the texts on yoga

***Niyama* according to Patañjali**	**Divine qualities according to *Bhagavad Gītā***
1. *Śauca* (physical, mental, external, internal cleanliness)	1. *Sattva saṁśuddhi* (purity of mind and intelligence) *Śauca* (cleanliness)
2. *Santoṣa* (contentment, satisfaction)	2. *Dama* (desirelessness) *Śānti* (calmness)
3. *Tapas* (austerity, penance, discipline to burn impurities of body and consciousness)	3. *Tapas* (austerity) *Apaiśunam* (non-abuse)
4. *Svādhyāya* (study of scriptures, Self-study)	4. *Svādhyāya* (Self-study, study of scriptures)
5. *Īśvarapraṇidhāna* (to perform right action and surrender the fruits to the Lord)	5. *Tyāga* (dedication, sacrifice) *Nātimānitā* (*Nā + atimānitā* -free from egoistic approach)
Additional *Niyama* according to Svātmārāma	(We repeat *tyāga* and *nātimānitā*, they correspond both to *Īśvarapraṇidhāna* and *āstikya*).
6. *Āstikya* (belief in scriptures, faith in the Supreme)	6. *Tyāga Nātimānitā*
7. *Dānam* (charity)	7. *Dānam* (charity)
8. *Siddhāntavākyaśravaṇam* (listening to established doctrines and truth)	8. *Śṛti* (scriptures, vedas)
9. *Hṛi* (modesty, humbleness in spite of being accomplished)	9. *Hṛi* (modesty) *Nātimānitā* (free from egoistic approach)
10. *Mati* (faith in confirmed knowledge and devotion to it)	10. *Jñāna Yoga Vyavasthiti* (steadfastness of intelligence) *Achapalam* (non-fickleness)
11. *Japa* (continuous recitation of *mantra* or the name of the Supreme)	11. *Japa* (recitation)
12. *Vṛta* (observance of vows)	12. *Yajña* (sacrifice)

These principles uphold, sustain and support one throughout the yogic journey. *Yama* and *niyama* are not to be considered as forced or imposed disciplines. They are truly speaking, *dharma* (righteous way of living). *Dharma* is the science of right duty. We human beings are presented with one more, an extra sense called *antaḥkaraṇa* or *dharmendriya* or the sense of conscience. In order to reach *dharmendriya* one has to tame the desires and passions by following *yama* and *niyama*. This is how *yama* and *niyama*, *śama* and *dama* go hand in hand. The desires and passions tend to lead one towards *bhoga* whereas desirelessness and passionlessness lead one to develop divine qualities.

It is interesting to see how *yama* and *niyama* of Patañjali and Svātmārāma are very close to the divine qualities explained by Lord Krishna in *Bhagavad Gītā* (see Tables n. 3 and 4):

The disciplines of *yama* and *niyama* are like the churning rod with which we have to churn our consciousness *(citta)* in order to bring the cream of divine qualities which are hidden within us.

According to Lord Krishna, fearlessness, purity of mind, steadfastness in pursuit of knowledge, charity, restraint of senses, sacrifice, self-study, austerity, uprightness, harmlessness, truthfulness, absence of anger, generosity, relinquishment of desires and wrong habits, serenity of mind, restraint from abusing others, compassion to living beings, aversion from sensuous objects, softness of heart, absence of revengeful thoughts and acts, freeing oneself from shameful thoughts and acts, absence of fickleness and oscillation of mind, smartness and sharpness of intelligence, forgiveness, fortitude, purity, absence of treachery and humility in place of egoism are all meritorious and divine qualities.

Patañjali's *yama* and *niyama* are well known to one and all. Apart from them, Patañjali gives his followers a few more remedial devices to increase the morale by developing certain qualities with the cultivation of a favourable mental disposition. They are:

Table n. 5 – Devices for practitioners for the development of a favourable mental disposition

1. *Śraddhā*	reverential faith, trust, confidence
2. *Vīrya*	vigour, physical, moral, mental power and spiritual strength
3. *Smṛti*	memory, recollection, firmly established intelligence
4. *Samādhi-Prajñā*	profound meditation where one loses one's consciousness and remains in the awareness of the real core of the being
5. *Maitrī*	friendliness towards all
6. *Karuṇā*	compassion towards those who are in sorrow
7. *Muditā*	gladness, joy towards those who are virtuous
8. *Upekṣā*	to be indifferent and dispassionate; to look at things with disinterest

If *yama* and *niyama* lead to moral wealth, then these eight types of virtuous wealth lead to the development of spiritual achievements and hence, are to be worshipped and adored. At the same time we have to find the means to avoid carefully the poisons and intoxicants, like lust and greed which rises up in the consciousness.

The afflictions are *avidyā, asmitā, rāga, dveṣa and abhiniveśa.*

Table n. 6 - *Kleśa* or affliction

Affliction	Demonic Quality	Enemy of Consciousness
1. *Avidyā* (ignorance)	1. *Ajñāna* (ignorance, want of knowledge)	Root cause of six enemies is *avidyā*
2. *Asmitā* (pride)	2. *Dambha* (hypocrisy, fraud) *Darpa* (ego, pride, passion)	*Moha* (infatuation) *Mada* (pride)
3. *Rāga* (attachment)	Forceful enticement	*Kāma* (desire) *Lobha* (greed)
4. *Dveṣa* (aversion)	3. *Krodha* (anger) *Paruśya* (harshness)	*Krodha* (anger) *Mātsarya* (malaise, envy)
5. *Abhiniveśa* (clinging to life, fear of death)	*Anurakta* (love of life)	*Lolatā* (fondness to life)

These are accompanied by six enemies *(śaḍripus)* of consciousness are nothing but toxins and poisons of the mind. *Avidyā* and *asmitā* are the poisons of the head and *rāga, dveṣa, abhiniveśa* are the poisons of the heart.

Āsana and *prāṇāyāma* are *artha* – the means – through which we develop endurance to bear aches, pains, problems and afflictions, and face all hindrances and obstacles without losing heart. If *āsana* is the head, then *prāṇāyāma* is the heart of *aṣṭāṅga yoga*. The head is the seat of consciousness and the heart is the seat of the subconscious. When the intelligence's of the consciousness and subconscious meet and help each other, the turmoil of head and heart is conquered and the intellectual and emotional centres are balanced.

Prāṇāyāma has two components – *prāṇa* and *prajñā*. *Prāṇa* is the vital energy and *prajñā*, the conscious intelligence. The moment *prāṇa* leaves the body, *prajñā* too leaves and death is inevitable. If *prāṇa* is vitiated then *prajñā* also is vitiated. If *prāṇa* is ignited then *prajñā* also is ignited. *Prāṇāyāma* teaches how to use the vital *prāṇa* in order to penetrate *prajñā* so that the wisdom of intelligence, or discriminative intelligence begins to shine.

Uparati is the cessation of sensual enjoyments. It is the intelligence, which leads one to discipline the mind. *Pratyāhāra* strengthens this spiritual quality. *Prāṇāyāma* and *pratyāhāra* work like 'twin-effects' in which the mind is disciplined and the intelligence flourishes, leading towards *dhāraṇā* and *dhyāna*. In *prāṇāyāma* the *prāṇa* and *prajñā* are strengthened, whereas in *dhyāna*, the *jñāna* and *śraddhā* are strengthened. This *śraddhā* is not mere faith, but a ripened revelation through experience. If *śraddhā* fails at this stage, the downfall is certain. Let me explain this with the following example. A wealthy person always has fear that a theft or robbery may occur and he may lose everything that he has gained. A practitioner of yoga also has to remember at this stage that a robbery may occur and he may lose his spiritual wealth. The accomplishments and achievements play like demonic qualities at this stage. These accomplishments and achievements overpower his spiritual growth and make him a slave of powers by stealing his spiritual wealth. If the *sādhaka* has a profound faith that his *prākṛtic sampat* is meant for Self-realisation and not for accomplishments, then *ātmadarśana* is certain. Otherwise, he will be caught in *āsuri sampat*, the demonic qualities such as arrogance, ostentation, conceit, indulgence, anger, harshness, ignorance and so forth. These disqualify one from the spiritual path. That is why Patañjali warns one against indulgence in achievements and attainments and reminds one to aim at *samādhi* or *samādhāna* for Self-realisation. He demands spiritual absorption and not material absorption.

Lord Krishna says:

Daivī Sampad Vimokṣāya
Nibandhāyāsurī matā
(*B.G.*, XVI.5)

Divine qualities are conducive to freedom whereas demonic qualities make for bondage.

Dhāraṇā, dhyāna and *samādhi* fulfil the third aim of man, *kāma*. For example the spiritual accomplishments or achievements are gained by integration of concentration, meditation and absorption which may tempt even the spiritually advanced yogi towards *kāma*. *Kāma* covers both sensual satisfaction as well as spiritual achievements *(siddhi)*. If one indulges in it, the gate of liberation *(mokṣa)*, the fourth and main aim, will be closed. Therefore, one has to solidify and strengthen *śraddhā* to gain spiritual property – *samādhāna*. *Jñāna* and *dhyāna* give *samādhāna* to proceed towards *samādhi*. *Samādhāna* sets the mental attitudes and energies in the right mode. Therefore, it is *samādhāna* which has to direct the energy of consciousness towards liberation and not accomplishments *(siddhi* or *vibhūti)*. A true yogi is one who goes beyond these four *puruṣārtha*.

The eight aspects of yoga explained by Patañjali lead one ultimately towards liberation by fulfilling the four aims and finally makes one devoid of the four aims when one establishes oneself in one's own nature. Then *svarūpa* and *svadharma* become one. Our *svarūpa* is Self and our duty – *svadharma* – is the realisation of the Self. Self is the goal (Table II).

The body is the *kṣetra*. The Self is the *kṣetrajña*. This *kṣetra* (with twenty-four elements or evolutes) is a *dharma kṣetra* as well as a *kuru kṣetra*.

It is a *dharmakṣetra*, if one uses it for the yogic practice to reach *kṣetrajña* – the owner and the master. The body is the known seer; the Self is the unknown seer. The known seer leads towards the unknown seer.

It is a *kurukṣetra* since the good and the divine qualities have to combat with the evil and the demonic qualities. The yogic wealth has to combat with *bhogic* wealth. As every human being fights for his rights and material wealth, so too every *sādhaka* has to fight within for his right to have spiritual wealth.

Lord Krishna brought Arjuna's chariot to the centre of the *dharmakṣetṛa* – *kurukṣetra* to watch and judge the strength of both the armies. Similarly, while treading on the yogic path, we have to watch the strength of both the armies, ourselves remaining in the centre.

The body is the chariot. The soul is the owner of the chariot. The intelligence is the controller holding the reins. The mind is the reins. The organs of action and senses of perception are the horses. Sitting in the chariot we have to watch. Are we able to fight the enemy or are we avoiding obstacles? Is the charioteer taking us in the right direction?

These are the questions to be asked and answered by ourselves through the practice of yogic disciplines. Yoga has to be worshipped to make ourselves spiritually wealthy. Yoga is meant to churn our consciousness so that the cream of spiritual qualities surfaces to amass spiritual wealth. *Saṁyama* that results from the integration of *dhāraṇā, dhyāna* and *samādhi (trayamekatra saṁyamaḥ)* leads to the integration of body, consciousness and self.

Let us adore, worship and pray to the Supreme to bless us with moral and mental health, spiritual and divine prosperity.

YOGA FOR HEALTH AND HAPPINESS*

The prime concern of each and every individual is health. But what is health? It may be broadly defined as that state of being wherein all the systems of the body function in unison without disturbing the growth of the body or impairing the development of the mind and intelligence. Each and every fibre of the body and each and every process of thinking are kept pure, clean and clear so that the individual experiences an unalloyed joy and happiness. In such a state, the intelligence urges one to stretch beyond that state of joyousness and to live in a state of divine poise and harmony. This state being the need of everyone, can yoga help us to attain this health, this happiness?

There is a popular misconception that yoga is only for those who have power of concentration. But all of us are not endowed with the power of concentration. A careful study of texts indicates that yoga can be practised by any one; be he a *kṣiptā* (wandering *citta); mūḍa* (forgetful and dull *citta*); *vikśipta* (oscillating *citta); ekāgrata* (one-pointed *citta);* or *niruddha* (restrained *citta).*

Yoga is like an ocean. The more one penetrates, understanding grows deeper and thereby one gains the insight to experience beyond the pale of the human intelligence.

Yoga is a fine art, and like any other fine art it seeks to express the artist's abilities to the fullest, but with one difference. Most artists need instruments like the violin or a painting brush or ankle bells as aids for their artistic expression. A yogi's sole instruments are his body and his consciousness.

Yoga is a science, which is based on physical, mental, intellectual, moral and spiritual techniques and well-tried evolved principles. It is a science, which shows how to commune with the body, the consciousness and the Self. It establishes a highly intelligent communication, or rather, a perfect communion between the body and the consciousness, and the consciousness

* Also published as: *Is Yoga for One and All? Bhavan's Journal*, October 17, 1971.

and the Self. It thereby brings a thorough understanding of one's nature so that one lives a profoundly positive life. Such an individual is at peace with himself and with his fellowmen. By regular practice of yoga he attains mastery over himself. Consequently, he is a master and not the victim of circumstances.

Patañjali, being highly sensitive, supremely intelligent and ever watchful, observed the nature of man and the norms of society. Then he enumerated systematically his findings in the form of aphorisms, known as *Pātañjala Yoga Sūtra*.

The aphorisms of *yama* and *niyama* remind one of a parent teaching the child what to do and what not to do. Just as parents teach their children what to do and what to say, what not to do and what not to say, allow them to do what is good and prohibit them from doing what is evil, Patañjali lays down codes of social morality for seekers of the truth, such as non-violence, truthfulness, non-stealing, celibacy and possession only of things essential for one's growth. After laying down a code of personal morality, he emphasises cleanliness in body, mind and speech, contentment, right actions, study in understanding of one's own nature and the self, and surrendering all to God. Patañjali considers these codes essential for men and women of thoughtful and perceptive intelligence.

He then observes the need for the body to be healthy, strong and tough. Just as parents encourage their children to participate in sports, games and physical exercises to strengthen and toughen their young bodies, he wants every aspirant to practise *āsana* and *prāṇāyāma*, not only for health and happiness, but also for a thorough development of the body to enable one to withstand strain and stress and thereby remain a true friend of the Self.

A devotee takes a bath, enters a temple, concentrates on his *Iṣṭa-Devatā*, focusing his mind on his subject of worship; similarly, if a yogic devotee wishes to make his body a fit abode for his soul, he too must purify and keep his body clean. This is possible only if he practices the third and fourth limbs of yoga: *āsana* and *prāṇāyāma*.

Disease and discomfort are the major impediments in our search for truth or reality. One must therefore remove these obstacles which come in the way of both physical and mental health. This is possible through *āsana* and *prāṇāyāma*. Health cannot be purchased, but is to be earned by hard and sincere effort day in and day out; then one is free from body-consciousness and a new light dawns which enables one to pursue and go beyond the awareness of the body. This is the beginning of spiritual *sādhanā*.

Āsana are said to be countless. Being countless, doubts arise in the mind of the beginner. He is confused as to where he is to begin and how. Knowledge of the alphabet is required if one wants to read and write, so one needs to know the fundamentals of each *āsana*. There are all kinds of *āsanas* like *Utthita Trikoṇāsana*, *Vīrabhadrāsana*, *Uttanāsana*, *Sālamba Śīrṣāsana*, *Sālamba Sarvāṅgāsana*, *Halāsana*, *Paśchimottānāsana*, *Padmāsana*, *Vīrāsana*, *Matsyendrāsana*, *Ūrdhva Dhanurāsana* and so on. But there is not a single textbook on yoga which definitely and categorically states which to do first and why and when, or which *āsana* to avoid and why and when. In these books, *āsana* has been dealt with in such a way that it needs an intelligent adaptation and adjustment for the requirements of the practitioner, depending upon his physical and constitutional fitness, strength and weakness of the whole body as well as different parts of the body, size of the body, defects, if any, and diseases which the individual might be suffering from. It is only then that this great and noble art can assist in eradicating the impurities of the body and make it a fit instrument for enjoyment of life without abusing it. It is only then that the body can be a fit vehicle to lead one towards enlightenment.

After thirty-five years of devoted and uninterrupted practice, I have worked out a synthesis of *āsana* and *prāṇāyāma* in accordance with the anatomy of the human body and the structural pattern of *āsanas* and *prāṇāyāma* for better results. I worked on how each *āsana* and *prāṇāyāma* aids and develops various parts of the body by opening a new horizon for the mind so that the *sādhaka* can practise them without fear of harm. I have discussed this in detail in my book *Light on Yoga*. This book has proved to be of value to individuals and institutions teaching yoga. They have found the system explained in the book a great assistance in achieving their objectives.

It has been demonstrated beyond doubt that *āsanas* tone all the systems of the body and maintain them in a healthy state making the body fit to be the temple of the Self.

Prāṇāyāma is a method, which regulates the flow of energy in man and oxygenates the whole system. Though some textbooks on yoga have classified *prāṇāyāma* into *Sūrya Bhedana*, *Ujjāyī*, *Śītakāri*, *Śītali*, *Bhastrikā*, *Bhrāmarī*, *Mūrchhā* and *Plāvinī*, Patañjali does not give any names but merely mentions five basic techniques of performing them. These are inhalation, inhalation-retention, exhalation, exhalation-retention and retention without a thought of inhalation or exhalation. The first two retentions are practised deliberately but the last one is non-deliberate and non-intentional. This is not possible for beginners. They must be adepts in the first two types of retention before attempting the last. Inhalations and exhalations should be slowly prolonged, and made subtle, sweet and delightful.

The practice of *prāṇāyāma* quietens the consciousness and makes it a fit instrument for meditation as it burns all the defects which appear in the form of *guṇa* and opens the gates for true knowledge to dawn on the *sādhaka*. Therefore, the *Upaniṣads* and yoga texts proclaim that "there is no purificatory action higher than *prāṇāyāma*. Through the destruction of impurity, purity is secured and the light of knowledge shines".

The kingdom of the body is a mysterious empire. *Ātmā* – the soul, is the Emperor. Breath is the Prime Minister and the consciousness is the Deputy Prime Minister. Breath is superior to consciousness. Unlike the consciousness, which takes various forms according to the inclinations of the emotions and the swaying of the senses, *prāṇa* (breath) does not change at all. Therefore, *prāṇāyāma* is very important for a yogi.

If the two limbs of yoga, *āsana* and *prāṇāyāma*, are followed regularly along with a proper diet, health and happiness is assured to the *sādhaka* in abundance. Otherwise, the body becomes a dwelling place for the demons of pain, misery, sorrow, suffering, strife, hatred, jealousy and envy throughout his life. The former path is the royal road for the path of *mokṣa* (freedom from the sheaths of body and consciousness), leading towards the state of a *jīvan mukta* (freedom of life in the state of the present living), whereas the latter way is the path towards the bondage of the soul or *ātma bandhana*.

Dhāraṇā and *dhyāna* follow automatically. They are experiences felt by the consciousness and are difficult to express in precise words. When all these are grouped together in one's yogic *sādhanā*, yoga brims in him fully and totally.

YOGA AND PEACE*

Before speaking on peace, I should admit that *yoga* and *śānti* were both existent before Patañjali. Probably we would not have known the ways to gain peace, if he had not given us a clear treatise on yoga. Hence my prayers to Him:

> *Yogena cittasya padena vācām*
> *Malaṁ śarirasyaca vaidyakena*
> *Yopākarottaṁ pravaraṁ munīnāṁ*
> *Patañjaliṁ prāñjalirānato'smi*
> *Ābāhu puruṣākāraṁ*
> *Śaṅkha cakrāsi dhāriṇam*
> *Sahasra śirasaṁ svetaṁ*
> *Praṇamāmi Patañjaliṁ*

Let us salute Patañjali, the incarnation of the King Cobra, the couch of Lord Vishnu, who gave us grammar to use right words, *āyurveda (āyu* means life, *veda* means knowledge) the Indian way of medicine, to preserve health and longevity and gain peace of mind through the practice of yoga. He holds the sword of knowledge to destroy *avidyā* and blesses practitioners with his hand.

Today the word *śānti* (peace) is uttered as 'peace' but spells 'war'. In the name of peace wars are taking place. We have landed on the moon, but we have not yet landed in our own hearts. Yoga is the method for exploration of the bright sun, the Self, that blazes in each individual so that the human brain may come closer to the conscience of the heart; then men can come closer to each other transcending individualistic personalities. Hence I feel that yoga is a subject of the 21st century. Many scientific and technological discoveries may disappear but yoga shall not. It is the only subject that can uplift, maintain, sustain, support and build up the growth of mental health in each individual to come closer to each one's heart.

* A talk given in Barcelona, Spain. October 26, 1986. Published in *Dīpikā*, Iyengar Yoga Institute London, no. 15 - Winter 1986; also in Victoria Yoga Centre Society, *Newsletter* - April 1988.

Yoga is a word with several connotations and meanings. It is synonymous with *samādhi*, meaning *śānti*, emancipation, liberation, freedom and beatitude. In the fourth chapter of the *Haṭhayoga Pradīpikā*, Svātmārāma mentions sixteen synonymous words and expressions for *samādhi*.

THE SERVANTS OF THE SELF

I would like to clear some misconceptions regarding the term *rāja yoga*, because there is a great deal of confusion about this. The *Haṭhayoga Pradīpikā*, the principal text on *haṭha yoga*, states that the senses are controlled by the mind and the mind is controlled by the breath. The text says:

Indriyāṇām hi mano nāthaḥ manonāthasya mārutaḥ /
Mārutasya layo nāthaḥ sa layo nādamāśritaḥ // (IV.29)

The lord of the senses is the mind; the lord of the mind is the breath; the nerves having softened the flow of breath, control the senses and subdue the mind.

The mind, the master of the senses, has to be poised by the flow of energy – *prāṇa*. The person who knows how to channel the breath is able to channel the consciousness and through this channelling brings the organs of action and the senses of perception under control.

You have heard of the zodiac and the nine major and two minor planets, which according to the laws of Hindu astrology, control the universe. They are the commanders of the Lord who has given them certain functions.

The *Kaṭha Upaniṣad* (V.1) considers the human body as *puram ekādaśa dvāram* (city with eleven gates).* These gates are the seven openings in the head (two eyes, two ears, two nostrils and mouth), three openings in the trunk (the navel, the excretory and genital organs) and the crown of the head or *brahma randhra*.

Similarly, there are five organs of action and five senses of perception, and the eleventh is the mind. These eleven gates are outlets of the emotional feelings of man. The yoga *sādhanā* is meant to close these ten apertures from any external contact and to divert them towards the eleventh sense, the mind. In this way, all eleven senses work in harmony to know the vessel – the consciousness. Then the Self, which is covered and hidden by consciousness, is revealed and brought to the surface.

* The *Śvetāśvatara Upaniṣad* (III.18) and *Bhagavad-Gīta* (V.13) give nine gates. They don't count the navel and *Brahma-randhra*. See also p. 114.

As the eleven planets of the external world are the servants of God, similarly, the eleven planets of our system are the servants of the seer, the *ātmā*.

CONSCIOUSNESS ENTICING THE SELF

According to Patañjali, *vṛtti sārūpyaṁ itaratra*, the uncultured *citta* (consciousness), which has not been disciplined, comes in contact with the eleven planets through the senses of perception and the organs of action. The seer gets attached to them and loses his path of peace, poise and tranquillity. (*Y.S.*, I.4).

When the *ātman* is not resting in its own abode, it is drawn by the eleven planets to become attached to them and it moves with them. According to Patañjali, the body is *tamas* or inert. So, one has to break the shackles of inertia of the body through *kriyā* or action which is a *rājasic* state, in order to become illumined in the conscience *(dharmendriya)*, and realise the true state of being, which is beyond the three *guṇa*.

The consciousness has two branches, one that is divine and pure, the other prejudiced with attachments and aversions.

The first one is experienced in sleep, as there is freedom from the contact of objects. In sleep there is tranquillity. Sleep refreshes the mind to work with freshness in our everyday life. Sleep rests the brain and mind with no movements in thoughts, words or deeds. Hence, one feels fresh after waking up from sleep. This freshness is not cultured tranquillity, as it does not evolve the mind or the intelligence or consciousness. The mind that you experience in sleep is not disturbed by thoughts. It has no branches or leaves and no waves. It is insomnia, when there are waves in the mind at the time of sleep. When the waves come to an end and thought ends, there is no activity, then sleep sets in.

The second one is that consciousness (which is the sprout of the Self) grows into a tree with several branches. The Self is the root, the trunk is the consciousness, branching into ego and intelligence as absorption and observation. Coming in contact with objects in various directions, it becomes like a tree with twigs and leaves. The waves of consciousness are like the movement of the leaves *(citta vṛtti)*.

In chapter IV, Patañjali explains that the consciousness comes in contact with objects felt by the senses of perception and gets attached to them. This disturbs inner peace and becomes *nirmita citta*, or fabricated consciousness. In sleep there is no fabrication. (*Y.S.*, IV.4).

We form opinions when we come in contact with each other. Today I am your friend, tomorrow an enemy; today you like me, tomorrow you may dislike me. Why? Because the consciousness comes in contact with ideas and gets prejudiced or biased.

If you can culture the intelligence, it comes to a state of *nirmāṇa citta*, cultured consciousness. This cultured consciousness cannot be acquired in a day or two. It has to be cultivated day in and day out.

In the *Yoga Sūtra*, Patañjali explains the functions of the brain very clearly. (*Y.S.*, I,17). The uncultured brain comes in contact with whatever it experiences. It becomes cultured and develops four characteristics: *savitarka, savicāra, sānanda* and *sāsmita*. Patañjali, a great scientist, knew about the hypothalamus, the seat that imprints happiness or pleasure and pain. He divided the brain into four parts, the analytical *(savitarka)* at the front, the discriminative *(savicāra)* at the back, blissful, elated *(sānanda)* at the base, the hypothalamus, and the auspicious 'I' *(sāttvic ahaṁkāra* or *sāsmita)* at the pineal gland or head of the brain. He speaks of *sāsmita prajñā samādhi*, or *samādhi* which stems from the seat of individual consciousness.

The auspicious state of 'I' or 'self' *(sāsmita)* is followed by the state of emptiness or void (*virāmapratyaya*). In this state, the aspirant, devoid of his ego, remains like a person lost at a crossroad. This is the state where the Self alone can save the Self as a friend, or the Self alone become the enemy of the Self. (*B.G.*, VI.5). To come out of this spiritual complacency, the *sādhaka* has no other means than pursuing his practice with trust, confidence, intense vigour, keen memory and power of absorption, (*Y.S.*, I.20), to experience the True Self. (*B.G.*, VI.6).

The brain is a thousand petalled lotus *(sahasrāra cakra)*. The petals of the lotus open when the sun rises and close at sunset. Similarly, the petals of the lotus of intelligence get closed in sleep and open in the wakeful state.

The yogi consciously simulates the experiences of sleep in *Śavāsana*. *Śavāsana* is done to experience the state that comes in sleep, by remaining passively in a pensive and quiet state. *Śavāsana* is equivalent to non-attachment.

Patañjali has given us what it means to be free from attachment. He says, *"Maitrī karuṇā muditā upekṣāṇāṁ sukha duḥkha puṇya apuṇya viṣayāṇāṁ bhāvanātaḥ cittaprasādanam"*. (*Y.S.*, I.33): Friendliness, compassion, gladness and indifference are the characteristics of non-attachment. As you learn to diffuse the consciousness evenly, through these four means in all states and moods, it leads towards non-attachment. From this cultivation you develop discrimination and discernment. The true detachment comes through discernment and not by forceful renunciation.

Discernment requires tremendous positive development of intelligence. ("I do not like you, so I avoid you," – that is not non-attachment). From non-attachment one comes to discernment, from discernment to detachment, and from detachment comes renunciation.

Similarly, you cultivate yourself in order to control all the planets of the Self, then you quieten to sublimate them after. The second chapter of the *Yoga Sūtra* says that the mind and the senses are there to serve their master, the Self. If that discrimination is not there, the senses and the mind become masters of the Self and this leads to pleasures and pains. If they are controlled and sublimated, then they have done their job; they do not interfere with their master – the Self. This is *kaivalya* or a state of aloneness. This is intuition, where the instincts are brought to the conscious surface. These instincts are cultured to become intuitive, as it is direct from the core of the being. Here, the seer is the seeker and the seeker is the seer. The difference between the seeker and seer disappears.

According to Patañjali, the consciousness has no light of its own but shines through the borrowed light of the seer. (*Y.S.,* IV.19). You should analyse this very carefully to understand the difference between the seer and the consciousness. He says that the light of the Self is reflected on the consciousness and consciousness works on the reflected light of the Self. Having been cultured it becomes civilised and realises that "I have no light of my own, I exist not by my volition, but on my master's command". This is the sublimation of the consciousness.

You all say that the great scientist Newton was the first to discover gravitational force. You will be interested to know that Patañjali knew this law. He states "When the consciousness is ripe, it rests on the lap of the seer due to the gravitational pull of the seer *(prāgbhāraṁ cittam).* When consciousness is ripe, it is drawn strongly towards the seer or the Self". (*Y.S.,* IV.26). The moment the consciousness is attracted towards the seer, it merges in the seer. Then one's body becomes pure, one's actions become pure and one's life remains totally pure.

THE VEHICLES OF THE SELF

You all say that Patañjali has not dealt with the body, but how many of you have read *sūtra* 47 of the third chapter, describing the wealth of the body?

"Rūpa lāvaṇya bala vajra saṁhananatvāni kāya sampat" (*rūpa* = form, beauty; *lāvaṇya* = grace; *bala* = strength; *vajra* = diamond; *saṁhananatvāni* = hardness; *kāya* = body; *sampat* = wealth).

"The beauty of form *(rūpa)*, grace of movement *(lāvaṇya)*, strength *(bala)* or magnitudinal extension when performing the *āsanas*, and the magnitudinal strength and awareness when breathing and meditating, compactness, firmness and brilliance of a diamond *(vajra saṁhanana)* and softness of a petal, constitute the wealth of the body."

He also says that when the yogi has cultivated and cultured his senses of perception, mind, intelligence, consciousness and conscience, these develop the speed of the seer and move as fast as the seer. (*Y.S.*, III.49).

Many of you say that *āsana* practice is physical, but where does Patañjali say this? While writing the commentary on Patañjali, Vyāsa explains thirteen *āsanas*. *Haṭhayoga Pradīpikā* states sixteen *āsanas* and signifies further *āsanas*.

This is the 'International Year of Peace Conference' and we, as yogis, are quarrelling on 'physical' and 'mental' yoga. Where is the peace, when the yogis have not understood the basics of yoga but speak ill of each other? It is unfortunate, but true.

There are three *sūtras* of Patañjali dealing specifically with the discipline of *āsana:*

Sthira sukham āsanam. (*Y.S.*, II.46) *(sthira* = steady and stable body; *sukham* = contentment and poise of mind; *āsanam* = posture).

Āsana is perfect firmness of body, steadiness of intelligence and benevolence of the self.

Prayatna śaithilya ananta samāpattibhyām. (*Y.S.*, II.47) *(prayatna* = persevering effort; *śaithilya* = relaxation; *ananta* = infinite; *samāpattibhyām* = completion).

Perfection in an *āsana* is achieved when the effort to perform becomes effortless and the infinite within is reached.

Tataḥ dvandvāḥ anabhighātaḥ. (*Y.S.*, II.48) (*tataḥ* = thence; *dvandvāḥ* = dualities; *anabhighātaḥ* = cessation of disturbance).

From then on, the *sādhaka* is undisturbed by dualities.

While learning *āsana*, *prāṇāyāma* or *dhyāna*, when the effortful stage changes into an effortless stage, then you are one with infinity where dualities disappear. When there is no duality, there is stability and oneness. When the posture is stable *(sthira)*, there is poise in the mind *(sukham)*.

How many of you have gone into the meaning of this *sūtra?* You sit cross-legged for ten minutes – you feel uncomfortable and change – is this stability? Yoga is disciplined poise and peace, not interrupted poise and peace. Disciplined freedom is a yogic code of conduct *(anuśāsanam)*. When you discipline your behaviour, you experience freedom and beatitude. By forgetting the first *sūtra*, we do not know to what extent we have murdered our living cells and brought sorrow to the soul of Patañjali.

To have *śānti*, peace, you have to have freedom. Take the analogy of a forest. One tree grows straight, another angular, one has a swollen trunk, another a thin one. On the same tree one branch grows in one direction, another branch in another direction; one branch is doing *Śavāsana*, another *Bhujaṅgāsana*, yet another *Tāḍāsana*. The trunk is the same, but the branches vary. Similarly, various *āsana* have been given for the seer may move in the tree of the body with its various branches without impediments and obstructions.

Patañjali has given a list of thirteen distractions:

Vyādhi (physical disease), *styāna* (langour, mental laziness, sluggishness, lack of interest), *saṁśaya* (doubt, disbelief, indecision), *pramāda* (negligence, carelessness), *ālasya* (physical laziness, idleness), *avirati* (self-indulgence, sensual gratification), *bhrāntidarśana* (living in the world of illusion, mistaken notion, erroneous views), *alabdhabhūmikatva* (missing the point, failure to reach the aim), *anavasthitatva* (backsliding, inability to maintain the progress achieved, inability to maintain steadiness in the practice). These are the causes of mental distractions *(citta vikṣepa)*. (*Y.S.*, I.30). Pain *(duḥkha)*, dejection *(daurmanasya)*, tremor of the body *(aṅgamejayatva)* and irregular, laboured or heavy inbreaths and outbreaths *(śvāsapraśvāsa)* are the companions *(sahabhuva)* of mental distractions. (*Y.S.*, I.31).

These are the obstacles enumerated by Patañjali, from physical disease to tremors of the body (today we call this Parkinson's disease), heaviness of breath and cardiac diseases.

If there is rheumatism in any part of the body, the intelligence cannot flow in these areas. For this reason the yogis traced different *āsanas* so that the trillions of cells in the body, which are born in a split second and die in a split second may have fresh blood brought to them so that they are fully activated. Today these are lifeless stillborn cells because we do not use them.

A lady may be pregnant for seven, eight or nine months and all of a sudden the child does not kick, there is no movement, no life. So she goes to the doctor and delivers a stillborn child. Similarly, the cells in our body, that generate life, become worthless because we do not use them properly. For this reason they die an unnatural death. *Āsana* practice creates potency in the cells for them to do their duty and then die peacefully. The length of life increases because *āsana* activates and supplies the blood to the cells of the body.

The *Varāha Upaniṣad* talks of *ratna pūrita dhātu* – blood filled with pearls, i.e. jewels of the life force. In today's language it is called hormones. When blood is filled with jewels of the life force, then there is buoyancy of life, benevolence of heart and peace. If I do not have any peace within myself, how can I speak of peace to others?

Patañjali speaks of *abhyāsa* and *vairāgya* – a positive approach to cultivate the consciousness. What to do is *abhyāsa* and what not to do is *vairāgya*. Thus, *abhyāsa* and *vairāgya* develop an undisturbed peace and poise in the consciousness of the *sādhaka*. *Abhyāsa* is practice and *vairāgya* is not to do that which disturbs the practice. *Abhyāsa* and *vairāgya* of Patañjali are mentioned in the *Haṭhayoga Pradīpikā* as *ha* (the sun) and *ṭha* (the moon). *Ha* means positive practice *(abhyāsa)*, *ṭha* is negative practice *(vairāgya)*. What one has to relinquish is *vairāgya*.

Unfortunately, all over the world yogis have explained the *Haṭhayoga Pradīpikā* at a physiological level and not on a psychological or spiritual level. This has created a vacuum. They say that *Haṭhayoga Pradīpikā* is physical and Patañjali's *Yoga* is spiritual. In physics, *ha* represents solar energy and *ṭha* lunar energy. *Ha* is the sun *(sūrya)*. The sun never fades, it is stable, it burns for all the twenty-four hours. It represents the seer, the core of the being, which is always bright and stable. The earth makes a complete turn every twenty-four hours, day after day, year after year. If the earth does not rotate, the rays of the sun shed over the same spot and the life force in us gets burnt. The energy of the moon *(candra)* is nothing but the energy drawn from the sun; the moon neutralises the heat of the sun's light.

In our body we have these same systems, the solar (the sympathetic nervous system) and the lunar (the parasympathetic nervous system). They are known in yogic terminology as *piṅgalā* and *iḍā*. The central nervous system is *suṣumṇa*. *Iḍā* and *piṅgalā* supply energy to *suṣumṇa*. When these two do not work, then we suffer from loss of energy. There are six chambers or *cakras* or storehouses of energy in *suṣumṇa*. In these chambers, the energy is accumulated by the practice of *āsanas* and *prāṇāyāma*. When you want energy, they provide you with their reserve energy. The seventh chamber or *cakra* is the *sahasrāra cakra*, where *prakṛti* and *puruṣa* unite.

Why is a lunatic so called? His mind is like the moon, which waxes and wanes. His mind is sometimes attentive, sometimes not. All of a sudden, after being bright, he fades.

Like the moon, which borrows its light from sun, the consciousness borrows its light from the Self. Control of consciousness by the practice of *āsana* and *bandha* makes the consciousness lose its identity so that it merges in the divine Self or universal consciousness.

Haṭha means 'will'. So, *haṭha yoga* is the science of will over matter. The *Haṭhayoga Pradīpikā* says that there are four evolutionary stages in the practice of yoga. The *Yoga Sūtra* also describes four types of student, *mṛdu* (mild), *madhya* (average), *adhimātra* (keen) and *tīvra* (intensely intense). (*Y.S.*, I.21-22).

EVOLUTIONARY STAGES OF THE *SĀDHAKA*

Haṭhayoga Pradīpikā and *Śiva Saṃhitā* describe four evolutionary stages in the practice,* starting from the gross and ending with the finest of the fine:

1. *Ārambhāvasthā:* The beginning state, where one 'scratches the surface' (*H.Y.P.*, IV.70-71; *Ś.S.*, III.28). This stage corresponds to *mṛdu* state of study in the *Yoga Sūtra* – that is the stage of anatomical analysis. After 'scratching' comes the second stage:

2. *Ghaṭāvasthā: Ghaṭa* means a pot – the body is like a vessel or a pot (*H.Y.P.*, IV.72-73; *Ś.S.*, III.55-59). After scratching the first surface or layer of the body, comes the study of its inner functions, the circulation of blood, the function of the vital organs, the movement of breath and so forth. This is *ghaṭāvasthā*. In modern scientific terms *ghaṭāvasthā* is known as the physiological functioning of the human body. The *sādhaka* begins to feel how the internal anatomical action produces a physiological reaction. This state corresponds to *madhya* or average type of study.

   From this physiological reaction, a new awareness is developed in the mind. Suppose you think psychologically to flex the biceps more, or turn more; or extend the liver, strengthen the floor of the bladder and so on, you have to understand that the effect of *āsana* is not merely physical or physiological, but psychological also. *Āsana* practice strengthens the inner body.

   What is this inner body? The inner body is the mind – this is the third stage of growth in *āsana*. The mind feels; but cannot discriminate, so it takes and consults its friend, guide and philosopher: the intelligence and acquaints it with the body.

---

* See also the author's *Light on Prāṇāyāma*, p. 16. Harper Collins, London

3. *Paricayāvasthā* (*H.Y.P.*, IV.74-75; *Ś.S.*, III.61-65): *Paricaya*, literally means 'acquaintance'. Here the intelligence is made to come closer in contact with the functioning of body, senses and mind. This is the state of intimate knowledge, where the mind acts with the intelligence as a public relations officer between physical and organic body. If I am not introduced to you, then you do not know me. When I am introduced to you, you come in close contact and then come to know of my intelligence and me. Similarly, mind takes the intelligence to the various parts of the body and introduces to the anatomical body, physiological body, the physical organs and senses of perception, by bringing the intelligence closer to the various systems of the body. Once this introduction is done then the intelligence, the mind, the physiological organs and the anatomical body function as a co-ordinated single unit.

   In this stage, the intelligence integrates the surface body and the inner body step by step to the core of the being, for the being to permeatê. This state corresponds to the *adhimātrā* state of the *Yoga Sūtra*.

   Finally, comes the last evolutionary stage, that of emancipation.

4. *Niṣpatti avastha* (*H.Y.P.*, IV.76-77; *Ś.S.*, III.66f): The state of accomplishment or consummation, where the consciousness and body (anatomically, physiologically, psychologically and intellectually) become one. When they become one, dualities or differences between body, mind, intelligence and consciousness disappear. When the dualities disappear, then all actions are done intuitively and directly by the core of the being and not by its agents. When this state is reached it is *niṣpatti*. He is in a *tīvra saṁvegin* or *adhimātrataman* (supremely intense) category of yoga *sādhaka* (see Table n. 7).

To conclude with this topic, we can say that during the first two evolutionary stages (*avasthā*), *sādhanā* is more on the level of gross senses (organs of action, senses of perception and mind) and the means used for *sādhanā* are the external limbs. This is called *ārambhāvasthā*, as it corresponds to *bahiraṅga sādhanā*, while *ghaṭāvasthā* corresponds to a transitory state between *bahiraṅga* and *antaraṅga sādhanā*.

During the third stage or *paricayāvasthā*, a great refinement takes place. Here a total synchronisation of intelligence and consciousness takes place. The gross organs co-operate fully with the pair of intelligence and consciousness. This is *antaraṅga sādhanā*.

In the last stage, *niṣpatti avasthā*, the body and consciousness are completely purified and reach the level of purity of the Self. Now, the Self acts directly. This is *añtarātma sādhanā*.

Please note that *ātmā* cannot be a *sādhaka* and has no *sādhanā*. It is due to our misunderstanding of the Self that we use the terms such as *ātma sādhanā*.

ONENESS OF THE *HAṬHAYOGA PRADĪPIKĀ* AND THE *YOGA SŪTRA*

You all think that dress is important. But dress beautifies only the outer body, whereas yoga postures tone and beautify the inner body, making each and every part tidy, neat and clean. Then you need not dress up for external display. If dress beautifies the external personality, yoga beautifies the inner personality. By yoga you enjoy yourself by feeling the beauty of control and action without division. By the practice of *haṭha yoga*, the various vestments of the Self are uncovered one by one till the *ātman* reveals himself as naked as the body. That is the essence of *haṭha yoga*.

The *Haṭhayoga Pradīpikā* has four chapters *(prakaraṇa)*. The first is on *āsana*, the second on *prāṇāyāma*, the third on *bandha* and *mudra* and the fourth on *samādhi*. When the author himself speaks of *samādhi* and *kaivalya*, how foolish we are to say that this yoga is physical yoga.

Patañjali's *Yoga Sūtra* consists of four chapters. The first is *Samādhi Pāda*. Do you mean to say that you and I can reach that state of civilisation which existed at the time of Patañjali? An average man could then understand the movement *(citta vṛtti)* and character of consciousness. Because of this he started the first chapter with *citta vṛtti* and finishes it with seedless *samādhi* *(nirbīja samādhi)*, that is reached when the sheaths of the *ātman* are one with the *ātman*, the seedless seed.

Then why did he write the second, third and fourth chapters? It is wrong for people to say that the later three parts of the *Yoga Sūtra* are an addition, added by others. Nothing is farther from the truth. He realised that people would fall from the grace of that intelligence, so he introduced the second chapter, *Sādhanā Pāda*, as a *bahiraṅga sādhanā* (external quest). Why did he go from internal quest to external quest? Because he knew that the intellectual level would fall.

In the first chapter he deals with the five fluctuations and disturbances of the consciousness. In the second chapter he speaks of five types of afflictions causing miseries or pains. They are on a gross level. Why did he not speak of pains in the first chapter? Because pains can be experienced at once by an ordinary person, whereas fluctuations cannot be experienced by one easily. He explains that the consciousness fluctuates due to pains. By working on the pains, the fluctuations cease and we are led from the external to the internal.

Table n. 7 - The evolutionary stages *(avasthā)* in *sādhanā*, according to the three main texts on yoga*

Bhagavad Gīta	*Yoga Sūtra*	*Haṭha Yoga Pradīpikā*	Type of *sādhanā*	Type of *sādhaka*	*Yogāṅga*	*Śakti*	Elements of *prakṛti* involved
Karma mārga	*TAPAS*	*Ārambhāvasthā*	*Bahiraṅga*	*Mṛdu*	1. *Yama*	***Prakṛti śakti***	1. Behaviour *(ācāra)* Character *(śīlam)*
					2. *Niyama* 3. *Āsana* 4. *Prāṇāyāma*	*Pṛtvī* (earth) *Āp* (water)	2. Organs of action Senses of perception 3. Mind *(manas)* 4. Breath *(prāṇa)*
		Ghaṭāvasthā	Transitory state from *Bahiraṅga* to *Antaraṅga* (turning point)	*Madhya*	5. *Pratyāhāra*	*Āp* (water) *Tej* (fire)	5. Mind directly controls the senses of perception
Jñāna mārga	*SVĀDHYĀYA*	*Paricayāvasthā*	*Antaraṅga*	*Adhimātra*	6. *Dhāraṇā*	*Vāyu* (air)	6. Intelligence *(buddhi)* Ego *(ahaṁkāra)* Consciousness *(citta)*
			Antarāṅga and *Antarātma*		7. *Dhyāna*	*Ākāśa* (ether)	7. Conscience (*Dharmendriya Anthkāraṇa*)
Bhakti mārga	*ĪŚVARA PRAṆIDHĀNA*	*Niṣpattyāvasthā*	*Antarātma*	*Adhimā-trataman (Tīvra saṁvegin)*	8. *Samādhi*	***Puruṣa śakti*** *Ojas śakti* (the light of the soul)	8. Soul *(ātmā prasādana)*

* Please note that this table contains a further and more refined explanation of the resume given in the table 4 (p. 84) of my book *Light on the Yoga Sūtras of Patañjali.*

If you read the 3rd *sūtra* of the second chapter and the 5th *sūtra* of the first chapter with attention, you will find a clear analogy and a deep connection between the two.

Avidyā asmitā rāga dveṣa abhiniveśāḥ kleśāḥ. (*Y.S.,* II.3).

The five afflictions which disturb the equilibrium of consciousness are: ignorance or lack of wisdom, pride of the ego or the pride of 'I', attachment to pleasure, aversion to pain, fear of death and clinging to life.

Vṛttayaḥ pañcatayyaḥ kliṣṭā akliṣṭāḥ (*Y.S.,* I.5).

The movements of consciousness are fivefold. They may be cognisable or non-cognisable, painful or non-painful.

Patañjali explains:

Te pratiprasavaheyāḥ sūkṣmāḥ (*Y.S.,* II.10),
Dhyānaheyāḥ tadvṛttayaḥ (*Y.S.,* II.11).

Subtle afflictions are to be minimised and eradicated by a process of involution. The afflictions which are not eradicated become the subject of focused attention and get transformed into *vṛtti.*

A careful analysis of these two *sūtras* shows that when *kleṣa* in any form is not taken care of in due time, they penetrate deep into the self and become *vṛtti.* Similarly, if *kliṣṭa vṛtti* is not restrained, an imbalance in the physiological body takes place and mentally disturbs one.

This makes us understand the necessity of practice as Patañjali so strongly emphasises in *Y.S.,* I.1,2 and *Y.S.,* II.1, with the code of yoga and the control of thought-waves of consciousness. Please note that the *kleṣa* (affliction) continue to exist till one reaches the stage of *pratyāhāra.* Only when *pratyāhāra* is mastered, the *kleśa karma* ceases to exist. The *akliṣṭa vṛtti* (non-painful fluctuation of consciousness) begins to shine from *pratyāhāra* onwards.

As I explained earlier, *Haṭhayoga Pradīpikā* enumerates four evolutionary stages of practice, of which the second one is the understanding of the functions of the body and unveiling its covering, until the Self shines on its own.

In the chapter on accomplishment *(Vibhūti Pāda),* Patañjali deals with the effects of *sādhanā* on one who reaches the higher levels of evolution. He presents a detailed list of thirty-five supra-natural powers or accomplishments; but warns that due to intoxication by these achievements, pores or fissures may develop between the consciousness and the Self (*Y.S.,* IV.27).

In chapter four Patañjali explains the ways and means to keep the consciousness without pores. Living in the world, doing one's duty, how can one be free without attachments? We have heard the *śloka "Yogaḥ karmasu kauśalam"*, (*B.G.*, II.50): "Yoga is skilfulness in action". Does anyone refer to Patañjali for equivalent terms? Possibly not.

Patañjali explains what is skilful action. In (IV. 7) he says that average persons have three types of actions – white, black and mixed. A yogi has neither white, nor black nor mixed *karma* but goes beyond these three. His actions do not bear any ambition for fruits. That is *yogaḥ karmasu kauśalam*. This does not come to you and to me. Only when intelligence is civilised *(samskṛta citta)* and ripened *(paripakva)* do the *vṛttis* dissolve *(kṣīṇa)*; then it is *yogaḥ karmasu kauśalam*. To maintain that pure ripened state, you have to continue the discipline of yoga. Nowhere does he say that when you reach *samādhi*, the practice of yoga ends. He cautions that even the state of *samādhi* is lost if the practice is discontinued.

Many people say that the *Haṭhayoga Pradīpikā* does not mention *yama* and *niyama*. Please read *sloka* 16 of the first chapter where *yama* and *niyama* are given. This shows that we do not read the textbook carefully. As the *sādhanā* in the *Haṭhayoga Pradīpikā* starts directly with the study of *āsana*, it is called *ṣaḍāṅga yoga*, whereas Patañjali's yoga is *aṣṭadaḷa or aṣṭāṅga yoga*. *Haṭhayoga Pradīpikā* is called yoga of six limbs *(ṣaḍāṅga)*: Probably morality was in vogue and everyone was practising it, so *āsana* became the first part which is why we read immediately of the effects of *āsanas*. Nevertheless, please note that in spite of explaining the *āsana* as the first limb, not only does Svātmārāma speak of *yama* and *niyama*, but adds five more *yama* and five more *niyama* than Patañjali (*H.Y.P.*, I.16).

The body is dull, *tāmasic*. *Āsanas* are given to bring the body to the level of the vibrant mind *(manas)*, which is *rajō guṇa*. From the inertia of the body the author wants the body to be as vibrant as the mind and then to practise further to change the vibrant body, mind, intelligence and consciousness to become *sāttvic*, so that one joins the unfading light of the Self, which is beyond the *guṇa*. This is the effect of *āsana*. Peace has to come from this. If the essence of yoga is lost, peace is lost. Each cell of the body has to have peace for the consciousness to experience peace.

I am citing the meaning with just three *sloka* from chapter IV of the *Haṭhayoga Pradīpikā* for all of you to know what the essence of *haṭha yoga* is:

Salile saindhavaṁ yadvat sāmyaṁ bhajati yogataḥ I
Tathātmamanasoraikyaṁ samādirabhīyate II

First is water and salt: Take a glass of water and mix in salt. Stir the water. When it has been stirred, taste the water from the bottom, middle or top; the salty taste is the same at all levels. Similarly, by the mastery of *haṭha yoga* the body appears as Self, the consciousness appears as Self, Self appears as Self and the whole being appears as Self. The same Self is tasted everywhere. (*H.Y.P.*, IV.5).

Antaḥ śūnyo bahiḥ śūnyaḥ śūnyaḥ kumbha ivāmbhare |
Antaḥ pūrṇo bahiḥ pūrṇaḥ pūrṇaḥ kumbha ivārṇave ||

Second is vessel and sea: Take a vessel and put it on the sea. If it is empty, it floats. We say it is empty, but the *Haṭhayoga Pradīpikā* says it is filled with air. If you press the vessel into the sea, it is filled with water – so whether it is empty or full, know that it is always full either with air or with water. Similarly, with yoga practice; when the body and consciousness come in contact with the Self, they become the Self. Self penetrates the body like the water or air of the vessel. The rivers of the body and mind, and the rivers of intelligence and consciousness, join the sea of the Self. (*H.Y.P.*, IV.56).

Karpūramanale yadvat saidhavaṁ salile yathā |
Tathā saṁdhīyamānaṁ ca manastatve vilīyate ||

Third is camphor and flame: Camphor and flame are separate. Strike a matchstick and bring it to the camphor; the camphor and flame become one, the camphor dissolves. In the practice of *āsanas*, the camphor of the body is burned by the flame of intelligence so that it dissolves and becomes one with the flame of the soul. (*H.Y.P.*, IV.59). Here the explanations of the *Samādhi Pāda* of Patañjali coincide with the *Samādhi Pāda* of *Haṭhayoga Pradīpikā*.

As in large cities we have two-way traffic, in our nervous systems also, we have afferent nerves and efferent nerves. The afferent nerves or sensory nerves carry the message towards the brain, while the efferent nerves or motor nerves receive the message from the brain for action. *Śiva Samhitā* uses the terms *jñāna nāḍī* and *karma nāḍī*. The very words convey that *jñāna nāḍī* stands for knowledge and *karma nāḍī* for action. *Jñāna nāḍī* carries the impressions of actions to the brain whereas the *karma nāḍī* receives the orders from the brain and acts accordingly.

The yogis knew the functions of the afferent and efferent nerves long ago before the medical scientists discovered them. The actions of *karma* and *jñāna nāḍī* have to be understood as 'inner and outer penetration'. Inner penetration is the action through which the body and consciousness get wedded to the Self. Outer penetration is the action through which the Self comes in contact with the consciousness and body and gets married to them. They are married both ways. When the vessel on the sea is up, it is married to air; when it is drowned in water, it is married to water.

The true balance of the *āsana* is when the head of muscle fibres does not poke the nerves of the skin; for this the *sādhaka* has to create space between the afferent and efferent nerves so that the brain receives the messages felt and sent by these nerves. This is known as the dual carriageway or dual avenue. Using these two conduits, *āsana* has to be practised for sending messages from the muscles to the skin and vice versa, for the intelligence and consciousness to feel the balance, harmony and delight. Conative actions are just done by impulse or volition, which is purely the function of the organs of action. When the actions of the motor nerves sends messages through the anatomical body for the cognitive senses of perception to feel, the actions become cogniseable. According to Patañjali, when the *āsana* and *prāṇāyāma* are done with conative actions and cognative feeling, they are external quests. When these two, the conative action and cognitive feeling, come in contact with each other, the mind enters there to act supramentally (in the terminology of Shri Aurobindo). The contact of conative action and cognitive feeling brings double attention. At that time the *āsana* is mental, because the mind is automatically brought there. The mind gathers information and approaches the intelligence to discriminate, reason and judge the position whether it is right or wrong. This involvement of intelligence is the beginning of spiritual *sādhanā* in *āsana*, where the difference between cognitive and conative action comes to an end. When all actions, be they mental or supramental come to an end, then all presentation is from the supreme intelligence, which in turn comes from absolute consciousness. This is *vivekaja jñāna* or exalted intelligence. (*Y.S.*, III.55). This is the zenith. This exalted intelligence is equal to the insight of the Self. In the *Yoga Sūtra* it is said that there comes a balance, where the exalted intelligence is equal to the intelligence of the Self; the *sādhaka* is in *kaivalyam* and the search for realisation comes to an end. (*Y.S.*, III.56). Then one is a yogi. Till then, he is a yoga practitioner. The same principles are applied to *prāṇāyāma* practice. Then this type of practice makes one merge into *dhyāna*, or meditation.

I am again reminding you of the five aspects that are involved in our practices: 1) conative action; 2) cognitive feeling; 3) mind that gathers information; 4) intelligence that reasons and decides what to do, what not to do; and 5) culmination; attaining divinity, peace.

The *Haṭhayoga Pradīpikā* explains this in depth, whereas Patañjali summarises it in one brief *sūtra*, that "the effortful effort becomes effortless". When the effort ceases, the divinity of the *āsana* comes at that moment. Non-divinity is not peace, external peace is not peace. Divinity is peace and peace is dynamic, as love is dynamic. Love without lust is pure and love with lust is not love. We love our children, our wives and our friends, but there is a difference in these. One may experience lust when one looks at one's wife; one may adore one's children; and may feel love with equanimity for a friend. So we create a mixed peace. Peace without attachment is real peace; it is peace without becoming proud. Peace in each and every cell exists in the form of self. Then there is peace everywhere and we look at each other in peace. Peace is positive. Peace is a property of yoga.

Yama, niyama, āsana, prāṇāyāma are evolutionary practices. *Pratyāhāra* is a plateau for stabilisation. It is a transitory state between the evolutionary practices and involutionary disciplines. *Dhāraṇā, dhyāna* and *samādhi* are involutionary disciplines. Thus, the eleven planets (five organs of action, five senses of perception and the mind) have to be involuted. Involution is the flow of energy towards the core. Evolution is the growth from the core towards the body.

THE WHEEL OF PEACE

The eight petals of yoga bring the fruit of poise and peace in us, peace in body and poise or harmony in mind. Unless there is peace in the body, there is no poise in the mind. Patañjali shows that heaviness in mind and body comes through *kleśa*. After experiencing that peace, we should express that peace to our neighbours and to society.

We are two-legged violent animals. We are violent not only within ourselves but with our neighbours also. We mistrust each other and try to cut the other's throat. There is competition. I know that I am using strong words, but there are healthy and unhealthy competitions.

I have conducted classes for three days. I showed improvement in some people, weakness in others. I had to ignite fire in order to bring weaker ones to the level of the others. This type of encouragement is healthy competition that brings peace all around. In cut throat competition there is only a fight and a flight.

Today we have two hundred people gathered here to cultivate that quality of non-attachment, through friendliness and compassion instead of anger. We are here to learn when to be friendly and when to be indifferent so that we all become strong with a positive attitude to develop the characteristics of a true human being.

Those who have attended my classes experienced a state of poise and peace. Did you not have peace of mind in these three days of classes? Didn't you experience peace after *Uttānāsana?* Wasn't your brain cool, calm and serene?

If all of us enjoy these experiences, why do we not take the message of yoga to others and do a service for our fellow beings? God has given us this great subject. So make life worthwhile by spreading civilised peace and cultured peace. Experience this peace and pass it on to your friends. Express it to your neighbours, to the community, then the human race will be the happiest in the Universe. Let us do this before the close of the 20th century.

The World Health Organisation declared that the 21st century would be the healthiest one. The 21st century begins in thirteen years. In order to make the 21st century generation delighted and happy, we should take all children between six and thirteen years and educate them in yoga. Due to the seed of yoga imbibed in them, their intelligence becomes fertile and cultured; then there is the possibility to see health and happiness in the world, as predicted by W.H.O. for the 21st century. What is the use, if it remains only on paper?

Up to now, science has advanced to make unhealthy people healthy. No science has advanced to keep healthy people healthy. Yoga is the only science which makes not only unhealthy people healthy, but also keeps healthy ones healthy. If health is built up from now on through yoga, the people of the 21st century will be kept healthy. Yoga helps each and every cell of the body to be born with potency, made to serve with potency and allowed to die with peace. This is health and health alone is the foundation of peace.

Science has offered a negative health and not a positive health. As life is dynamic, so is peace and yoga is the science of charging life into serene dynamism. Patañjali calls this the flow of tranquillity *(praśānta vāhinī)*. (*Y.S.*, III.10). It is this serenity and health, which we would all like to see everywhere in the 21st century. It cannot come unless we work for it.

In yoga, *yama* and *niyama* are traditional. They are in all people's blood. Don't you tell your children what to do and what not to do? What not to do is *yama*, and what to do is *niyama*. It is all in our blood. It exists from the moment we are born. This is known as *pūrva sādhanā*, or the fruit of our previous evolution. *Āsana*, *prāṇāyāma* and *pratyāhāra* are called *uttarōttara sādhanā* (progressive practices). *Prāṇāyāma* washes away the impurities of the mind and brain, and *pratyāhāra* ripens the mind for meditation. (*Y.S.*, III.2).

From the above *sūtra* you can understand that *yama*, *niyama*, *āsana*, *prāṇāyāma* and *pratyāhāra* are the real practices of yoga.

Dhāraṇā, *dhyāna* and *samādhi* are not practices, but the wealth of yoga. If you progress well in your practice and *sādhanā* is ripe, the fruit blossoms on its own.

So, if you pursue with zeal your practice of *āsana*, *prāṇāyāma* and *pratyāhāra*, with the principles of *yama* and *niyama*, then *dhāraṇā*, *dhyāna* and *samādhi*, the wealth of yoga, are in your hands. A tree never says, "I want fruit now", because the natural end of the tree is the fruit.

Similarly, the natural end of yogic *sādhanā* is *dhyāna*, the real peace and poise.

These days, we do not believe in God who created man, but we believe in man-created God – the political Gods. We are in a very unfortunate situation. We should revolutionise ourselves and not follow these gods. If we adjust according to what they say, then we are cowards and we will have no peace.

God bless you all. You carry this message of yoga to your neighbours, family and community. Let us have a new world.

LET US BE YOGIS.

YOGA – A WAY TO MAINTAIN PEACE

You turn your back on persons you dislike and you don't like to face those that you do not like or relish. But have you seen your back except by chance in a mirror, or possibly while dressing? If you have, it was not with a direct mind. Have you tried it any time or thought it worth the while to think about your back as you breathe in and out with your lungs, or holding the breath when you try to lift something?

There is an ancient story, which is full of wisdom. There are two brothers who stay very close to each other in the neighbourhood. But they have never met nor seen each other, though not because they are hostile to each other or are on inimical terms. Our two eyes are placed like these two brothers in the neighbourhood. Eyes act as organs of action as well as senses of perception. They feel and partake of our joy, happiness and pleasure. They become sad and suffer when we are morose. Since the nature of *prakṛti* has placed them in a particular position, the only avenue for them to meet is through the inner eye. If you close both the eyes, they meet each other and enjoy the bliss of that meeting. Man could be proud of having landed on the moon in an effort to explore the vast expanse of the universe. How many of us have thought of exploring our own consciousness, our own inner being? Unfortunately, we leave this job to psychoanalysts, psychologists or psychiatrists to tell us what we are and what exactly our mental, emotional and psychological conditions and problems are. Then we ask them to guide us on the way to tackle our problems or cope with tensions and stresses. To cure our bodily ailments, physical and physiological troubles, pains, afflictions, illness and diseases, we run to doctors and physicians. Few among us believe that we have spiritual problems and seek a treatment in the holy books, like *Bhagavad Gītā*, the Koran or the Bible, the Old and New Testaments. But has your back turned its back on you? No! It makes its presence felt almost constantly. According to reliable sources, at least five million Americans suffer from back and lower back pain. This is second only to the sore throat, from which every second American suffers.

In addition to the above problems, artificial pollution and modern life styles invite troubles and tension. Back pain snowballs innumerable miseries. Working women cannot provide the near and dear ones well-balanced and nutritious meals. They cannot put in their best at their office work for lack of concentration. What is more, backache puts them out of the mood for socialising and meeting people. They are confined to the house fretting and fuming. They are neither in nor out of the house. Males have to curb and curtail their outdoor activities.

The back is basically the fulcrum of the human body structure. It is the spine which decides about the rate of inhalation, exhalation and retention of the breath. You hold the breath when you lift something.

We mentioned about sore throats, which make life equally unbearable and take the spice away from life. It implies that you need better lungpower to resist cold, foul air, and toxins discharged by industrial plants and factories with smoke belching out from their tall chimneys. Besides all these, a lot of viruses carrying a variety of infections are in the air. Those with better immune power or resistance can neutralise the effects of these viruses and spare themselves from disease and ill health. A common man needs sturdier lungs than a mountain top hermit or a Himalayan yogi who breathes pure and life giving air.

Before explaining how yoga can help to face these afflictions of our modern life, let us see first what yoga is.

Without going into the philosophy or esoteric aspects, yoga signifies unison of the three principles that constitute the human being. They are the body, the consciousness and the individual self *(jīvātmā)*. The working of all three in concord leads to integration. This paves the ground for merging the *puruṣa* and *prakṛti* – the seer and the seen. The *puruṣa* is lame and cannot move and *prakṛti*, which is mobile, is blind. Together they can do wonders.

Yoga is a factual subject, based on direct perception. Yoga is an experimental and experiential art and science.

The *āsana* or posture works to combine physical action and insight, with balance, strength and endurance, and then go further to explore the inner depth of our being, keeping its vehicles intact. It is work and relaxation. *Āsana* moves joints and various muscles by supplying sufficient blood and charging and recharging them like a battery. *Āsana* is meant for *'snāyu vṛtti nirodha'.* From this perfection of body, it proceeds towards the consciousness, uncovering its layers with space and focussed silence.

The stress of modern life pressurises the emotions, creating disturbances in the glandular system. The adrenal glands secrete adrenaline and pour it into the blood. The constant use of these glands and their hormones for less important purposes can ruin the body. The secretions of adrenal glands cause the small arteries to contract. The other glands also get affected on account of our emotional imbalances and our irregular ways of living. These are mainly: 1) improper diet, 2) excessive diet, 3) eating of over-refined foods, 4) lack of physical exercise, and 5) irregularities. All these combined together lead to further physical ailment and mental tension.

Prāṇāyāma is meant for *prāṇa vṛtti nirodha,* i.e. control of the vital flow of energy. In *prāṇāyāma,* the breath that we draw in fuses the element of fire and water in our system, and produces a new energy known as bio-energy. This is produced by elongating the inhalation and exhalation between pauses.

Pratyāhāra controls the fluctuations of *manas* or mind *(manovṛtti nirodha).* The mind or *manas* being considered as the eleventh sense *(indriya), pratyāhāra* completes *indriyavṛtti nirodha* (restraint of the senses of perception, organs of action and mind), which is primarily realised through *yama* and *niyama.* In *pratyāhāra,* the mind is distinctly controlled.

As the practice of *āsana* deepens, it leads to breath awareness. *Prāṇāyāma* oxygenates blood and energises the body. However, excessive *āsana* practice results in strained muscles, while excessive *prāṇāyāma* practice leads to a serious energy disruption. The sedate and sober message is: 1. Respect your capacity, 2. Practice regularly, 3. Create self-discipline, 4. Begin where you are.

The eight-petalled yogic practices cannot be dissociated in one's life. Yoga is not like choosing to switch on one of these at the cost of others. Meditation and silence is a yogic process of providing deep rest to the system by allowing the consciousness to achieve a quiet state. The meditation gradually extends beyond the sitting practice to build a foundation for compassion and creativity in all departments of life. It endows the practitioner with a capacity to resolve the conflicts of life by peaceful methods. Meditation aims at stilling the consciousness and catching a glimpse of the inner core of our being. This produces a constant and a full state of awareness. By learning and cultivating love and kindness towards others, man faces any situation in his life with intelligence and compassion. It is essential to be attentive, as *citta* is quick to move towards the enjoyment of pleasures that continue to wet the appetite for both life and *citta. Āsana* is therefore meant to experience *śauca* (cleanliness) and *santoṣa* (contentment), whereas *svādhyāya* (Self-study) leads to understanding of the Self.

To keep and maintain a perfect balance and well being on physical, mental, emotional and psychological levels, yoga will be a true friend and a great guide. By yogic practice, a quiet peace settles in you from the core of your being to each part and parcel of your body and from each part of your body to the core of your being. In this state peace settles within yourself and around yourself.

YOGA AND MIND CULTURE

Yoga starts not only with the analysis of sorrow but also helps trace the root cause of sorrow. Sorrow is termed as *kleśa* (affliction). They are either visible and recognisable or invisible, hidden and non-recognisable. The afflictions are: 1. nescience 2. egoism 3. attachment to lust and greed 4. aversion, hatred or malice; and 5. selfishness or the fear of losing the joys of life.

Avidyā and *asmitā* (1&2), are intellectual defects, *rāga* and *dveṣa* (3&4) are emotional defects and *abhiniveśa* (5) is an instinctive defect. These defects confirm that man is made of head, heart and life. He has to use his discriminative power for clarity in intelligence, emotional stability in the upheavals of day to day life and transformation of the instinctive fears of life into a fearless state.

Yoga controls and sublimates these defects through direct perception, imagination and analyses them to distinguish facts. It explains the reactions of these afflictions, throws light on the causes of sorrow and offers practical means to eradicate them and makes the practitioner experience pure unalloyed bliss.

As affliction, joy and pleasure, belongs to the movements of the consciousness, the sublimation of consciousness with conscious effort is the key to release the self from sorrow and joy.

Yoga is defined as the cessation of all forms of thinking (*Y.S.,* I.2), whether internal or external, that sprout with or without volition.

What is *citta?* We normally use the word 'mind' to mean several things. For example inspiration, aspiration, drive, will power, intelligence, reason and consciousness are the stuff of the mind. But in yogic terms, *citta* stands distinctly for three things braided together. They are mind, intelligence and the 'I', which ascertains that 'I know'. Mind has the power of gathering and feeling. It has no determinative power. Intelligence discriminates, reasons and comes to determinative knowledge. Hence, the Indian sages call the mind *manomaya kośa* and intelligence *vijñānamaya kośa* whereas the Western scholars consider both these sheaths as a psychological sheath.

Buddhi or intelligence, being the nearest vehicle to the self, prides itself as true Self. This creates egoism. All these three vehicles: the mind, the intelligence and the 'I' or 'me' originate from the *citta* and revolve around it. By controlling the vibrations of *citta* they cease to function. Then the SELF shines on its own as a WITNESS without getting caught in the turmoils and upheavals of life.

Today we use the word 'mind' for *citta*. The mind is the means, which classifies, co-ordinates and channelises the impressions gathered from the external world through the senses of knowledge and experiences from the organs of action. These experiences create various and divergent thought-waves, attracting the mind towards sensual enjoyment and attachments. Gradually these satisfactions hanker for more and more and the mind becomes an instrument to gratify them. If these are uncontrolled they bring chains of sorrow such as fear, suspicion, indecisiveness and oscillation. They remain immature, ending with failures, pains and delusions creating a fickle and weak mind.

If these oscillations are well guarded by a disciplined mind, happiness is the result. To get the best out of the mind, one has to know how it functions and how it thinks.

By nature the mind is split. Mind on the one side is caught up with the pleasures of the world and on the other seeks freedom from them. Several factors split the mind further. They are physical ailments, lack of mental disposition, illusion, isolation, pains, miseries and despair.

In order to conquer all the obstacles, which come in the wake of training the mind from the state of *mūḍa* (dull) to the state of *niruddha* (refinement), the ethical disciplines, the physical disciplines, the mental disciplines and the intellectual disciplines are dealt with. These disciplines train the mind to come to a single state so that the emotional, intellectual and instinctive defects are eradicated and transformed into pure intuitive knowledge.

Thus the dual state of mind *(dvaita)* is channelled to a monistic state *(advaita)*, which is dynamic, positive and clear in its approach to life. The practitioner of yoga sees evenness *(viśiṣṭādvaita)* in all things – whether animate or inanimate – as the creation *(līlā)* of God and surrenders himself to that Supreme Soul.

Besides the practice of the eight aspects of yoga, Patañjali enumerates other qualities, which are required for development of a quiet mind. They are friendliness, compassion, gladness and indifference towards failures. Here, one should be delighted to be with one's master and show contempt when it becomes an instrument of abuse. Then he wants us to build up faith, courage, memory and a single-pointed awareness. Thus the mind is cultivated and taken away from *avidyā* (ignorance) to *vidyā* (knowledge), from *vidyā* to *savidyā* (right and auspicious knowledge), from *asmitā* (egoistic self or self-esteem – *rājasic* by nature) to *sāsmitā* (pure self – *sāttvic* by nature) and from *sāsmitā* to *nirāsmitā* (Self or *puruṣa*).

Only the mind, civilised qualitatively by the culture of yoga, may experience this state where all the vehicles of man become pure, eternal and beautiful.

YOGA AND *DHARMA**

INTRODUCTION – WHAT IS YOGA?

We are caught in the web of words. Hence, it is rather hard to define the term yoga and *dharma*, and satisfy everybody. Nowadays people from East, West, South and North, are attracted towards yoga and *dharma*.

First let me explain what yoga means. Yoga is derived from the root *yuj* meaning to bind, to join, to attach and to yoke, to focus one's attention on, to use and to apply. Yoga means the yoking of the body, the senses, the mind and the intelligence together in order to bring the *jīvātman* (the individual soul) to commune with the *Paramātman* (the Supreme Soul). This yoking together is achieved by firm discipline whereby one lives in a pure, perfect and divine state of consciousness in which there is no feeling of 'I' or 'me' or 'mine' or 'yours'.

So, the practice of yoga begins with yoking, joining and using the different components of body and consciousness, and proceeds towards the integration of the entire human being in order that he or she can experience the unalloyed eternal bliss of *samādhi*.

Yoga is one of the foremost and most refined forms of Indian art based on an extremely subtle science, the science of duty of the body, of the consciousness and of the self. It is the wealth of wisdom that shows the right way to live and sometimes enables one to have an insight into one's innermost being. As *dharma* is universal, it may be considered as the highest philosophy, covering the ethical, physical, mental, intellectual and spiritual duties of man.

WHAT IS *DHARMA?*

According to the Mahābhārata, *"Patitam patantam patiṣyantam dhārayati iti dharmaḥ. Dhāraṇat dharmaḥ ityāhaḥ". "Dharma* is that which supports, sustains, upholds those who have fallen physically, morally or spiritually, or those who are falling, or those who are about to fall".**

---

* Also published as: *Yoga and Religion*.

** Patañjali does not offer a direct definition of *dharma*. Vācaspati Miśra discusses in detail about *dharma*, defining it as "that which becomes the cause of enjoyment of heaven" (*Tattva Viśāradi*, II.12).

Dharma has no denomination and no frontier. *Dharma* is that which is revealed and realised through divine inspiration. The moment *dharma* is translated into religion, then it strikes one as religion of the Hindus, Zoroastrians, Jains, Buddhists, Christians, and so on. The truth revealed to the Buddha is called Buddhism. The truth felt by Jesus Christ has come to be known as Christianity, that of Mohammed became Islam, that of Mahāvīr became Jainism, and so on. *Vedic dharma* is known as *sanātana dharma*, that has no founder. This *sanātana dharma* is wrongly interpreted as Hindu *dharma*. The word 'Hindu' is a polluted form of the word 'Sindhu'. This was the name given to the inhabitants of the eastern bank of the Sindhu river. "The *Veda* is the source of *dharma*" *Vedo' khilo dharma mūlam*" (). *Sanātana* means eternal *(nitya)*. The word *veda* comes from root *vid* (to know). Both *veda* and *sanātana*, have neither a beginning nor an end. *Sanātana dharma* is a divine exposition *(apauruṣeya)* and not a man-made code. *Dharma* also means the science of duty. *Dharma* is a code of conduct, a guide to live in the right direction. It is prescribed by the *Vedas* as one of the four motifs of human existence, namely, *dharma* (duty), *artha* (means of livelihood, prosperity), *kāma* (pleasure) and *mokṣa* (liberation).

VARṆA

The *dharma* of every individual depends upon one's social order, way of life, one's stage in life and individual aspirations. The very nature of the individual is known as *varṇāśrama-dharma* (duties of communities). *Varṇa-dharma* was established as a division of labour according to one's physical capacity, intellectual calibre, personal traits and behavioural tendency and so forth for the benefit of society. The word *varṇa* literally means 'colour', 'cover' or 'quality'. As such, the *varṇa* of the person was decided according to the *guṇa* and the latent imprints of the past *karma*. Thus, the four classes are:

1. Those who attend to the spiritual needs of the people are called *brāhmaṇa;*
2. Those who defend the country and govern are called the *kṣatriya* or martial class;
3. Those who look after the economic growth and prosperity of the nation are known as the mercantile class or *vaiśyā;* and lastly,
4. Those who provide service and manpower for the growth of the nation are known as the labouring class or the *śūdra*.

Today, *varṇa dharma* is ceasing to exist.

Table n. 8 - Divisions of *dharma*

DHARMA

- I. *Puruṣa dharma* (the science of soul)
  - A. *Jīvātma dharma* (the science of individual soul)
  - B. *Paramātma dharma* (the science of Universal Soul)
- II. *Prakṛti dharma* (the science of nature)
  - A. *Acetana prakṛti dharma* (science of inanimate or unconscious nature)
    1. *Mṛṇmaya dharma* (science of earth element)
    2. *Annamaya dharma* (science of food)
    3. *Vāyumaya dharma* (science of air element)
    4. *Nābhasa dharma* (science of celestial elements)
    5. *Tejasa dharma* (science of fire element)
    6. *Raktamaya dharma* (science of blood)
    7. *Asthimaya dharma* (science of bones)
    8. *Bījamaya dharma* (science of seed)
  - B. *Sacetana prakṛti dharma* (science of animate or conscious nature)
    (division according to way of procreation the species take)
    1. *Tiryak dharma* (science relating to animals and birds)
    2. *Atiryak dharma* (science relating to non-animal beings)
       - A. *Mānuṣa dharma* (human *dharma*)
         1. *śārīaka* (related to body)
            - a) *yogika* (yogic)
            - b) *māllika* (wrestling, etc.)
            - c) *dhānuṣya* (archery)
            - d) *nāṭya* (dance)
            - e) *sāngītika* (music)
            - f) *vyāvahārika* (concordance of speech and action, behavioural pattern of *kāya, vācā* and *manasā)*
         2. *mānasika* (related to mind)
         3. *ātmika* (related to soul)
         4. *rājakīya* (political)
         5. *sāmājīka* (social)
         6. *ārthika* (financial)
         7. *laukika* (public affairs)
         8. *daivika* (spiritual practice)
         9. *vārṇika* (related to *vārṇa)*
         10. *āśramika* (related to each *āśram)*
       - B. *Amānuṣa dharma* (non-human *dharma*)
         1. *rākṣasa dharma* (inhuman, demons)
            (born to Kāśyapa from his wife Dithī, and from groups of angels also)
            - a) *daitya*
            - b) *dānava*
            - c) *āsūrika*
         2. *devatā dharma* (celestial, angels)
            (born to Kaśyapa from his wife Adhithī)*
            - a) *yakṣa* (semi-gods)
            - b) *gandharva* (celestial musicians)
            - c) *kinnara* (semi-gods attached to the service of Kimpuruṣa, having a head of horse and a *vīṇa* in their hands)
            - d) *kimpuruṣa* (semi-god attached to the service of Kubera.)

Mahabhārata, Ādi Parva III.66

ĀŚRAMA

Though *varṇa dharma* is disappearing, *āśrama-dharma* holds sway on society irrespective of creed.

Āśrama dharma has four stages. They are meant for the evolution of human beings from material towards spiritual needs. The first is *brahmacarya* – the period devoted to the study of the scriptures. The second is the stage of *gṛhastha* or the life of a householder – at the root of family and society. The third is the stage of *vānaprastha* or preparation of the mind for retirement from objects of the world. Lastly is the stage of *sannyāsa* or renunciation of the material world in order to pursue the spiritual goal. It involves complete suspension of all activities of the *citta* and devotion on *Īśvara*, the Lord and the Architect of the Universe.

PURUṢĀRTHA

As I said in the beginning of my talk, each human being in each moment of his life pursues a motif. The sages of yore divided these motifs into four categories in order to guide man towards a right understanding of the motifs of his existence. They are: *dharma*, *artha*, *kāma* and *mokṣa*. These *puruṣārtha* are common and applicable to every human being on earth, to whatever *āśrama* or *varṇa* he may belong to.

Dharma indicates the way of life and yoga takes one to the art of living in a perfect life. Both yoga and *dharma* are refined after thorough discipline, defining each movement in action, thought and word for the betterment of the individual as well as humanity. *Dharma* has its own scientific techniques like yoga, showing ways and means to move from *avidyā* (ignorance) to *vidyā* (knowledge), from *tamas* (darkness) to *jyoti* (light), from *apūrṇā* (immaturity) to *pūrṇā* (maturity) and from *mṛta* (mortality) to *amṛta* (immortality).

Man is blessed with having hands, heart and head, which correspond to *karma* (work), *bhakti* (worship) and *jñāna* (wisdom).

As yoga is one, so is *dharma*. They are, however, interpreted according to the prevailing conditions, time and place.

Aṣṭadaḷa yoga leads one to achieve seven states of consciousness which Patañjali speaks of as *saptadhā prāntabhūmikā prajñā*.* (*Y.S.*, II.27). These are control of body, organs of action, senses of perception, breath, mind, intelligence and consciousness.

---

* See also the author's *Light on the Yoga Sūtras of Patañjali* (pp. 130-133). Harper Collins, London.

DIVISIONS OF *DHARMA*

Dharma is divided and subdivided into several aspects (see Table n. 8). First of all there is the division of *dharma* into *puruṣa dharma* and *prakṛti dharma*.

The former is divided into *jīvātma dharma* and *paramātma dharma*, whereas the latter is branched into *acetana prakṛti dharma* and *sacetana prakṛti dharma*. *Acetana prakṛti dharma* comprises *mṛṇmaya, annamaya, vāyumaya, nābhasa, tejasa, raktamaya, asthimaya* and *bījamaya*. *Sacetana prakṛti dharma* is subdivided into *tiryak* (relating to animals and birds) and *atiryak dharma* (relating to non-animal beings). Animals and birds belong to the *tiryak*, while *atiryak* covers *mānuṣa* and *amānuṣa dharma*. *Amānuṣa-dharma* belongs to *rākṣasas* (goblins) and *devatās* (Gods), which again branches off as *daitya, dānava* and *āsūrika* on the one hand and *yakṣa, gandharva, kinnara, kimpūruṣa*, on the other.

Mānuṣa-dharma is mainly of three parts. They are *sārīraka, mānasika* and *ātmika* besides *rājakīya, sāmājīka, ārthika, laukika, daivika, vārṇika* and *āśramika*. This *mānuṣa dharma* covers *varṇa dharma* and *āśrama dharma*.

Table n. 9 - Divisions of *sādhanā*

TYPE OF *SĀDHANĀ*	THE METHOD TO REALISE IT	THE *YOGĀṄGA* CONCERNED
1. *Bahirañga sādhanā*	1. Ethical discipline	1. *Yama* 2. *Niyama*
	2. Physical-mental discipline	3. *Āsana* 4. *Prāṇāyāma*
2. *Bahirañga - Antarañga sādhanā*	3. Pure mental discipline	5. *Pratyāhāra*
3. *Antarañga sādhanā*	4. Intellectual discipline	6. *Dhāraṇā*
	5. Experience of cosmic consciousness	7. *Dhyāna*
4. *Antarātma sādhanā*	6. Experience of the grace of the soul	8. *Samādhi*

Śārīra dharma is of *yogika (yogic)*, *mallika* (athletic exercises, like wrestling, etc.), *dhānuṣya* (archery), *nātya* (dance), *sāngītika* (music) and *vyāvahārika* (concordance of speech and action).

IMPORTANCE OF *ŚĀRĪRA-DHARMA* IN YOGA

The body is the main instrument to follow the *dharma* of man. Kālidāsa says, *"Śarīramādyam khalu dharma sādhanam"* (the health of the body is the root for all *dharma sādhanā*). According to *Muṇḍakopaniṣad*, (III.2.4), *"Nāyamātmā balahīnena labhyaḥ"* (a weakling can not reach the Self). These two quotations amply illustrate the great importance of physical well being not only for enjoyment *(bhoga)* but also to be free from *bhoga*. A weakling cannot realise *ātman*, neither is any *sādhanā* possible without peace in the body and poise in the consciousness. In order to have both poise and peace, the yoga *dharma* has been placed in the first order. Yoga has no nationality, caste, time, age, sex or dogma. It is a universal culture, as it is for all human beings on the earth. *Dharma* is the culture of the self and so is yoga. It makes its *kṣetra* (the field or the body) pure and holy for the *kṣetrajña (puruṣa* or the Self) to dwell in.

Yoga is divided into four types of *sādhanā*, according to the physical and intellectual calibre of the practitioner. They are *bahiraṅga sādhanā*, *bahiraṅga* cum *antaraṅga sādhanā*, *antaraṅga sādhanā* and *antarātma sādhanā*. *Bahiraṅga sādhanā* comprises ethical practices in the form of *yama* and *niyama*, physical and mental practices in the form of *āsana* and *prāṇāyāma*. In *bahiraṅga* cum *antaraṅga sādhanā* the earlier disciplines are brought to maturity by *pratyāhāra*. *Antaraṅga-sādhanā* is the discipline that is cultivated by *dhāraṇā* for intellectual stability while in *dhyāna* the consciousness is purified. In *antarātma sādhanā* the consciousness is sanctified and purified for the grace of the Self to shine in *samādhi* (see Table n. 9).

One who pursues knowledge of the Self should not neglect the body. Is it not the abuse of the Self, if a part of the Self, viz. the body, is neglected? Is it not necessary to be completely aware of the body if one wishes to be totally aware of the Self?

By practising yoga, a *sādhaka* acquires the light of the Self, which leads towards God-realisation.

The observance of *dhārma* also leads one towards the true realisation where life and death are experienced as one. Yoga causes the consciousness to experience a state of stillness and silence without any fluctuations, any divisions or dualities between subjective and objective thinking. Both *dharma* and yoga lift the *sādhaka* from the state of being towards the state of becoming, to experience and live in a pure and unalloyed state of existence.

Yoga is commonly known as *aṣṭāṅga yoga* which consists of *yama, niyama, āsana, prāṇāyāma, pratyāhāra, dhāraṇā, dhyāna* and *samādhi*.

Yama is a collective name comprising non-violence, truthfulness, non-covetousness, continence and freedom from greediness. These constitute social ethics where class, time and place play no part. They are universal principles for all.

Niyama as individual discipline has five aspects: internal and external purity, contentment, burning zeal or passion to pursue the goal of the spiritual life, study which enlightens the intelligence for Self-knowledge and surrender of all our deeds at the feet of the Lord.

The body has been given to us as the abode of Brahman. Through it, the Self expresses itself like a pure crystal. It is *adharma* to treat the body as something untouchable. It is a known fact that the body wears out and is discarded. Nevertheless it is the only instrument for attaining realisation and as such it has to be kept in perfect condition. To keep the abode of the *ātman* pure, *āsana* and *prāṇāyāma* are practised.

The intelligence controls the mind and directs the organs of action and senses of perception to reach its destination: the Self. By yogic practice, the *sādhaka* makes the body strong, healthy and harmonious and move away from desires, leading towards freedom from afflictions and fluctuations.

IMPORTANCE OF *MĀNASIKA DHARMA* IN YOGA

God has form and He is formless also. He is concrete as well as abstract. He is in all and in every form. Realising this, the *sādhaka* performs *āsana*, placing the self in the position of that *āsana* as his chariot, salutes and surrenders himself with humility to God. With this attitude of surrender, the *sādhaka* transports himself from the physical and mental planes towards the spiritual plane. Here, the *bahiraṅga sādhanā* is converted into *antaraṅga sādhanā*. Where he drops the identity of the *ahaṁkāra* and cultivates *vinaya* (humility).

Prāṇāyāma develops the physiological and psychological sheaths by feeding the cells with life force. Its practice gives energy, strengthens will power, makes the brain alert and elates the *puruṣa*.

Prāṇāyāma has four facets. They are *pūraka* (inhalation), *antara kuṁbhaka* (inhalation retention), *recaka* (exhalation) and *bāhya kuṁbhaka* (exhalation retention). In this process worship or *bhakti* is involved.

In *pūraka* it is not the air inhaled, but the very Lord Himself who enters in the form of breath. The Lord is Infinite and as such, He is not too far to be felt. The Infinite Lord is outside our finite body as well as in the depth of the core of the body. The *sādhaka* inhales the infinite and holding it *(antara kuṁbhaka)* becomes completely merged with the *jīvātman* (individual soul). He does not allow any thought to intrude or create disturbance while the Infinite is communing with his individual self. In exhalation *(recaka)* the *sādhaka* adjusts his thoughts by allowing the self to surrender, through his outgoing breath, to the Lord. He places his very essence of life through the conditional process of exhalation as a devotee places the garland of flowers at the feet of his chosen deity *(Iṣṭa Devatā vigraha)*. In the exhalation-retention *(bāhya kuṁbhaka)* he waits for the Lord to accept his deep surrender and remains throughout that retention with humble serenity and oneness with Brahman.

Pratyāhāra is hidden in the very process of *prāṇāyāma*. The mind drawn by senses goes out and hankers for worldly pleasures. By the practice of *prāṇāyāma* the senses are drawn in the reverse gear and their energies are made to flow back towards the inner fullness of the mind so that they are detached from the objects of pleasure. in *pratyāhāra* the senses are trained to be yoked to the inner light that is ever pure, real, and one without a second.

ĀTMIKA DHARMA IN YOGA

Dhāraṇā (concentration), *dhyāna* (meditation) and *samādhi* (a state of existence without the feeling of I) are termed by Patañjali as *saṁyama* or integration. Integration proceeds from *sthūla* (the gross) to *sūkṣma* (the subtle). *Saṁyma* is of various kinds:

Table n. 10 – The stages of subjective integration (The inner world of man)

1. *Śarīra saṁyama*	(integration of body)
2. *Prāṇa saṁyama*	(integration of breath)
3. *Indrīya saṁyama*	(integration of senses)
4. *Manō saṁyama*	(integration of mind)
5. *Jñāna saṁyama*	(integration of objective knowledge)
6. *Buddhi saṁyama*	(integration of subjective knowledge)
7. *Citta saṁyama*	(integration of consciousness)
8. *Ātmā saṁyama*	(integration of the soul)

Bringing together and transforming all the eight petals of yoga, whether in the practice of the *āsana* or *prāṇāyāma* or while studying or during concentration or meditation, is *kaivalya* or *antarātma-sādhanā*.

Through a regular uninterrupted practice of yoga, the impediments, which affect the path of *antarātma sādhanā (Y.S.,* I.30-31), are discarded and a perfect communion between body and consciousness, consciousness and Self, is established. This is the aim of yoga as well as of *dharma*.

The *Yoga Sūtra* proclaims that the eight petals of yoga, when practised uninterruptedly with zeal and devotion, leads to the experience of the seven stages of consciousness or wisdom as explained in *Y.S.* II.27. But in modern language they are equated with the knowledge of the anatomical body, knowledge of the physiological body, knowledge of the mind, including both acquired objective knowledge and subjective experienced knowledge. These take one closer to the Self, to have insight into one's own being.

In *saṁyama*, the cogniser *(grahītṛ)*, the instrument of cognition *(grahaṇa)* and the object to be cognised *(grāhya)* are purified and united. Lord Krishna expresses *saṁyama* as the knower *(jñānaṁ)* knowledge *(jñeyaṁ)* and the object of knowledge *(parijñātā)*, all get united *(B.G.* XVIII.18). In this way diversity disappears and identities are dissolved. *(Y.S.,* I.41). The *sādhaka* then lives in that state of pristine purity, known as the divine state. In that glory of oneness, the body, mind, intelligence and consciousness are all submerged in the sea of the Self. Life and death are at a standstill; there is no movement or even the feeling of individual existence.

The nearest example is that of the ocean. The surface of the ocean is rough, but it is tranquil and quiet at the bottom. Though the yogi lives in the body and realises all his actions of the world, he remains calm and quiet. He discards one layer after another from the *sthūla* (gross), to *sūkṣma* (subtle), from *sūkṣma* to *kāraṇa* (cause) so that he lives in a state of *guṇātita* (free from the qualities of nature), as *jīvanmukta* or *mokṣa*, living and performing deeds as a normal individual. Is it not then the highest state of wisdom? Is it not the aim of *dharma* to live and experience *ātma sākṣātkāra*, as yoga points towards *ātma darśana mārga?*

If you compare the aims and methods of yoga with the aims and methods of *dharma*, you easily understand how both pursue the same goal.

As yoga leads from the cult of the body to the culture of the Self, from the individual to society, from society to the world at large, *dharma* too, like a gigantic tree, shelters the whole of humanity, leading one towards the path of righteousness. He who follows yoga as *dharma* (righteous duty) drinks the nectar of spiritual fragrance as the culmination of *dharma*, and yoga is the same.

Just as the spiritual fragrance of a tree is in the culmination of juicy and tasty fruits, so too the termination of yoga *sādhanā* and *dharma sādhanā* is *ātmānanda jīvana*.*

---

* Nevertheless, according to the *Yoga Sūtra* (*Y.S.,* IV.7), an accomplished yogi not only avoids *adharma* or black actions but even goes above the *dharma* or right actions. It is told in *Mahābhārata* that: "Abandon *dharma* and *adharma*, abandon truth and untruth and abandon (the mind) by which you abandon all."

"Leaving all duties of *dharma*, surrender and take shelter in ME. I will liberate you from all sins", says Lord Krishna in the Path of Self-Surrender (*B.G.,* XVIII.66).

YOGA DEMANDS EFFICIENCY IN *SĀDHANĀ* *

Today is *Patañjali Jayantī.* Many of you have asked me to talk on the *Sādhanā Pāda* of Patañjali from my own experience. You know, I am not a man of words but a man of action. My aim is to practise and to be in yoga. Talking is neither my aim, nor my habit, nor profession. It is very difficult for me to put experiences into words. In fact, the moment experiences are verbalised, they lose their potency. Words are loose, whereas experience is firm and solid. Experience makes one take a further dip in practice whereas words separate one from experiencing. Experiences are ocean-deep and sky-high. Words have limitations. Experiences take one towards the inner journey while words take one towards the outer world. *Sādhanā* must be done; it cannot be verbalised, as it is modest and silent. *Sādhanā* cannot make one talkative.

Talks are filled with *rajō dharma (rājasic* nature). Without *rajō guṇa,* it is not easy to talk. Experience is illuminative, *sattva dharma.* Therefore, I am forced to express the *sāttvic* experience through *rajō guṇa. Rajō guṇa* is expressive. It expresses thoughts, whereas *sattva guṇa* just illumines. Therefore, I have to depend upon *rajō-sattva,* so that I can express whatever I have experienced. While giving a discourse, I have to build up *rajō-sāttvic guṇa,* whereas at the time of practice I am *sattva-rajō dharmi.* To keep this balance is very hard.

Normally, those who give lectures find their voice very sweet. As a singer cultures, tones and tunes his voice, a lecturer with the practice of talking, makes his voice sweet and smooth. I have never cultured my voice, because I never thought that I would have to give lectures in my life. So I request you to forgive me for my harsh voice. But know that though my voice is harsh, my practices and experiences are sweet. I request you to accept, on this *Diwali* day, the sweet-dish of experienced knowledge acquired through my *sādhanā.*

Often, it is believed that *sādhanā* has to be attempted with closed eyes and it has nothing to do with action. First of all get rid of this misunderstood notion. Lord Patañjali's yoga is full of dynamic action *(sādhanā kriyā).*

---

* A talk given by *Gurujī,* on *Patañjali Jayantī* on 16th October 1990.

Patañjali's *Yoga Sūtra* is in four chapters: 1. *Samādhi Pāda*, 2. *Sādhanā Pāda*, 3. *Vibhūti Pāda* and 4. *Kaivalya Pāda*. People think that Patañjali has explained *sādhanā* only in *Sādhanā Pāda* and the rest of the *pādas* are mere philosophy. This is not true, as all four chapters are filled with *sādhanā*, from the grossest level to the most subtle. Hence all four are *sādhanā pādas* given according to the development and culture of the intelligence and consciousness of the *sādhaka*.

Indian philosophy is not just theoretical. It contains both theory and practice and these two go together, hand in hand. Even in the *Yoga Sūtra*, the *sādhanā kriyā* is present in all the four chapters. The *sādhanā* explained in these *pādas* are of different levels depending upon the intellectual and spiritual levels of the aspirants. The *sādhanā* is upgraded as the aspirant's intelligence gets upgraded. Besides these, there is an interrelationship and interdependency of *sādhanā* at different levels. One has to interlink the *sādhanā* explained in different chapters. According to the growth of each individual's intelligence, *sādhanā* differs in quality to enable everyone to recognise the level of the cultured nature of his consciousness.

As theory and practice go together, science, art and philosophy also go together. The science of yoga is adopted in an artistic way resulting in spiritual experience. Hence, yoga is *jñāna*, *vijñāna* and *prajñāna śāstra*. *Jñāna* is an acquired knowledge or cognisance. *Vijñāna* is the investigation through experiment to distinguish through judgement, the right from the wrong. *Prajñāna* is a distinctive intelligence, which comes with prudence and wisdom. *Prajñāna* is based on experiences, which are filtered and refiltered repeatedly.

In short, *jñāna* is just a collection of knowledge. *Vijñāna* is specialised knowledge attained by investigation and discrimination. When acquired knowledge and investigating knowledge are tested by *sādhanā*, it becomes *prajñāna*. Then, it is no more knowledge but wisdom.

Samādhi Pāda explains *jñāna* and *vijñāna śāstra*. *Sādhanā Pāda* connects through experience *jñāna* and *vijñāna*. *Vibhūti Pāda* covers the theory and practice of *vijñāna* and *prajñāna*. The fourth chapter guides on how to live continuously in that *prajñāna* state.

Let me put it in another way. *Samādhi Pāda* makes of the aspirant a *jñānī*. *Sādhanā Pāda* transforms an *ajñānī* (ignorant) into a *sujñānī* (a well informed person). *Sujñāna* is matured knowledge. *Vibhūti Pāda* makes one a *vijñānī* and prepares one to become the *prajñāni* as dealt with in *Kaivalya Pāda*.

When *jñāna-vijñāna-prajñāna* are linked and realised through a practical approach, it is called *sādhanā kriyā*.

Yogic method is full of *sādhanā* and Patañjali nowhere indicates the end of *sādhanā* except in the last *sūtra* of the text, where he uses the term *puruṣārtha śūnya* (devoid of fourfold aims of life). (*Y.S.*, IV.34). This indicates that the *sādhanā* ends when the *sādhaka* is devoid of all aims. This happens when he has achieved all that has to be achieved and nothing remains for him to realise. Therefore, I say that the *sādhanā* commences, according to Patañjali, from the very first *sūtra* and ends with the last *sūtra*.

To indicate *sādhanā*, Patañjali uses different terminology at different places:

In *Samādhi Pāda*, he uses the word *anuśāsanam* (discipline). The word 'discipline' indicates the practical approach. So *anuśāsanam* signifies application and administration and not pondering.

Another word used in *Yoga Sūtra* is *abhyāsa*. *Abhyāsa* is an effortful practice. It means repeating the practice again and again effortfully, skilfully and intelligently.

In *Samādhi Pāda*, Patañjali asks us to do *sādhanā* to reach *nirbīja samādhi*. He asks the practitioner to analyse and examine his consciousness *(citta)* with its fluctuations, modifications, afflictions and potentials. He asks the disciple to survey the quality of *citta* and its movement. He asks the disciple to gear up practice with faith, reverence, energy, vigour and valour. Patañjali asks the doer to develop memory and to purify it so that his awareness helps him to acquire real knowledge through intense contemplation. He even asks the disciple to develop devotion *(bhakti)*, towards the Supreme so that the Lord within *(Antaryāmin)* guides him. He explains *citta prasādanam* and gives several methods to diffuse the consciousness gracefully. He asks aspirants to purify their intelligence through *samāpatti* so that consciousness is made crystal clear, made favourable and conducive to contemplate on God.

The whole foundation for yogic practice is laid in the second chapter. That is why it is called *Sādhanā Pāda*. This chapter is considered as the commencement of yoga. A beginner or a neophyte is always caught in the web of doubt and laziness because of his ignorance. Doubt is in the head and laziness is in the body. He needs to be uplifted. The practice of yoga will uplift him from ignorance to the level of understanding, and from immaturity to maturity. It is like the guardians looking after a minor child, guiding him in a right direction, until he becomes mature.

In *Sādhanā Pāda*, Patañjali uses the word *kriyā*. This word indicates action. He knows human psychology. He knows that intellectuals are strong-headed and they are likely to convert the knowledge into logical structure without experiencing it for themselves. Often logic and practice seem to be drifting away from each other. One finds that whatever is logical most of the time appears impractical and whatever is practical seems to be illogical. It seems as though logical and practical knowledge are going parallel to each other never to meet again. *Kriyā yoga* is the blending of practice and logic, reasoning and feeling with the intelligence of the heart and intelligence of the head. Then this reveals to the *sādhaka* the facts as truth through experience.

Kriyā yoga is three-tiered yoga, which includes *tapas, svādhyāya* and *Īśvara praṇidhāna*. *Tapas* is self-discipline. The aspirant burns away his impurities with ambition to reach perfection by adopting certain disciplines. Here, he exerts discipline by his own will. *Svādhyāya* is Self-study. Here, he reflects on himself as well as on his behaviour. He watches the afflictions of *citta* and how he is caught in them. He realises that the afflictions of his consciousness keep him away from the Self. To discard these afflictions he is advised to correct his actions. All these procedures come under *svādhyāya*. Then comes *Īśvara praṇidhāna*. *Īśvara praṇidhāna* is love towards the Supreme Lord and to cling on to Him. As the *sādhaka* advances in the path of yoga, he finds impediments bedevil him. Therefore, Patañjali asks the *sādhaka* to have the foundation of *sādhanā* in *karma, jñāna* and *bhakti*, in order that these three pillars support him till the end. Thus, Patañjali expresses *karma, jñāna* and *bhakti* as *tapas, svādhyāya* and *Īśvara praṇidhāna*. This *kriyā yoga* or yoga of action is the key-point of *sādhanā* (practice). It is a master key, which is applied in every step of practice from the base to the zenith as the aspirant climbs up on the path of yoga.

Then comes the word *anuṣṭhāna*. *Anuṣṭhāna* is a word which indicates devotional practice with spiritual involvement. Patañjali is not asking the yoga of action to be followed merely as work for work's sake. The *kriyā yoga* has to be well established in the practice as *anuṣṭhāna*. *Aṣṭāṅga yoga* or eight-petalled yoga has to be practised devotionally on these three tiers.

Vibhūti Pāda (the chapter on accomplishments) is like higher education based on *dhāraṇā*, *dhyāna* and *samādhi*. The *siddhis*, which have been explained in the third chapter, are the result of *saṁyama* (integration). When the concentration, meditation and absorption are woven together into a single thread, it is integration. This leads towards supernatural powers. This process of integration comes under the category of *sādhanā*. There is *sādhanā kriyā*, but it is innermost. You cannot see it, show it, or express it.

The body of muscles and bones, the organs of action, the senses of perception, the five gross elements, the five subtle elements, and consciousness *(citta)*, mind *(manas)*, intelligence *(buddhi)* and ego *(ahaṁkāra)* are transformed to reach the state of refinement and purity. Patañjali explains this as *pariṇāma* meaning transformation. At this stage, the *sādhaka* totally changes in his behaviour both externally and internally.

Table n. 11 - The presence of *sādhanā* in four chapters of *Yoga Sūtra*

Chapter	The path	The layer penetrated	The restraint of	The fruit
I. *Samādhi Pāda* (chapter on absorption)	*Bhakti mārga* (the path of devotion)	*Vijñānamaya kośa** (intellectual body) (common to chapters I and III)	– All the vehicles of nature – from *karmendriya, jñānedriya,* mind, intelligence, consciousness, and "I" ness directly.	<u>*Vicāra śuddhi*</u> The purification of thought (through different *samāpatti*)
II. *Sādhanā Pāda* (chapter on *sādhanā*)	*Karma mārga* (the path of action)	*Annamaya kośa* (physical body) *Prāṇamaya kośa* (physiological body) *Manomaya kośa* (psychological body)	– Step by step, the *karmendriya* (the organs of action) – *Jñānendriya* (the senses of perception) – *Manas* (mind) are brought under control and stabilised	<u>*Ācāra śuddhi*</u> The purification of behaviour and character leading to purification of action
III. *Vibhūti Pāda* (chapter on accomplishment)	*Jñāna mārga* (the path of knowledge)	*Vijñānamaya kośa** (intellectual body) *Buddhimaya kośa** (the body of direct perception) *Ānañdamaya kośa* (the body of joy) *Cittamaya kośa* (the body of consciousness)	– *Antareñdriya* (subtle organs): • *buddhi* (intelligence) • *ahaṁkāra* (ego) • *citta* (consciousness) – *Dharmendriya* (conscience)	Transient state towards *Ātma darśana* (reflection of the soul)
IV. *Kaivalya Pāda* (chapter on emancipation)	*Vairāgya mārga* (the path of renunciation)	*Ātmamaya kośa* (the body of the Self)	Blended, integrated and culminated	*Vīrāṭa puruṣa darśana* (the reflection of shining splendid Self) (*citiśakti* or power of the Self)

* For convenience sake, *vijñānamaya kośa* and *buddhimaya kośa* are separated, though they are all encased in *cittamaya kośa* or the sheath of *citta*.

The fourth chapter is considered theoretical. Naturally, one feels as though there is no *sādhanā* in it. It is not true. Patañjali does not explain any *sādhanā kriyā* but guides one how to maintain purity in *sādhanā* without allowing it to become stale or polluted. He says that though the consciousness is drawn towards the seer, on account of carelessness and negligence and the past hidden impressions arising, fissures are created, separating the consciousness from the seer (*Y.S.,* IV.27). These fissures are removed only by *sādhanā* and an understanding of *dharmamegha samādhi* (*Y.S.,* IV.29).

I hope that it is clear now that *sādhanā* is not limited to *Sādhanā Pāda* alone. *Sādhanā* is stressed in all the four chapters. Only it becomes subtler, finer and deeper in the fourth chapter. The *ātma sādhanā* is the ultra-subtle form of all *sādhanā*.

To conclude, one may compare *Samādhi Pāda* to *bhakti mārga*, *Sādhanā Pāda* to *karma mārga*, *Vibhūti Pāda* to *jñāna mārga* and *Kaivalya Pāda* to *vairāgya mārga*. The first chapter is the path of devotion, the second is the path of action, the third is the path of knowledge and the fourth, the path of renunciation. But this categorisation is also at a gross level. At the subtle stage, they cannot be differentiated.

The *Samādhi Pāda* is the sublimation of all the vehicles of nature, the organs of action, senses of perception, mind, intelligence, consciousness and 'I' ness. Hence, the science of yoga begins from the periphery with the *Sādhanā Pāda*, for the conquest of organs of actions, senses of perception and mind. The explanation in *Vibhūti Pāda* is meant to conquer the *buddhi* or intelligence, *ahaṁkāra* or ego, *citta* or consciousness and lastly the conscience or *dharmendriya*. *Samādhi* is the highest state of yoga, which can be reached either directly through the pure consciousness or by following, step by step, from the periphery of the body. Therefore, the *Sādhanā Pāda* begins from *annamaya*, *prāṇamaya* and *manōmaya kośa* to penetrate *vijñānamaya kośa* as explained in *Samādhi Pāda* and connects both *pāda* to the *Vibhūti Pāda*, to penetrate from *vijñānamaya kośa* further towards *buddhimaya kośa*, *ānandamaya kośa* and *cittamaya kośa*, while *Kaivalya Pāda* leads us to penetrate *ātmamaya kośa* (see Table n. 11).

Samādhi Pāda invites the attention to be focused on thoughts so that they are cleansed and filtered. This purification of thought is called *vicāra śuddhi*. The different types of *samāpatti* are meant for this purpose.

Sādhanā Pāda draws the attention to purify the behaviour and character so that the action is purified. This is called *āchāra śuddhi*. The *Vibhūti Pāda* draws the attention to experience the divine glories of *jīvātman*. The *siddhi* (accomplishment or achievement) are proofs of divinity within us. That is why the chapter is named *Vibhūti Pāda*. As Lord Krishna in the tenth chapter of

Bhagavad Gītā profiles His own glory, so too Patañjali emphasises in this chapter that the divinity lies within us. But he does not forget to remind us that glories of *jivātman* are not as expansive as the glories of *paramātman*. So comes the fourth chapter.

This chapter ponders over *kṣetra* and *kṣetrajña*, the field and the knower of the field. Patañjali makes us realise the difference between *puruṣa* (seer), *prakṛti* (nature) and the Lord who is above all. In this sense, *Kaivalya Pāda* corresponds to *viśvarūpa darśana* (the vision of the Cosmic Form) of the Lord or the cosmic form of the Lord. Patañjali expresses *citiśakti* (the power of the Self). *Citiśakti* is the light, which guides us. *Paramātman* is *citiśakti*. He is omniscient, omnipotent and omnipresent. This is *virāṭa puruṣa darśana* (the reflection of shining splendid Self).

Diwali is the festival of lights. Let the light of the Lord lead you to reach Him.

SECTION III

PATAÑJALI AND HIS YOGA SYSTEM

THE *YOGA SŪTRA* OF PATAÑJALI – GEMS OF WISDOM*

Patañjali's gems of wisdom are a treatise on man's quest for the sight of the Self. It is divided into four chapters: *Samādhi Pāda, Sādhanā Pāda, Vibhūti Pāda* and *Kaivalya Pāda.*

In the first chapter, the purpose of life is explained. The second deals with essential and methodical discipline for evolution in oneself. The third takes us further towards an intricate and intensive *sādhanā* for sighting the Self, whereas the fourth sings the song of the Self, to savour its nectar.

SAMĀDHI PĀDA

(Chapter on Total Absorption)

I.1 The treatise on the discipline of yoga for enlightenment begins now, with auspiciousness.

I.2 Yoga is the cessation of movements in the consciousness.

I.3 When consciousness is silent, the seer *(ātmā)* radiates in his own grandeur.

I.4 At other times, the seer becomes entangled with the objects seen by the consciousness.

I.5 Consciousness has fivefold waves, painful or non-painful, cognisable or uncognisable.

I.6 The fivefold waves of consciousness are caused by correct knowledge, incorrect knowledge, imaginative knowledge, sleep and memory.

I.7 Correct knowledge is dependent upon direct perception, inference and authoritative scriptural testimony.

I.8 Incorrect knowledge is mistaking the identity of one thing for the other or one object for another.

I.9 Fanciful or imaginative knowledge is that which is devoid of substance.

I.10 Sleep is the non-feeling of mutations in the mind.

I.11 Memory is the recollection of expressions and experiences without colouration.

I.12 Practice *(abhyāsa)* and detachment *(vairāgya)* are the means to still the consciousness.

* The readers are requested to go through this translation or parts of it in one stretch. This will offer them a clear insight on the author's exposition of *Yoga Sūtra.*

I.13 Practice is an effort to still the mind's fluctuations in order to silence the consciousness.

I.14 Long, uninterrupted, alert practice is the firm foundation for stabilising the consciousness.

I.15 Keeping the consciousness detached from desires helps one to practise with perseverance.

I.16 When the intelligence of the head and the intelligence of the heart are clean and clear, one develops to reach true renunciation.

I.17 Practice and renunciation develops four types of awareness in the consciousness. These are *vitarkā, vicāra, ānanda and asmitā.* I have prefixed *sa* (auspiciousness) for the *sādhaka* to use the facets of intelligence auspiciously: *savitarkā* (self-analysis), *savicāra* (reasoning and reflection), *sānanda* (the feeling of delight) which is not just pleasurable *(preya)* but spiritual *(śreya)* and *sāsmitā* (the pure and divine state of being).

I.18 When pure consciousness is developed by practice, hidden impressions may shoot up and disturb the purity of the consciousness.

I.19 Pure consciousness brings a bodiless state or a merging into nature, leading towards stagnation in practice and/or isolation.

I.20 Pursue yogic discipline with faith, vigour, memory, keen intellect and power of absorption to experience the absolute consciousness.

I.21 For one who is sharp and extremely vehement in practice, the goal is instant.

I.22 For those whose practices are mild, average or intense, it becomes time-bound.

I.23 Several ways are offered to restrain the consciousness. One is total surrender of oneself to God.

I.24 God is defined as ONE who is untouched by reactions of actions or by cause and effect.

I.25 God is the seed of all knowledge.

I.26 He is the first and foremost preceptor of all preceptors, unconditioned by time.

I.27 He is represented in *āuṁ,* which is termed as *praṇava.*

I.28 This *āuṁ* must be constantly uttered while feeling its full significance.

I.29 This develops pure consciousness and minimises or eradicates obstacles.

I.30 The causes which obstruct serenity and purity of the consciousness are: disease, doubt, carelessness, laziness, sense gratification, living in the world of illusion, inability to persist in what is undertaken and being unable to maintain the achieved progress.

I.31 Besides these nine obstructions, sorrow, despair, depression, tremor of body, nervousness and laboured breathing run concurrently, distracting the consciousness further.

I.32 Single-minded effort is the only way to overcome these obstacles.

I.33 The effort begins in cultivating consciousness so as to become favourably disposed, serene and benevolent through cultivation of friendliness, compassion, gladness and indifference respectively, towards joy and sorrow, as well as virtue and vice.

I.34 Or/and by maintaining the quiet psychological state of consciousness that is felt after exhalation;

I.35 Or/and by concentrating on an object that helps to maintain steadiness;

I.36 Or/and by meditating on a sorrowless, luminous, effulgent light;

I.37 Or/and by contemplating on enlightened beings who were and are free from attachment;

I.38 Or/and by reflecting on the knowledge obtained while one is in a sleepy, dreamy or wakeful state.

I.39 Or/and by contemplating on an object or on an idea that is conducive to yogic practice.

I.40 By following the preceding various alternative methods of practice, according to one's physical, mental and intellectual capacity, one develops the power to penetrate from infinitesimal particles to infinitely great objects.

I.41 The practitioner experiences that the knower, the known and the instrument used to recognise the knower is himself – the seer. He develops sensitivity, stability, choicelessness, stainlessness and purity like a pure transparent jewel.

I.42 For him the word, with its meaning and with its knowledge, is moulded to shine forth as new knowledge *(savitarkā samādhi).*

I.43 Consciousness loses its identity when memory is cleansed and purified. It becomes non-analytical *(nirvitarkā samādhi).*

I.44 Contemplation on subtle aspects of the elements of nature *(tanmātras),* whether deliberate or non-deliberate, becomes *savicārā* and *nirvicārā samādhi.*

I.45 The subtlest component of nature is consciousness. When it dissolves on its own in the seat of the Self, it is free from stain.

I.46 All these above mentioned methods of concentration and contemplation are with a seed or support. They are known as *sabīja samādhi.*

I.47 Proficiency in non-deliberate contemplation leads towards the knowledge of the seer.

I.48 When consciousness dwells in wisdom, there dawns direct spiritual perception.

I.49 This matured, truth-bearing wisdom is first-hand knowledge, or intuitive knowledge. (It does not depend upon *sūtra* I.7 from now on.)

I.50 With this new truth-bearing wisdom, a new life begins.

I.51 This has also to be relinquished to experience the seedless state of *samādhi (nirbīja samādhi).*

SĀDHANĀ PĀDA

(Chapter on Practice)

II.1 Discipline, study of the spiritual scriptures and surrender to God are the fountain for yogic *sādhanā*, termed as *kriyā yoga*.

II.2 Through *kriyā yoga*, afflictions get reduced and it helps as a precursor to *samādhi*.

II.3 Lack of understanding, pride, attachment to attractions, aversion to pains and fear of death are the five afflictions.

II.4 The mother of all afflictions is want of understanding. It may remain dormant or attenuated, interrupted or fully active.

II.5 Accepting mundane things as permanent, impure things as pure and sensual pleasures as spiritual, is lack of knowledge.

II.6 Assuming that the ego is the seer, is pride.

II.7 Pleasure breeds desire.

II.8 Distress breeds hatred.

II.9 The urge for self-perpetuation and fear of death are the subtlest of all afflictions.

II.10 These afflictions have to be minimised and eradicated.

II.11 Brooding on afflictions leads to psychosomatic diseases. These thoughts get washed out by meditation.

II.12 The latent imprints of accumulated actions form the 'cause and effect' in life.

II.13 The fruits of actions of previous lives shape the present birth, the span of life and the things to be experienced.

II.14 Good or evil actions in the past qualify one for pleasant or non-pleasant experiences in the present life.

II.15 The wise man knows that pleasant experiences have tinges of sorrow and keeps aloof from them.

II.16 The pains that are yet to come can be prevented.

II.17 Association of the seer with the seen is the cause of distress. Avoidance of union between them is the remedy for distress.

II.18 Nature, with its three *guṇa (sattva, rajas* and *tamas)*, exists for the enjoyment of pleasures, or for the emancipation of man.

II.19 Nature has four divisions. They are differentiable and undifferentiable, phenomenal and noumenal.

II.20 Though the seer is pure, he witnesses nature without being reliant on it.

II.21 Yet nature exists only to serve the seer so that he abides in his own pure state.

II.22 Nature is meant for the emancipation of the seer. The relationship ends when nature's job is fulfilled, whereas it continues to affect ordinary souls.

II.23 Nature reminds the seer to discover his true Self.

II.24 Lack of spiritual understanding is the cause of the false identification of the seer with the seen.

II.25 When the seer is separated from the seen, want of knowledge is vanquished. Emancipation or *kaivalya* is explained.

II.26 All pains are avoided through uninterrupted awareness of discriminative knowledge.

II.27 This discriminative knowledge develops seven states of awareness: conquest of body, senses, energy, mind, intelligence, consciousness and self.

II.28 Practice of yoga removes the cause of afflictions so that the crown of wisdom radiates in its own glory.

II.29 Yoga is an eight-petalled discipline. These are *yama, niyama, āsana, prāṇāyāma, pratyāhāra, dhāraṇā, dhyāna* and *samādhi.*

II.30 Moral injunctions *(yama)* are non-violence, truthfulness, non-stealing, continence and freedom from greed.

II.31 The above five components of *yama* are universal vows unconditioned by place, time, class or concept of duty.

II.32 Observance of cleanliness, contentment, discipline, spiritual study and devotion to God are *niyama.*

II.33 Principles that run contrary to *yama* and *niyama* are to be encountered with knowledge and awareness.

II.34 Pain are of three degrees – mild, medium and intense, caused by three types of behaviour – direct indulgence, provoked and abetted. They are motivated by greed, anger and delusion and they have to be countered and corrected with right knowledge and behaviour.

II.35 Non-violence in word, thought and action causes one to abandon one's hostile nature.

II.36 When one is established in truth, whatever one says happens.

II.37 Precious jewels come to one who is free from covetousness.

II.38 Spiritual knowledge flows through the observance of continence.

II.39 Knowledge of past and future lives shines like a mirror when one is free from greed.

II.40 Cleanliness develops disinterest in the pleasures of the world.

II.41 A cleansed body with a purified mind becomes a fit instrument for self-awareness.

II.42 Contentment brings an unmeasurable delight.

II.43 Self-discipline *(tapas)* eradicates the impurities of body and mind and kindles the sparks of divinity.

II.44 Self-knowledge *(svādhyāya),* Understanding of oneself, leads towards God-realisation.

II.45 Surrender to God induces *samādhi.* Or: *Samādhi* leads one towards God *(Īśvara praṇidhāna).*

II.46 Perfection in *āsana* brings firmness in body and benevolence in mind.

II.47 When the effort to perform becomes effortless, perfection in an *āsana* is achieved.

II.48 From then on, the practitioner is undisturbed by dualities and is fit to begin *prāṇāyāma.*

II.49 *Prāṇāyāma* is the regulation of the inbreath and the outbreath.

II.50 *Prāṇāyāma* has three movements – deep and fine inhalation, retention and exhalation. They are measured according to the space in the trunk, time and precision.

II.51 The fourth type of *prāṇāyāma* is a non-deliberate and an effortless one. It transcends the previous three types and restrains (all external and internal) thought movements.

II.52 *Prāṇāyāma* removes the veil covering the light of knowledge and heralds the dawn of wisdom.

II.53 Then, the mind becomes fit for concentration.

II.54 By this dawn of wisdom, the mind controls the organs of action and the senses of perception, and takes an inward journey towards the seer. This is *pratyāhāra.*

II.55 With this control, the mind turns ripe and avid to reach its maker – the seer.

VIBHŪTI PĀDA

(Chapter on Attainment)

III.1 Concentration *(dhāraṇā)* means focus of attention.

III.2 An uninterrupted flow of attention with awareness is meditation.

III.3 The merging of the meditator and the object of meditation is absorption *(samādhi).*

III.4 When concentration, meditation and absorption become one it is integration.

III.5 Lustre of wisdom and insight comes through integration of subtle senses: intelligence, 'I' and consciousness.

III.6 This wisdom can be used compartmentally or totally as needed.

III.7 Concentration, meditation and absorption of the later three subtle practices of yoga are internal, compared to the first five components of yoga.

III.8 Similarly, concentration, meditation and absorption are external compared to seedless *(nirbīja) samādhi.*

III.9 When he loses attention, the *sādhaka* has to return towards the restraint of consciousness. This is *nirodha pariṇāma.*

III.10 In between rising thoughts and restraints, the stream of tranquillity flows.

III.11 Alternation of attention takes place between one point and many points or vice-versa. Controlling this oscillation leads towards absorption. This is *samādhi pariṇāma.*

III.12 Maintenance of total attention without interruption is *ekāgratā pariṇāma.*

III.13 The transformations accrue on account of the culture of consciousness from the present potential state *(dharma)* towards a special significant development *(lakṣaṇa),* and then to reach its essence, the real state *(avasthā)* of the Self.

III.14 The changing quality of the consciousness derives from the characteristic properties of nature, namely, *sattva* (purity), *rajas* (energy) and *tamas* (dormancy).

III.15 Successive sequential changes cause the distinctive transformation in the consciousness.

III.16 By this distinctive transformation, the yogi integrates with himself and reads the past and future.

III.17 He will have the mastery of language by listening to sounds.

III.18 He knows all about his past and future lives.

III.19 He becomes a clairvoyant.

III.20 He develops the faculty of studying precisely the minds of others.

III.21 He acquires the ability to be invisible at will.

III.22 He will have the ability to stop the infrastructure of the elements without others knowing it.

III.23 He has the foreknowledge of his exact time of death.

III.24 He gains physical, mental and spiritual strength through friendliness to all.

III.25 He can be at will as strong as an elephant.

III.26 Concealed things that are near or far appear to him on their own.

III.27 He has the knowledge of the solar system.

III.28 He has the knowledge of the changing position of the stars.

III.29 He knows beforehand the cause and course of events.

III.30 He has perfect knowledge of the human system.

III.31 He acquires the power to overcome hunger and thirst.

III.32 He can remain immobile like a tortoise at will.

III.33 He gets visions of perfect beings.

III.34 He becomes the knower of all knowledge.

III.35 He has thorough knowledge of the functions of the consciousness.

III.36 He differentiates consciousness from the seer with ease.

III.37 He feels, sees, tastes, hears and smells without the help of the senses of perception.

III.38 These powers which appear natural to a yogi and super-natural to others, are hindrances to *samādhi.*

III.39 He can enter another's body at will.

III.40 He can walk on water, swamps and thorns.

III.41 He can blaze like fire.

III.42 He can hear divine sounds irrespective of distance or place.

III.43 He can levitate.

III.44 He can move outside his body.

III.45 He knows in full the gross and subtle mutation of nature.

III.46 He can reduce himself to the size of an atom or expand. He can become light or heavy. He has access to everything. He can pierce rocks and control anything and be a Lord of everything.

III.47 He acquires unsurpassed beauty, grace, strength and lustre.

III.48 He has mastery over nature and recognises the purpose of the conjunction without involving himself.

III.49 He subdues nature and moves faster than light and sound.

III.50 He gains lordship over all things; he becomes omnipresent, omnipotent and omniscient.

III.51 With all these successes, he should cultivate non-attachment, so that he may live in the abode of the Self.

III.52 Celestial beings try to seduce him and pull him down from this grace of yoga.

III.53 He must detach himself from these powers and concentrate his attention on the moment as well as the movement of moments (time) to gain an exalted knowledge without the feeling of time and place.

III.54 By this, he distinguishes faultlessly the differences in similar objects.

III.55 Such a yogi grasps anything and everything in an instant.

III.56 This exalted intelligence being equal to the purity of the seer, he has reached perfection in yoga.

KAIVALYA PĀDA

(Chapter on Absolute Liberation)

IV.1 Divine powers are the results of birth, herbs, incantations, self-discipline and meditation.

IV.2 Transformation takes place in these four types of souls due to the abundant flow of the potentialities of nature.

IV.3 As a farmer builds embankments to regulate the flow of water to his fields, the prudent yogi channels the potentialities of nature for spiritual development.

IV.4 Created intelligence of the head is *asmitā*, which forms bias and prejudice. It is the cause of pain and distress. When it is nurtured, it becomes ripe and leads the *sādhaka* to know the seer.

IV.5 The root mind is one, but it branches into numerous activities creating fluctuations, modifications and modulations.

IV.6 The restraining of these various activities brings the root mind to the surface.

IV.7 Actions are of four types: white, grey, black and that which is beyond these three. The yogi's actions are neither white nor black nor mixed. But for others, actions are either white, black or mixed.

IV.8 Performance of these types of actions leaves impressions, which manifest when conditions are favourable and ripe to reach the goal of Self-realisation.

IV.9 Though life is interrupted by species and lineage, place and time, memory and impressions exist uninterruptedly to connect them to the present life.

IV.10 Impressions and desires are beginningless and endless for an average person.

IV.11 Though life is bound by desires and subliminal impressions *(saṁskāras)*, culturing of intelligence and consciousness puts an end to desires and fades out the subliminal impressions in a gradual process.

IV.12 Existence of past and future is as real as the present. The past has been experienced, it has lost its flavour. The future is yet to manifest, while the present is a moment. The movement of moments creates past and future and affects the consciousness.

IV.13 The qualities of nature and time interweave with consciousness in both gross and subtle forms.

IV.14 The rhythmic mutation of *sattva, rajas* and *tamas* is the cause for action, reaction and effects.

IV.15 The essence of objects remains the same but appears different according to the movements of qualities of nature in the consciousness.

IV.16 The essence of an object is not dependent upon one's consciousness. If the consciousness fails to recognise an object, the object has not stimulated the consciousness. It does not mean that the object does not exist.

IV.17 The essence of objects reflects according to the state of the consciousness whether it is tainted or pure. They remain unknown if the consciousness does not ponder on them.

IV.18 As the seer is changeless, he is aware of the mutation of the consciousness.

IV.19 Consciousness cannot perceive its own nature, as it is not self-luminous.

IV.20 Consciousness cannot comprehend both the seer and the seen at the same time.

IV.21 If the consciousness were both perceiver and perceived, things would end in confusion because of its multiple state.

IV.22 Consciousness distinguishes between its own light and that of the seer. It develops purity and leans towards the changeless seer.

IV.23 Consciousness realises that it has no light of its own but it borrows the light from its source, the seer. Hence, its sense of comprehending all comes to an end.

IV.24 Consciousness is equipped to act equally in conjunction with the seer or the seen on account of its proximity to both of them.

IV.25 But the intelligence cultures the consciousness to develop purity to dwell closer to the seer.

IV.26 On account of this purity, consciousness inclines towards the seer to experience the state of indivisible existence.

IV.27 With this progress, the force of past impressions may disturb its path towards emancipation.

IV.28 The yogi has to relinquish all powers. Otherwise, he will be caught in the web of afflictions at once.

IV.29 By this relinquishment, virtue pours forth, washing away all subliminal impressions and afflictions in the consciousness. From then on, a seedless state of cleanliness and clarity are experienced.

IV.30 In this state, the cycles of reactions of afflicted actions come to an end. Freedom flows like an unruffled river.

IV.31 Henceforth, all other kinds of knowledge appear insignificant compared to this virtuous knowledge which is free from all impurities.

IV.32 By this the *guṇa* retire in nature, having fulfilled their duties.

IV.33 On account of this, the uninterrupted cycle of moments is comprehended.

IV.34 From now on, the yogi is devoid of all aims of life. He is free from the qualities of nature and lives in the state of *kaivalya* (emancipation).

Here ends the spiritual journey of yoga after this teaching.

Here end the Gems of Wisdom of Sage Patañjali.

YOGA OF PATAÑJALI

Patañjali's *Yoga Sūtra* are in four chapters. The first deals with the science of duty *(dharma)*, guiding one to learn spiritual knowledge. It teaches the *sādhaka* how to use his life after acquiring knowledge. This chapter is called *Samādhi Pāda*. The second deals with the way of life *(artha)*. This is to put in practice what has been learnt *(Sādhanā Pāda)*. In the third chapter *(Vibhūti Pāda)*, he explains how the views and ways of life bring a wealth of knowledge, which blossoms and showers achievements on the practitioner. In the fourth chapter *(Kaivalya Pāda)*, Patañjali explains that the spiritual realisation is superior to all the above mentioned attainments and advises the *sādhaka* to renounce them and continue practice, aiming at the final goal, emancipation.

The first chapter speaks on ethics and morality, right action and the ways of cultivating virtue *(śīlatā)*. It shows ways of transforming the uncultured consciousness into a cultured consciousness.

The first chapter explains yoga as a universal religion and guides one to become a religious person in that sense. It shows how the principles of yoga guide one to move from the pleasures of the world towards the eternal auspicious state of being.

'Self' is a pure cultured entity. Yoga is the root subject, which on its own teaches one to reach the Self.

Yoga shows the ways to cultivate, within the practitioner, the art of diffusing the root mind, known as seer *(draṣṭā)*, in the field of his body, to feel the divinity from inside out and outside in.

It not only covers the four classes *(varṇa)*,* four stages of life *(āśrama)*,* four qualities *(guṇa)*, four aims of life *(puruṣartha)* but also four types of *sādhanā*, viz. *bahiraṅga* (external), *bahiraṅga-antaraṅga* (the transient state between external and internal), *antaraṅga* (internal) and *antarātma* (innermost) to feel the core or the Self *(ātmānubhava)*.

---

* cf. Yoga and *Dharma*, p. 159.

Yoga first works on body, senses and energy, then on the mind, bringing stability in intelligence *(buddhi)* and consciousness *(citta)*. Afterwards it takes one to commune with the Self *(ātmanivedana)*.*

The first *pāda* speaks of cultivating the mind and consciousness to develop cheerfulness *(samādhāna)* free from worldly sorrow or discontentment. Mind and consciousness can bind or liberate man. Therefore, yoga begins with the culture of the mind, the outer layer of the consciousness as it is tainted with the *tāmasic* (inertia), *rājasic* (vibrancy) and *sāttvic* (luminosity) qualities of nature. Conquest of these three qualities of mind is *samādhāna citta*. So the end of *samādhi* is spiritual *samādhāna*.

The mind that gathers knowledge through the help of senses of perception and organs of action, gets coated through direct perception *(pramāṇa)*, misperception *(viparyaya)*, misconception *(vikalpa)*, sleep *(nidrā)* and memory *(smṛti)* (*Y.S.*, I.6). These five oscillating states of the mind are checked and controlled by practice and detachment of the *aṣṭadaḷa* (eight-petalled) *yoga* of Patañjali (*Y.S.*, I.12).

Yoga sādhanā involves uninterrupted, devoted, long practice (*Y.S.*, I.14), while detachment cultivates the mind to discard those thoughts that are not congenial towards the practice of yoga (*Y.S.*, I.15).

Practice is of four types: mild *(mṛdu)*, average *(madhyama)*, keen *(adhimātra)* and vehement *(tīvra)* (*Y.S.*, I.21-22), whereas detachment is of five types: disengaging the senses from action *(yatamāna)*, keeping away from desires *(vyatireka)*, control of mind *(ekendriya)*, mastery of desire or bringing the desire under control *(vaśīkāra)* and vanquishment of pride or ego by supreme detachment *(paravairāgya)*.**

Hence, yoga is a two-fold path. The first four petals of *aṣṭadaḷa yoga* are evolutionary practices and the last three are involutionary while the fifth one is a transitional state.

By following these aspects of yoga, the wandering or roving mind gets stabilised and conditioned to think and analyse things and thoughts clearly *(vitarka)*. Differentiating through reasoning *(vicāra)* between sensual and spiritual bliss, helps the *sādhaka* to come closer to the individual self *(asmitā)*. As he comes closer to the individual self, he gets elated and experiences ecstasy or *ānanda* (*Y.S.*, I.17). In this state of ecstasy he may forget his yogic discipline: here

---

* Complete, pure and direct surrender to the Lord.

** cf. the author's *Light on the Yoga Sūtras of Patañjali*, pp. 62-63. Harper Collins, London.

Patañjali particularly emphasises that the *sādhaka* must not stagnate in that state, but go back to *sādhanā* with trust, vigour and rigour, memory and attentiveness (*Y.S.*, I.20) in order to reach the highest or absolute state of aloneness *(nirbīja samādhi)*.

Patañjali deals with two types of approach. One with support and the other without support. He begins with devotion to God, the *Guru* of all *gurus* (*Y.S.*, I.26), who is free from afflictions and reactions of actions (*Y.S.*, I.24), and who is the seed of all knowledge (*Y.S.*, I.25).

Then he advises the cultivation of friendliness, compassion, indifference to good and bad and to be glad whatever our temperamental problems might be (*Y.S.*, I.33). Besides this, he suggests the practice of *prāṇāyāma*, emphasising pensive retention after exhalation (*Y.S.*, I.34), or total involvement in the chosen practice, (*Y.S.*, I.35), or to understand the meaning of the sorrowless light of knowledge (*Y.S.*, I.36), or to contemplate on spiritual personalities as guides in life, (*Y.S.*, I.37), or to contemplate on the knowledge of sleep and the knowledge of dream, (*Y.S.*, I.38), or to meditate on any pleasing object conducive to steadiness of consciousness. This pleasing object must be chosen in the frame of *yogābhyāsa*. (*Y.S.*, I.39). These various suggestive techniques, advocated by Patañjali, offer a close study of *citta (citta parikrama)*. Persistent following of such a *sādhanā* he says, brings crystal clarity in mind that the seeker, the seer and the search for the seer are one and the same. (*Y.S.*, I.41). The confusion of seeker, seeing and seer is created by memory and mind as separate entities. The mind *(biṁba)* and memory *(pratibiṁba)* are not two separate entities, but they are one and the same.* Such a *sādhanā* makes one reach a state of matured intelligence and have the insight of the seer.

The subject is vast, but time is short. So, let me deal with other chapters before closing my talk.

Patañjali deals with five afflictions, (*Y.S.*, II.3), and five fluctuations, (*Y.S.*, I.5), of body and consciousness.** They are caused by desires *(vāsanā)* and invite physical, physiological, emotional, intellectual and spiritual diseases. These diseases boomerang on life and hence he emphasises the importance of yoga.

Patañjali divides yoga into three tiers: *tapas* (burning zeal), *svādhyāya* (study of one's self from the body to the core) and *Īśvara praṇidhāna* (surrender of the individual force to the cosmic force) (*Y.S.*, II.1). Patañjali guides us in the practice of yoga to develop a cultured head, a cultured

---

* Vāchaspati Miśra, *Tattva-vāiśāradī*, II.17.

** cf. Essence of the *Yoga Sūtra* of Patañjali, p. 200.

cleanliness and purity in the heart so that the intelligence grows vertically and horizontally to live in peace and poise; peace in the cells and poise in mind. The human and divine qualities hidden in the *sādhaka* come to the surface and he lives then fully.

Patañjali terms this quality of intelligence as *vivekaja jñāna* or exalted intelligence. Very often, when this exalted state of intelligence sprouts, the eight supernatural powers *(aṣṭa siddhi)* come to him and tempt him to use them. Then he gets tainted and intoxicated with pride.

The eight powers are 1) *aṇimā* (becoming very small); 2) *mahimā* (increasing one's own size at will); 3) *garimā* (becoming heavier); 4) *laghimā* (becoming weightless); 5) *prāpti* (power of obtaining everything); 6) *prākāmya* (attainment of every wish); 7) *īśatva* (supremacy over all); and 8) *vaśitva* (power of subjugation over anyone or anything).

One has to renounce all these powers so that the crystal clear state of intelligence remains close to the ever fresh attentive core of being. The union of *buddhi* and *ātmā* is the end of yoga. With this union, consciousness dissolves and rests in the abode of the Self. This is the culmination of the yoga of Patañjali.

YOGĀMṚTA – YOGA IMMORTAL

Yoga touches man at all levels of life: physical, mental and spiritual. It is a practical method for making one's life purposeful, useful and noble.

Honey is sweet from whichever end of the honeycomb it is sipped. So is yoga. Yoga enables one's organs of action, senses of perception, mind, intelligence, consciousness and the trillions of cells of his body to get attuned to the conscious essence of the seer. Yoga enables the *sādhaka* to perceive directly and to experience the world within and around himself to gain insight and to feel the divine joy of all creation and to share the ambrosia *(amṛta)* of divine wealth and happiness with his fellow-beings.

The *Yoga Sūtra* are specifically compiled to cover different facets of life, exploring them in depth. Patañjali, the composer of the *Sūtra,* shows the ways of adopting and adapting the principles of yoga to everyone, whether one is initiated or uninitiated, intelligent or unintelligent. One can plunge deeply into the reservoir of the *Sūtra* and tasting the nectar of integrity, shine with purity and divinity.

Yoga is a friend to those who embrace it. It uplifts compassionately its practitioners from the clutches of pain and sorrow and enables them to enjoy life with delight and joy. It makes the lazy body active and vibrant like the mind, then leads both to be in harmony with the Self.

Patañjali was a master of yoga. He is referred to as a *svayaṁbhū* (*svayaṁ* = one's own accord; *bhū* = existent), incarnated by his own will. He is considered as an immortal being. He adjusted himself to the human level and experienced the sorrows and joys of humans and found ways of overcoming them. This resulted in his treatise on yoga. In this treatise, he explains clearly and unreservedly the ways of surmounting afflictions of the body and fluctuations of the mind for man to enjoy unbiased bliss and felicity. His divine words and ideas are precise and original. Even after centuries his immortal words remain ever fresh, fascinating and absorbing.

The *Yoga Sūtra* is a distillation of human wisdom by a supreme master, considered as a master of masters. Just as a jeweller strings the pearls together on a thread to form a necklace,

Patañjali composed the yogic *sūtras* like gems of knowledge woven together as a garland of illuminative wisdom for its practitioners. They help the sincere and serious practitioners to become deeply cultured, highly civilised and worthy human beings.

There are a hundred and ninety-six *sūtras* in all. They begin with the code of discipline for culture of the mind so that it is tuned to the excellent luminosity of the Self.

The practice and study of yoga, with the help of the *Yoga Sūtra*, lead the *sādhaka* to face and perceive his true nature. As each note is essential to form a musical composition, each word of the *Sūtra* conveys the wealth of thought and understanding of the depth of nature and life, in order to experience emancipation and freedom. They ignite the hidden divine fire of man and make him drink the nectar of life, flowing with friendliness and compassion towards his fellow beings.

The text begins with the word *anuśāsanam*. *Anuśāsanam* means the codes of conduct to build one's character for better living and higher thinking. This character building is known as the science of duty *(dharmaśāstra)*. The path of *dharma* leads to the gateway of *kaivalya*. *Kaivalya* is freedom from the contact of worldly things and thoughts. It is freedom from mundane existence. The orderly science of duty is instilled in the *aṣṭadaḷa yoga* of Patañjali in the *sūtras*. The *aṣṭadaḷa* discipline of yoga, followed with dedication and devotion, helps practitioners to become stable in their minds and to live with equipoise in all circumstances.

The first chapter, *Samādhi Pāda*, deals with the ways of cultivation of religiousness in life. In this *pāda*, the *sādhaka* learns to know the Supreme Soul *(Brahman)*. He is advised to live truthfully in word, thought and deed. Naturally, doubts may arise in the minds of the readers as to why Patañjali suddenly began his treatise on the realisation of Brahman.

Samādhi means the way of tracing the source. This source is the essence of consciousness expanded and diffused impartially and evenly *(adhyātma prasādanam)* in body, senses, mind and intelligence.

Hence, Patañjali must have commenced his *sūtra* with spiritual contentment to lure and influence high intellectual souls to reach *samādhi* instantaneously and at the same time tempt the non-gifted and non-initiated with glimpses of the essence of being, so that sooner or later they too undertake the journey to the goal of life – the sight of the Self.

The second chapter, *Sādhanā Pāda*, explains the ways and means to move from the base towards the zenith in yoga. This *pāda* describes to a novice the practical means to achieve the purpose of life. By following the prescribed practices of yoga, he gains physical and mental health and enjoys the pleasures of the world with contentment.

All those who attempt to learn yoga may not be spiritual seekers. Patañjali encourages them to practise yoga so that they may one day become interested and follow the spiritual aspects of life (see *B.G.*, VII.16).

The third chapter, *Vibhūti Pāda*, explains super-natural powers. These super-natural powers may tempt one towards lust. To avoid this lust, Patañjali teaches non-attachment to the practitioner, so that he may live without lust for power but proceed further towards freedom and beatitude. Super-natural powers are all alloyed with the three qualities of nature. These three qualities of nature are the three cosmic egos or personalities of nature hidden in the first principle of nature, the cosmic intelligence *(mahat)*. Patañjali wants us to follow his gems of advice to experience the effortless, indivisible state of a pure being. This state of pure being is the state of absolute consciousness or absolute aloneness, where the seeker and the seer are united into one.

Let your body, mind and Self, blend into one to lose their identities as do the three rivers Gangā, Yamunā and Sarasvati at their confluence. This blending of three into one is Yoga immortal or *Yogāmṛta*.

May Patañjali's grace fall on all through the illuminative rays of yoga, so that the light of yoga penetrates all to live in poise and peace.

May the wisdom of yoga in you all bring the nectar of peace in your body, poise in the cells and serenity in your mind.

YOGA OF ACTION

The chorus of the song today is that life is full of stress. Life is becoming painful. None in the affluent countries, the Third World developing countries or those plunged in hunger, want, malnutrition, or nations ravaged by war and strife, are happy.

Man is arrayed against himself. Insecurity and fear haunt and daunt the people. We are in the Centenary Celebration year of Swami Vivekananda's Universal Vedantic Message delivered by him in the first Parliament of World Religions held in Chicago in 1893. Even after a century of his clarion call for peace, one finds the world is caught in turmoil. Humanity is at the crossroads of history.

I sensed the feeling of turmoil of mankind during the American Iyengar Yoga Convention at Ann Arbor, Michigan.* It was not different in the Canadian Iyengar Yoga Conference, Toronto.** And at the European Iyengar Yoga Convention, thousands of kilometres from Toronto, at Crystal Palace Sports Centre, London,*** it was the same. The blanket of unhappiness cutting across barriers of religion, history, geography, language, race and ethnic considerations is the same on the human mind.

Why such turmoil of insecurity, distrust and fear of each other? Through self-alienation, man is set against himself and the world at large. I tried to ponder and analyse the cause for this deep universal sorrow and misery. Humanity is being dragged into a life of sorrow instead of towards human values and well being.

Swāmi Vivekānanda gave his call for action in Chicago in 1893. Humanity needs the message imbued in spiritual discipline like the message of Lord Krishna in *Bhagavad Gītā* to Arjuna to "fight on":

---

* 6-14 August 1993.
** 16-20 August 1993.
*** 24-30 August 1993.

Sukhadḥukhe same kṛtvā
lābhālābhau jayājayau /
tato yudhyāya yujyasva
nai'vaṁ pāpam avāpsyasi //
(*B.G.*, II.38).

Hold alike pleasure and pain, gain and loss, victory and defeat, and get ready for battle; then you will not incur sin.

The *Kaṭha Upaniṣad* epitomises the present world scenario stating: "Fools dwelling in darkness, wise in their own conceit and puffed up with vain knowledge, go round and round, staggering to and fro, like blind men led by the blind".

I often wonder that the world is too much with us. We tend to take trifles of life too seriously but only at the level of thinking and brooding, devoid of meaningful action. The human body is a playground of *jīvātmā* as the world is the playground of the Lord. The body, the mind and self all come into play with five senses of perception, five organs of action, five elements (earth, water, fire, air and ether) and their qualities (odour, taste, shape, touch and sound). The mind is the coach and the intelligence is the arbitrator.

The playground should be proper and the player must be fit to play the game. Playing the game for the human being means to live fully with vitality. Sage Patañjali in his wisdom chartered out for all of us the game plan, the qualities needed by the player to play the game with vigour, energy and optimism. The key of the game is to use our wits, to strike a balance between the body, mind, emotions and the self. The elements are made to play the game within their judicious limits, set by nature, to do their best towards the progress of man. This is not a competition for supremacy between nature and *puruṣa*, but a friendly game in which both do their best. The vital difference between the games in which we normally participate and the yoga *sādhanā* is the realisation of the Self. Though we compete and play, in yoga we are not looking for victory or triumph. We go on playing till our last breath or as long as the Almighty wishes.

Many questions are raised as to why Swami Vivekananda chose the Chicago Congress for his message to the West. In India and in the East where the *vedic* religion thrived and flowered, he advised the youth to play football instead of reading the *Bhagavad Gītā*. With the philosophy of abnegation of self and self-denial, the masses were misled to look inward while the poverty and subjection were calling for action.

He wanted to ensure that the masses did not turn to the retiring life of a 'recluse'. He stirred up the people at home into action by his call to "rise and awake", as he knew that 'spirituality' was not a means to attain material well being and mundane needs that the body cannot be fed by spiritual practice alone. The West had possibly too much of material prosperity but its spirit was languishing.

Patañjali with his immense prowess over yoga and language codified the entire *yoga darśana* in 196 *sūtras* (aphorisms). The world is too ill at ease, and virtually going berserk in the pursuit of *bhoga* (enjoyment) at the expense of the Self. Patañjali's *Yoga Sūtra* provides the seed for the total evolution of the human being. The world, which has gone full circle in pursuit of material and mundane pleasures, is now turning back to yoga with.millions practising yoga for physical health, mental calmness and emotional poise.

Yoga is for overall health, irrespective of caste, creed, age or sex. Health and contentment, are the best acquisitions. Whether it is in pursuit of duty *(dharma)*, or to earn a livelihood *(artha)*, or for enjoyment of life and worldly pleasures *(kāma)* or for liberation and emancipation *(mokṣa)*, it is a MUST. The *Upaniṣads* proclaim that a weakling cannot enjoy the pleasures of life *(bhoga)* or liberation *(mokṣa)*. Carakācārya says: "Health is the most important foundation in order to follow the four aims of man": *dharma, arṭha, kāma* and *mokṣa ("dharmārtha kāma mokṣāṇām ārogyam mūlamuttamam")*.

Pain or suffering is of three kinds:

1. *Ādhyātmika* (self-inflicted and invited): it is up to us to reduce or eliminate it by keeping the balance of fitness of body, mind and Self working in co-ordination.
2. *Ādhidaivika:* affliction or disease *(roga)* caused by genetic factors over which humans have not been able to gain control or find a cure.
3. *Ādhibhautika:* afflictions that arise out of the disturbances of the ratio of the elements in the body. Pain, sorrow, harassment, agony, misery, distress, discomfort, torments, grief, worry, vexation, disease, torture and annoyance are the afflictions with their source in ignorance. The other sources of pain and misery are egotism, attachment, aversion and too much caring for one's own existence.

What human beings need is a look into the 'interior' of their own Self and see within. Man is a triune of body, mind and Self. The body is called the *kṣetra* or the field and the 'inner man', the dweller in the body, is called *kṣetrajña (Bhagavad Gītā)*.

Patañjali's *Yoga Sūtra* is the seed for total evolution of the human being. The aim is to culture the body, mind, emotion and intelligence to reach the superconscious state hidden in all. Yoga is essentially a spiritual science *(mokṣa śāstra)* and the gain of physical or mental health are only its pillars.

The four chapters *(pāda)* of the *Yoga Sūtra* are *Samādhi Pāda, Sādhanā Pāda, Vibhūti Pāda* and *Kaivalya Pāda.*

Samādhi Pāda discusses the ways and means for purifying the mind and cultivating the *citta. Sādhanā Pāda* offers methods and means to enrich *citta* by removing lack of understanding. *Vibhūti Pāda* signifies the plentiful gift of yoga but with a caution, that the use of these gifts for self-gratification can backfire and temptation to use the powers could bring about the downfall of the yogi. *Kaivalya Pāda* leads the *sādhaka* to the state of liberation.

The principle of yoga is to observe the ethical, physical, mental and intellectual disciplines for character building. This stress of discipline must be of right means. *Yama* (moral and mental restraint) and *niyama* (physical and mental observance) are rules of moral values and codes of behaviour relating to oneself and society. They are individual disciplines as well as social disciplines. The growth of civilisation is marked by culturing the mind. Yoga cultures the body and the consciousness.

Suffering *(kleśa)* is an inevitable component of life and has to be borne. We have ourselves invited suffering. We have saturated the mother earth with all kinds of toxins, dumping nuclear waste in the sea and on the land. We have polluted the natural resources, the water we drink, and we have released huge volumes of poisonous gases in the air through our factories and industries. Are these the true needs of mankind or are they due to the greed of man to acquire more and more material comforts? Have they brought us any mental peace though our lives have become easier, leaving us with leisure time? In affluent homes, children, women and men get bored. They do not know how to use their leisure time to attend to their bodies to keep them healthy and strong and to stabilise their mind in order to nurture the Self. They all seek to escape by watching movies, which are full of violence, murder, mystery, fiction, crimes, sex orgies and drunkenness.

New York, Chicago and many other cities of the world have become insecure and unsafe. In these cities, you cannot enjoy normal life out of doors and even living within the confines of the house is insecure. It is the same in all the countries around the world. In Japan, one of the world's industrial and economic giants, the rate of suicide has crossed the danger mark. Why and what to live for is the bogey before the youth and those fit to work. The old are dying uncared for in homes for the aged. Surviving as vegetables without zest, they raise their hands in despair towards the heavens to lift them from this world, from the 'living mortuary'.

Did I not point out in my book *Light on Yoga* what we were coming to, as far back as 1966? "These yogic commandments are the rules of morality for society and the individual; when not obeyed they bring chaos, violence, untruth, stealing, dissipation and covetousness".

Reap as you sow. We have a surfeit of it; violence, ill health, disease, hunger, malnutrition, starvation, strife, discord, fighting and infighting, right from the affluent and advanced nations to the impoverished third world countries. Are we not aware of the havoc we are playing with our environment and depleting the mother earth? *Yama* and *niyama* are great universal commandments not limited by geographic, regional or ethnic considerations. Non-violence (*ahiṁsā*) of Patañjali connects us to the root of love. Truthfulness *(satya)* deals with the culture of the mind. *Brahmacarya* is for moderation of sex for all, youth, men and women. Is not accumulation *(aparigraha)*, hoarding far beyond our needs and means, irreligion in yoga?

Yoga is for us, here and now. These are not matters of superconsciousness or spirituality. Western philosophy and modern psychology are not clear in their concepts of *citta* of *vedic* philosophy. Mind, intelligence and consciousness cover the different aspects of the human being. When mind dominates the entire brain, the intelligence and consciousness are compressed. At times the intelligence swamps the brain and the mind is compressed. You must have realised this when you are totally involved and absorbed in something, a ray of illuminating light of consciousness appears shining from the Self. The fluctuations in consciousness sprout from the *asmitā*. Direct thought-waves create a disturbed state of mind. In misperception *(viparyaya, Y.S.,* I.8), the sense perception deceives us while in misconception (*vikalpa, Y.S.,* I.9), the senses work correctly but the mind cannot conceive correctly.

It is intriguing why Swami Vivekananda exhorted the youth to play football rather than read the *Bhagavad Gītā*, a descent from the high platform of immortality of the soul to the average intelligence. He wanted militancy in action and the fighting spirit more than sermons on philosophy.

His desire was to fire the imagination of the inert masses, which were smothered in inaction. A wrong message had gone to the people from the saints and philosophers. The messages like *Jaganmithya* (the world is illusion) which spreads despair and gloom. At the turn of 1993, just one hundred years after the Chicago address, the world and particularly India, needs the message of 'arise and awake' to arouse the masses into action, to 'play the game', to engage in the battle.

"Hato va prāpyasi svargaṁ jitvā vā bhokṣyaśe mahīm", says Lord Krishna to Arjuna: "If you are slain you will go to *svarga* (heaven), and if victorious in this battle, you will enjoy the sovereignty of the earth, the pleasures of the world".

Mankind must shed unworthy weaknesses. The brave do not get faint hearted. The world is in turmoil. Take the words of Swami Vivekananda to heart and resolve to fight. *"Tato yuddhāya yujyasva"*, engage yourself in the battle, which is going on between *kṣetra*, the field and *kṣetrajña*, the fielder. The solace and way is in the yoga of Patañjali.

When *ahaṁkāra* is subdued, consciousness disappears and then the light of the Eternal surfaces. This is the method that Patañjali offers to the human being to move from worldly pleasures towards emancipation and liberation *(kaivalya)*.

ESSENCE OF THE *YOGA SŪTRA* OF PATAÑJALI

I have been asked today to speak on Patañjali's *Yoga Sūtra*. Patañjali was an immortal soul and I am a mortal being. How can a mortal speak about the immortal words of an immortal soul? Patañjali's words are original and eternal. My words on him may be a duplicate or just a repetition. Hence, I feel that I am too insignificant and not worthy to speak on Patañjali and his work. Being myself on the first step of the ladder, or at 'A' in the alphabet of yoga, how can I utter 'Z', the last letter of the alphabet, the zenith of yoga?

PATAÑJALI

Let me tell you a little about the background of Patañjali. He is said to have been born some time between 500 and 200 BC. Nobody can give the exact date because in India the dates of the lives of the great sages were measured according to the grammer that was in vogue during their time.

Patañjali was a *svayaṁbhū* (born with one's own will power). Born of his own will like Lord Krishna or Lord Rama, he was a fully evolved soul, gifted to us by God. His words and sayings remain enchanting and fresh even now. I am sure it is going to be an all-absorbing subject for centuries to come. He had no parents and according to Indian mythology was the incarnation of Lord Ādiśeṣa.

Ādiśeṣa is a great King Cobra whose body is the seat of Lord Vishnu. It is said that once Lord Shiva, the king of dance, invited Lord Vishnu and other deities to see his famous dance, *tāṇḍava nṛtya*. As Lord Shiva danced, Lord Vishnu became absorbed in it. He began to vibrate with the rhythm of the graceful movements of Lord Shiva. Lord Vishnu was seated on Ādiśeṣa, the great cobra. The great King Cobra became breathless under the weight of the Lord, which was increasing, and began gasping for air. When the dance came to an end, Ādiśeṣa felt the lightness in the Lord's body. Amazed by this change of weight, he asked the Lord, "How is it that you were so heavy when Lord Shiva was dancing and as soon as the dance finished you became light?". Lord Vishnu replied, "I was so fully engrossed in His movements that my nerves and body vibrated as if I myself were dancing. That is why you felt it". Seeing how impressed Lord

Vishnu was with the dance, Ādiśeṣa decided to learn the dance himself.* However, Lord Vishnu predicted, "You must wait. Lord Shiva is going to ask you to do some work. At that time you will be incarnated on Earth and then you will learn dance". That time arrived and Lord Shiva asked him to write a commentary on grammar. Ādiśeṣa saw that his Master's prediction had been realised and was overjoyed with the words of Lord Vishnu and the grace of Lord Shiva. He began looking for a mother who was both a *yogini* and a *tapasvini* (a woman who had done much yoga and fervent penance). He meditated and waited to find the right mother to accept him as a spiritual child and to allow him to realise his aspirations. After some time he found Gauṇika, who had no children and who had done penance for several years. She was praying to the rising sun, saying. "My time has come to an end and whatever knowledge I have gathered it was only through you, O Sun God. As I have no son or daughter to pass it on to, I return my knowledge to you". She took some water to offer as oblation, closed her eyes and prayed. As she opened her eyes to offer the water to the Sun God, she saw a very tiny snake moving in the water that she was holding in her palms. At first she was terrified and said, "What polluted water I have taken!". As she was saying this, the tiny snake at once assumed human form, prostrated and begged her to accept him as her son. She accepted him as her son and named him Patañjali – *pata* means fall and *anjali* means the folding of the hands during prayer. He is also known as *Gauṇikā putra* (son of Gauṇikā). Thus, Patañjali means "fallen into the palms at the time of prayer".

As the young boy grew, Gauṇika became more and more impressed by him and transmitted her knowledge to him.

Eventually Patañjali completed his first duty, the commentary on grammar.** Then he decided to learn dance. As he was learning dance the idea struck him that the various movements of the body could be used for understanding the functions of the body. He studied the system of the body, using the knowledge of matter, the elements and their qualities. Through the study of the outer and inner body he brought out the system called *Āyurveda*. *Āyuḥ* means life and *veda* means knowledge, so *āyurveda* is the knowledge of life, and not the knowledge of medicine, as it is understood now. There is an important distinction between understanding of life force and medicine. (Many scholars believe that the treatise written by Patañjali on medicine is the famous *Caraka Samhitā* and that Caraka was his pen name in his work on *āyurveda*.) Finally, he composed the aphorisms on yoga, known as the *Yoga Sūtra*.

---

* That is why many dancers in India pay respect to Patañjali as the father of dance.

** In present times, It is very hard to imagine how one man could be a master of grammar, a master of medicine and a master of yoga. Because of this, some western scholars have conjectured that Patañjali, the author of a treatise on grammar based on the work of the grammarian Pāṇini, must have been the son of Pāṇini. Neverthless, the Indian tradition considers that the three treatises on grammar, on medicine and on yoga are composed by the same Patañjali.

There are also stories on the teaching of sage Patañjali. It seems that he had one thousand students who wanted to learn and understand his knowledge and experiences. Patañjali consented to teach all the one thousand students at one time, but on one condition, that he would impart lessons sitting behind a large screen.

He had said that nobody should see or peep through the screen and if they did so, then all would be turned into ashes. The pupils agreed to his conditions and underwent training without seeing their preceptor. On a particular day, out of these one thousand pupils, one became very restless and inquisitive to see how one person could simultaneously teach one thousand pupils. He was so excited that in his eagerness he forgot to take heed of his master's words and peeped through the screen. At once all the disciples were reduced to ashes.

Fortunately or unfortunately, on that very day, one disciple did not attend the class. He later came to know that all his colleagues were reduced to ashes. As this pupil had not taken his master's permission for his absence, Patañjali cursed him and he became a *Brahma Rākṣasa* (the ghost of a *brahmin* who in his lifetime indulges in disdainful spirits).

The master was also happy that at least one of his pupils escaped this terrible fate. Realising his mistake the pupil approached the master with humbleness. He apologised to his master for his absence and begged him to forgive his mistake. The sage was happy that at least one of his disciples had escaped this dreadful fate. He blessed the disciple so that he could later return to his original human form. Then he guided his disciple to the secrets of yoga philosophy. In this way the whole knowledge, which was going to be lost, was preserved and transmitted by at least one disciple.

THE STRUCTURE OF *YOGA SŪTRA*

The *Yoga Sūtra* contains 196 aphorisms, classified into four *pāda* or chapters.

With his highly evolved state of intellect Patañjali begins his *Sūtra "citta vṛtti nirodhaḥ"*. We are nowhere near the consciousness or the source of consciousness *(ātmā)* to know its waves. He starts from the finest and minutest particle of *prakṛti* or nature to embrace *puruṣa* (Self).*

In the first chapter, Patañjali explains the states and qualities of consciousness and shows the ways to eradicate all fluctuations or movements through mental discipline *(manō*

---

* The soul is vast. Unless the skin and the self are brought closer to each other through intelligence, the comprehension of this principle of Patañjali will remain difficult. So, your practice has to become worthy.

sādhanā). In this chapter he deals specially with evolved souls. He teaches them how to maintain and sustain their evolved states of consciousness in order to experience the state of aloneness *(kaivalya).*

It also gives methods for disciplining the consciousness (mind, intelligence and ego). As Patañjali begins this chapter with the culture of the *citta* (consciousness), many call his method *rāja yoga. Rāja* means a king. *Citta* being considered the king of the body, organs of action and senses of perception, the yoga which deals with the consciousness is termed *rāja yoga.* Patañjali goes deeper than *citta* and makes one trace the king of the mind and consciousness – the seer.

In the second chapter, Patañjali comes down to guide unevolved souls. He explains the lower vehicles of the consciousness *(citta),* like the senses of perception and mind, showing the ways that they too can learn to become free and feel the Self. It is a chapter on action covering *abhyāsa* or effort in full.

In the third chapter, he speaks of the miraculous powers of yoga. These powers appear as a signboard, proving that one is having the right approach. *"Te samādhau upasargāḥ vyutthāne siddhayaḥ".* (*Y.S.,* III.38): These attainments are impediments to *samādhi,* although they are powers in active life. If the *sādhaka* is overwhelmed with the powers, he will be like a person who, running to avoid the wind, gets caught in the whirlwind. He cautions the *sādhaka* to be careful and remain non-attached to and uninterested in these miraculous powers and to continue his *sādhanā.* He gives examples of those who were caught in the web of these powers and those who were free from them. Nahūṣa, who belonged to the mortal world, became the Lord of Heaven. Due to the misuse of his powers, he fell from grace and was sent back to earth in the form of a snake. Urvaśī became a creeper. Ahalyā became a stone by Gautama's curse. The yogi reaches the pinnacle of life when he is uninterested in power. Nandī, the bull, reached Lord Shiva and became His vehicle. Matsyendra, the fish, became the greatest *haṭha yogi* on earth.

The fourth chapter explains the state of the *sādhaka* as a king amongst men. We learn through this chapter that yoga is a means, an effort, a restraint and integration. It is a means to practise what has to be practised and learn what has to be learnt *(abhyāsa).* Detachment is a method of restraint to avoid what should be avoided and restrain what has to be restrained *(vairāgya).* Here Patañjali shows the difference between *samādhi* and *kaivalya.* In *samādhi,* the *sādhaka* experiences a state of oneness between seer and seeker, subject and object, the observer and the observed, the doer and the observer. In *kaivalya,* not only does he express his experiences but lives a dynamic illuminative state of life, moving in the world and performing his day to day duties without himself getting involved in his work or with people.

SAMĀDHI PĀDA

In the first chapter *(Samādhi Pāda)*, Patañjali goes beyond the mind and explains that *citta* (consciousness) is like a box, which encases the mind, intelligence and ego *(ahaṁkāra)*. For the sake of convenience and quick understanding, I use the word 'mind' for *citta*. Mind is made up of *sattva* (luminosity), *rajas* (dynamism) and *tamas* (inertia). As our minds have three qualities, our actions too have three qualities: white *(sattva)*, grey *(rajas)* and black *(tamas)*. The yoga discipline takes one's mind and actions beyond these three qualities. They become neither white, nor black or grey.

Karma aśukla akṛṣṇam yoginaḥ trividham itareṣām (*Y.S.*, IV.7).

A yogi's actions are beyond white, black and grey. The actions of others are white, black or grey.

In that *guṇātīta karma* (action free from the qualities), the *puruṣa* appears in purity, making the yogi experience the perennial knowledge of wisdom. This state is called *samāpatti* or *samprajñāta samādhi*.

Samādhi is of two types, one is *sabīja* and the other is *nirbīja*. *Bīja* means seed. *Sabīja samādhi* is achieved by deliberate efforts with a support or seed to hold on. This is divided into *savitarkā*, *nirvitarkā*, *savicārā*, *nirvicārā*, *sānanda* and *sāsmitā* (see Table n. 12). *Savitarkā* and *nirvitarkā* are the ways of contemplating on gross things and *savicārā* and *nirvicārā* on subtle things. *Sānanda* is the achievement of control of subtle senses and *sāsmitā* is the mastery of the lower mortal self *(asmitā)*. *Nirbīja* is without a seed. This contemplation is an experience without deliberate efforts.

Table n. 12 - Classifications of *samādhi*

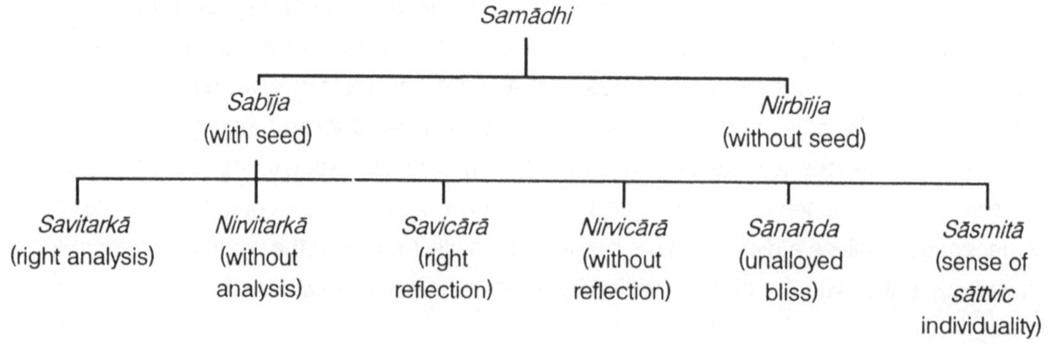

Each person has a particular quality of mind. The particular qualities of mind are five: dull *(mūḍa)*, lazy *(kṣipta)*, oscillating *(vikṣpta)*, steady *(ekāgra)* and the one beyond these four states *(niruddha)*. The mind, with its quality, moves and gets modified according to direct perception, misperception, misconception, sleep and memory. Memory is the art of maintaining and sustaining all the impressions of all above-mentioned supports. These movements and modifications may be painful or non-painful. The painful ones are felt immediately and the non-painful ones, which are hidden, may appear at a later time. Though *puruṣa* (Self) is pure, he gets caught and moves in the spokes of joy and sorrow like a spider living in its web and becomes a part of suffering.

What are these sufferings? One develops diseases, languor, doubt, carelessness, laziness, self-indulgence, living in the world of illusion, failure to reach the aim, inability to maintain a certain point after reaching it and dejection which may lead to negative thinking.

Avidyā (ignorance or want of knowledge and understanding) is the mother of all afflictions. Patañjali explains that right knowledge is earned either by direct perception *(pratyakṣa)*, or through inference *(anumāna)* or through testimony *(āgama)*. He concludes that the best way to right understanding begins when we put an end to trials and errors. This direct experience can be obtained through *abhyāsa* and *vairāgya*. *Abhyāsa* is of three types. It may be slow, middle or intense. It can be multiplied according to one's capability, energy and method of action.

Practice involves long uninterrupted effort with zeal and passion for the subject, faith, courage, steadiness, calmness, tenacity and perseverance. Just dragging on in life with negative thoughts is to be avoided as these thoughts revolve around the six spokes: desire *(kāma)*, anger *(krodha)*, miserliness *(lobha)*, infatuation *(moha)*, pride *(mada)* and jealousy *(mātsarya)*. If the *sādhaka* is caught up in these turmoils, he finds it very hard to distinguish between mind and self.

Patañjali shows ways in order to train the mind and to take it from negative health towards positive health. The universal method of ethics leads towards positive health of not only the body but also the mind. Hence, it is essential that the body is cleansed, the senses sublimated, the mind purified for joyful consciousness to realise the Self. The principles of *yama* and *niyama* are to be followed irrespective of class of birth, time, place or sex. When one follows *yama* and *niyama*, one begins to cultivate qualities such as friendliness, compassion, joy and indifference (when necessary). The proper judgement of these qualities helps to diffuse the *citta*, not only in one's behaviour with others, but also in society. Be friendly to one and all irrespective of their happy positions so that you cultivate freedom from jealousy. Be compassionate to those who are in need. Be joyous when someone is better than you are and be happy with yourself when you see that you are placed in a better position than many. If someone does a bad act, guide him and if he does not change, even with repeated guidance, then show indifference.

Patañjali shows ways of restraining the consciousness. First he advises one to surrender to God and he explains the characteristics and qualities of God. He says that God is free from all afflictions and untouched by actions or their fruits. He considers God as the "first teacher", "the teacher of all teachers" and wants the *sādhaka* to reach Him. God is unconditioned by time, place and space. He is represented by the sacred syllable *āuṁ*. This *āuṁ* should be known through *japa* (prayer), *artha* (meaning) and *bhāvanā* (feelings). This helps to release the mind from the intellectual and emotional upheavals and transforms one to experience the Self *(ātmānubhava: ātmā = Self, anubhava =* experience).

The mind gets filled with serenity and insight. The *puruṣa*, which remained as *avyaktan* (invisible Self), appears as a *vyakta puruṣan* (a visible Self). He is now in a seedless state (*Y.S.*, IV.29-30).

SĀDHANĀ PĀDA

In the second chapter *(Sādhanā Pāda)*, Patañjali explains the causes of unhappiness and concludes that *avidyā* is the source of all sorrows. Then he shows the ways for the conquest of *avidyā*.

As I have said earlier about the states, qualities and movements of the mind, Patañjali guides the practitioner in this chapter to climb from the lowest step of the ladder to reach the pinnacle or the highest state and to experience the unalloyed and untinged state of *samāpātti prajñā or samādhi*. He shows a method for this and calls it *kriyā yoga*. *Kriyā* is action or effort *(abhyāsa)*. He groups the eight-petalled yoga into three tiers of *tapas* (penance), *svādhyāya* (Self-study through direct perception and testimony) and *Īśvara praṇidhāna* (surrender to God).

He enumerates the five afflictions and says that they may be dormant, attenuated, repressed or active. These afflictions are either the result of the past *karmas*, or caused during the present life. The accumulated *karma* of past and present lives affects one later in this life or sows the seed for the future birth, as cycles of birth and death.

In order to burn out these deposits of *karma*, Patañjali shows the way through *kriyā yoga*.

Yoga texts speak of three types of pain. They are self-abuse *(ādhyātmika)*, disharmony in elements like tides, cyclones, drought and famine – either dry or wet *(ādhibhautika)* and genetic and allergic diseases *(ādhidaivika)*. The *ādhyātmika* pains are caused when the body comes in contact with the self. Patañjali advises us to be very careful to avoid the future pains. As joys breed desires and non-fulfilment of desires breeds grief, he wants us to understand the words 'going with' or 'against' the current *(pakṣa* or *pratipakṣa bhāvana)*. Evolution is *pakṣa* and involution is *pratipakṣa*. They are also called *prasava* and *pratiprasava*. *Prasava* means evolution or *pravṛtti mārga* and *pratiprasava* is the opposite of evolution, involution or *nivṛtti mārga*.

Evolution *(prasava)* is the process where the seer comes in contact with nature, nature with *mahat* or cosmic intelligence, cosmic intelligence with the individual as consciousness *(citta)*, the five elements: ether *(ākāśa)*, wind *(vāyu)*, fire *(tej)*, water *(āp)* and earth *(pṛthvī)*, and their qualities *(tanmātra)*: sound *(śabdha)*, touch *(sparṣa)*, form *(rūpa)*, taste *(rasa)* and odour *(gandha)*, the five senses of perception and five organs of action. Please know that *citta* covers the mind *(manas)*, intelligence *(buddhi)* and ego *(ahaṁkāra)*. The involution process *(pratiprasava)* is the return journey, i.e. body to mind, mind to intelligence, intelligence to the ego, ego to nature and nature to the seer. This stage of reverse journey is known as *dhyāna* or meditation.*

KRIYĀ YOGA SĀDHANĀ (THE PRACTICE OF THE YOGA OF ACTION)

Yama, *niyama*, *āsana* and *prāṇāyāma* are involved in *tapas*. *Yama* channels the organs of action and *niyama* disciplines the senses of perception. *Āsana* harmonises the body, which is made of five elements. *Prāṇāyāma* gives power over the special qualities of the elements; sound, touch, sight, taste and odour.

Pratyāhāra and *dhāraṇā* are the thread for self-study. *Pratyāhāra* is the area for stabilisation of intelligence and *dhāraṇā* is the reverse journey or the retreat of the organs of action and senses of perception, mind and intelligence, towards the Self. At this stage one begins to get a glimpse of non-painful movements *(vṛtti)*. These are:

- *nirodha vṛtti* (restrained stable state of consciousness),
- *praśānta vṛtti* (tranquil state of consciousness),
- *samādhāna vṛtti* (cheerful state of consciousness),
- *ekāgra vṛtti* (attentive state of consciousness), and
- *divya vṛtti* (pure state of consciousness).

* For more details, see the author's *Light on the Yoga Sūtras of Patañjali*, Table 9, pp. 124-125. Harper Collins, London

Citta being the minutest form of *prakṛti* has to be made to merge in *puruṣa*. This is *dhyāna*. Hence *dhāraṇā* and *dhyāna* are called *antaraṅga sādhanā* or the inner quest. These methods are the subtle aspects of yoga. Surrender of the self *(jīvātmā)* to the Universal Self *(Paramātmā)* is *Īśvara praṇidhāna* or the Innermost quest. Here one loses one's identity.

Thus the journey from *yama* to *dhyāna* ends in the river of tranquillity, without any ruffles, or like the sea without any waves. *Citta* is the sea and its *vṛtti* (movements), are the waves. In this river of tranquillity *(praśānta vāhinī)*, the *sādhaka* lives without variations; truth that is eternal *(dharma pariṇāma)*, without qualities *(lakṣaṇa pariṇāma)* and without changes in his own state at all times *(avasthā pariṇāma)*. Here, the consciousness is isolated and the Self is free of place, time or change.

By following the disciplines of the second chapter even the unskilled person reaches the highest knowledge – the splendour of illumination.

Thus Patañjali concludes touchingly, that the effect of this *kriyā yoga*, with all the steps of the yogic ladder, is that "not only are the impurities of the body and mind cleansed, but also the light of wisdom dawns and replaces arrogance or pride by innocence (humbleness)".

Yogāṅgānuṣṭhānāt aśuddhikṣaye jñānadīptiḥ āvivekakhyāteḥ (*Y.S.*, II.28).

SIDDHĪ (ACCOMPLISHMENT)

In the third chapter *(Vibhūti Pāda)*, after explaining *dhāraṇā*, *dhyāna* and *samādhi*, Patañjali deals with the miracles which come as by-products. It is said that a perfect yogi has knowledge of time, stars, planets and of the future. He knows the workings of the mind of others. He knows everything that is knowable. In this sense he is the all-knower, but he will not be the seed of knowledge. He gets *aṣṭa siddhi* or eight supernatural powers. He can become light or heavy, small or large. He can become powerful and acquire all possessions. He can be the Lord of everything and keep anything under his control.

Patañjali emphasises that the yoga *sādhaka* should put aside all these achievements, unmindful of these miracles if he wants to pursue his spiritual quest. He must understand this by living in the moment, without being caught in the sequence of moments, so that the intelligence becomes as pure as Self. Then, he experiences *kaivalya* or *tūriyāvasthā*. Otherwise, he is caught in the net of these powers and loses all. If that happens, then he has to restart yoga as a raw beginner.

KAIVALYA PĀDA

The fourth chapter *(Kaivalya Pāda)* explains the state of aloneness. In this modern world of science and technology, we speak of hybrid seeds and fine pedigrees. Patañjali says that the *kaivalya* state can be experienced through birth *(janma)*, drugs *(auṣadha)*, incantations *(mantra)*, burning zeal in efforts *(tapas)* and supreme meditation *(samādhi)*.

A farmer builds beds from one field to the other for the water to soak in and then takes the water to the adjoining field by breaking that bed. Man may make or mar his progress through *karma* good or bad. As weeds are removed from the land after ploughing for the crops to grow healthily, good action leads to a spiritual life and bad action binds one to the world.

Ego *(ahaṁkāra)* is the root cause *(mūlakāraṇā)* for good or bad actions. Yoga removes the weeds of the mind and leads one to trace its source. This source is the root mind. This root mind is the seat wherein all the latent impressions *(pūrva saṁskāra)* are stored and create various minds in one personality. When this source mind is traced by *abhyāsa*, the *sādhaka* is free from deposits. It is only the various facets of that single mind that makes one accumulate the imprints of actions. These actions rebound with reactions, as cause and effect, creating white, black or grey actions. When the single mind or the big mind is traced, the yogi is free from all the residues of *karma* and becomes a desireless person. There are no spokes left for aspirations or actions or fruits. He acts without movements, modifications or modulations. Everything comes to an end. He is a perfect yogi.

As the wick, oil and flame form into a light, all diversities cease to exist and unity settles between his word, work and wisdom. His knowledge becomes total and full. For others, the object may be one, experience may be another and words may be quite different as their knowledge and understanding change due to their limitations.

An accomplished yogi distinguishes the changing knowledge of the consciousness from the changeless understanding of the Self. He does the work of the world as a witness – uninvolved and uninfluenced. As rows of mirrors reflect the same object, the single mind perceives the objects and reflects them like a crystal. It is known as *bimba – pratibimba svarūpa (bimba* means a reflecting mirror and *pratibimba* means the re-reflection of the first mirror on the second mirror).* All speculations, deliberations and discriminations come to an end and liberation *(mokṣa)* is experienced.

---

* See Vācaspati Miśra, *Tattva Vaiśāradī*, II.17.

He lives in the experience of discriminative knowledge *(vidyā)* without any tinge of lust, anger, greed, infatuation, pride and malice. This is *ṛtaṁbharā prajñā* – truth-bearing knowledge and seasoned awareness that leads towards virtuous awareness or religious awareness *(dharmamegha samādhi).* This intelligence, which is free from the veil of all doubts, becomes eternal knowledge. This exalted intelligence and wisdom perennially flows in the yogi like torrential rain, without affecting him. This is *kaivalya* or the final emancipation of the yogi.

I conclude quoting from sage Vyāsa's comments on the *Yoga Sūtra:* "Yoga is the teacher to learn, start yoga to live in yoga, develop yoga by yoga and comprehend yoga through yoga".*

---

* *Vyāsabhāṣya.*

ANUŚĀSANAM *

I am good in observation, good in reflection, good in performance, but I am very bad at memorising things. As I am presenting for you from different angles the thoughts of Patañjali, I thought that I should quote him. Though I am not good at remembering quotes, I think that it may help you to follow the path of yoga with faith and vigour.

FOUR CHAPTERS OF *PATAÑJALI*

Patañjali's *Yoga Sūtra* is divided into four chapters:

1. *Samādhi Pāda* (chapter on the theoretical principles of yoga and superconsciousness),
2. *Sādhanā Pāda* (chapter on practice),
3. *Vibhūti Pāda* (chapter on attainments) and
4. *Kaivalya Pāda* (chapter on liberation).

I don't know why Patañjali chose these titles for each chapter. It is difficult to bring out the hidden meaning, because all the chapters are filled with some sort of *sādhanā kriyā* or the cleansing process or action. Not one chapter is devoid of *sādhanā*. The *sādhanā* with which he deals are given according to the development of one's intelligence and the culture of consciousness. This is how the beauty of various *sādhanā* glows in all the chapters.

Samādhi Pāda is a *jñāna vijñāna śāstra* (objective view with scientific experimentation). The yoga *sādhanā* of the first and the third chapter converts the objective views and experimental knowledge into experiential wisdom *(prajñā)*. The theory of the first chapter and the practice of the second and third chapters, when converted into science, art and philosophy, become *yoga śāstra*, *yoga kalā* and *yoga darśana*. Thus, when *jñāna*, *vijñāna* and *prajñāna*** are blended and integrated together, that knowledge becomes *viśeṣa jñāna* or *ṛtambharā prajñā*.

---

* Discourse given on *Patañjali Jayanti*, Tuesday 16th October, 1990, in Ramaamani Iyengar Memorial Yoga Institute, Pune.

** See - "Yoga Demands Efficiency in *Sādhanā*", p. 168.

The last chapter is called *Kaivalya Pāda*. As a master yogi, he utilises the subjective experience of *prajñāna* to churn out the fragrance of the inner core and to savour the taste of the *sat chit ānanda* (eternal truth, knowledge and bliss state).

The yogi who reaches this state lives dispassionately utilising his life in the upliftment of his fellow beings with the help of his exalted knowledge. This is how the four chapters are filled with *sādhanā*.

All *ācāryas* devoted their intellectual energies to building the path of *mokṣa*. They paid tremendous attention to the path of emancipation, but they did not attribute any importance to the pleasures of life or *bhoga*. *Bhoga* actually means worldly knowledge *(laukika jñāna)*. The *ācāryas* showed how to live in this world by transforming the worldly knowledge into spiritual knowledge *(ādhyātmika jñāna)*.

Our *ṛṣis* and *ācāryas* were not lacking in the *laukika jñāna*. They were using worldly knowledge as necessities, but their thoughts were only on the spiritual sight. Only Cārvāka – the materialist philosopher, said "Beg, borrow, steal, and enjoy life". He taught, "Survival of the fittest". However, he was a guide as well as an eye opener for other philosophers, who used the principle of Cārvāka as a foundation and discovered the ways of spiritual practice for man to evolve by minimising material needs, in order to reach the knowledge of the Self. Cārvāka refused to see beyond the seen and the other philosophers studied and worked to see beyond the seen.

Table n. 13 – The five traditional *kośa* and their corresponding elements

Sheaths of the body	Five gross elements	Five subtle elements
1. Physical sheath *(Annamaya kośa)*	Earth *(pṛthvi)*	Smell *(gandha)*
2. Physiological sheath *(Prāṇāmaya kośa)*	Water *(āp)*	Taste *(rasa)*
3. Mental sheath *(Manōmaya kośa)*	Fire *(tejas)*	Shape *(rūpa)*
4. a) Intellectual sheath *(Vijñānamaya kośa)* as well as b) Direct perceptive sheath *(Buddhimaya kośa)*	Air *(vāyu)*	Touch *(sparśa)*
5. a) The sheath of the consciousness *(Cittamaya kośa)* as well as b) The sheath of bliss *(Ānandamaya kośa)*	Ether *(ākāśa)*	Sound *(śabda)*
The Self or *puruṣa*	Beyond the gross and subtle	

THE ELEMENTS AND THE *KOŚA* OF THE BODY

Know that the body has eight *kośa* (layer or sheath): *annamaya* (physical layer), *prāṇamaya* (physiological layer), *manōmaya* (psychological layer), *vijñānamaya* and *buddhimaya* (intellectual and direct perceptive layers), *ānandamaya* (the layer of joy), *cittamaya* (the layer of consciousness) and *ātmamaya* (the layer of the Self). The first seven are connected to the five elements: earth, water, fire, air, ether (see Table n. 13). The seventh element is consciousness, which is the Universal cosmic intelligence transformed as individual consciousness. The eighth is the Self. Yoga *sādhanā* is meant for one to progress from the physical layer towards the Self.

Patañjali has spoken more of the inner person. He only speaks at a few places of the outer person. These five elements, as well as cosmic intelligence, are considered as the coverings of the eternal Soul. All these seven layers or sheaths have to be unveiled through yogic *sādhanā* as they are the microcosmic structure of a human being *(piṇḍānda)*.*

In order to cross the bridge between *piṇḍānda* and *brahmāṇda* (microcosm and macrocosm – man and Universe, the nature and Self), we must understand the macrocosmic energy. The first principle of nature in each individual is the consciousness *(citta)* with its three components. I have said that *citta* is the corresponding element in the microcosm of the macrocosmic *Mahat*. This is why I consider *citta* as the seventh layer, the eight being *ātmamaya kośa* or the Self.** So far as my knowledge goes, I think that these are the seven frontiers or seven areas that each individual has to uncover to reach the abode of *ātman*.

SĀDHANĀKRIYĀ

What is *sādhanā*? *Sādhanā* is an action done with observation, reflection and precise performance. The word *sādhanā*, which is the title of the second chapter, appears as *abhyāsa* in the first chapter. *Abhyāsa* means to practise repeatedly an action over and over again. Though the word *sādhanā* is the title of the second chapter, it is not mentioned even once in the fifty-five *sūtras* of this chapter. Is it not interesting to note that the word *sādhanā*, used in this chapter, conveys the idea of *kriyā* and *anuṣṭhāna*? (*Y.S.*, II.1 and II.28). How is it that Patañjali calls *Sādhanā Pāda*, and uses the word *kriyā* at the very beginning? *Kriyā* means action, where the blending of the

---

* *Piṇḍānda*, literally "lump egg", stands for human body or microcosm. *Brahmāṇda*, literally "egg of Brahmā", refers to the Universe, macrocosm *(Advayatāraka-Upaniṣad*, - 9). It is very interesting to note that Patañjali dedicates fourteen of the thirty four *sūtras* on *Vibhūti* to the *saṁyama* on the macrocosm *(brahmāṇda)* and its elements (*Y.S.*, III.16-29), nineteen *sūtras* to the *saṁyama* on the microcosm *(piṇḍānda)* and its elements (*Y.S.*, III.30-48) and one on the *saṁyama* both on macrocosm and microcosm (*Y.S.*, III.49).

** See author's *Light on the Yoga Sūtras of Patañjali*, pp. 133. Harper Collins, London.

intelligence of the head and the heart takes place. Hence the term *kriyā yoga* is used to re-emphasise the quality of the *sādhanā*. Similarly, the *anuśāsanam* of I.1 and *anuṣṭhāna* (reverential and devoted practice) of II.28, convey the same meaning, as all petals of yoga require *anuśāsanam*.

From this it appears that *kriyā, abhyāsa, anuṣṭhāna* and *sādhanā* are synonymous terms. Ideas behind all these words are similar; the stress is that one must intensify one's *sādhanā* to expedite and pursue the goal at the earliest time possible. Compare *"tapaḥ svādhyāya Īśvarapraṇidhānāni kriyāyogaḥ"*, (*Y.S.*, II.1): "Burning zeal in practice, self-study and surrender to God are the acts of yoga", of this chapter whereas *yogānuśāsanam* (*Y.S.*, I.1): "Begins an exposition of the sacred art of yoga with prayers for divine blessings". The precept, the demand and the action are given to the *sādhaka* to reach the highest aim of life. Hence, there is no difference in the content though the terminologies are different.

Kriyā or action is *tapas*. The idea of *tapas* and self-discipline is discussed in the seventeenth chapter of *Bhagavad Gītā*. Each one is afflicted with pains. We study how to overcome the pains or to lessen them. For persons like you and me, these pains are dealt with very clearly in the *Sādhanā Pāda* of Patañjali. The object of this chapter is to guide us to understand and to begin yoga from the gross level of consciousness. It is the understanding of different sheaths of the body (see Table n.13).

In all levels of consciousness, practice of *āsana* and *prāṇāyāma* deals essentially with cleansing or *śuddhi kriyā*. This cleansing process will take place from the physical and physiological sheaths towards the *ākāśa* or space, the vehicle of sound and life.

These sheaths of the body are involved in purification, self-discipline and austerity. The first discipline of yoga is austerity *(tapas)*. The second discipline is the study of the self *(svādhyāya)*, to wash out all the subliminal impressions. This *pāda* guides the practitioner to move from the known towards the unknown. *Īśvara praṇidhāna* (path of *bhakti*) is the third discipline. It has two qualities. One is subjugation or subduing the *ahaṁkāra*. The second is the surrender of oneself to God. These three tiers of yoga are meant for the purification of body *(kāya)*, speech *(vāca)* and thought *(manasā)*, namely, purity in actions, good speech and good thoughts. That is why yoga is filled with right action *(karma)*, right knowledge *(jñāna)* and surrender *(bhakti)*.

Therefore, I think this *Sādhanā Pāda* is for us all.

It is easy to begin the practice with the second chapter and then proceed to the other three chapters. In the second chapter, the *annamaya, prāṇamaya* and the *manōmaya kośa* are subdued. The disciplining of *vijñānamaya kośa, buddhimaya kośa, ānandamaya kośa* and *cittamaya kośa* is discussed in the first and third chapters. When these are accomplished, then one reaches the sheath of the soul through the discipline offered in the fourth chapter.*

KLEŚA (AFFLICTION)

Why do we have to practise *tapas, svādhyāya* and *Īśvara praṇidhāna?* Is *sādhanā* essential? We are all entangled in *avidyā*. We are caught in fluctuating thoughts, which may be from defective intelligence, mental or emotional upheavals or attachment to things seen or heard or desired which are not obtainable. The abode of emotional defects is the house of the heart, while defective intelligence is in the house of the head.

Obstacles *(antarāya)* sprout from *citta*. This leads each individual to search for the betterment of his life with its underlying functions despite all obstacles. Yet fear is the subtlest of all *kleśa*, which is difficult even for a wise man to conquer.

Thus, the *Sādhanā Pāda* aims to rid man from these three intellectual, emotional and instinctive defects. As I said earlier, the cause of defects is want of spiritual knowledge created by lust, anger and greed; they become the disturbing factors of the consciousness.** These in turn create fluctuations in one to act directly or indirectly, inducing an effect, which in turn brings permanent pain and permanent unhappiness. The pain may be mild, medium or intense depending on the degrees of action. *Kriyā yoga* is the way to control these disturbances of the consciousness.

Patañjali says throughout his expositions that afflictions can be minimised through meditation on God. Total contemplation and absorption on God is the remedy for conquering *avidyā*. He gives the five mental states or modifications, *"pramāṇa viparyaya vikalpa nidrā smṛtayaḥ"*, (*Y.S.*, I.6): They are: correct knowledge, misperception, misconception, sleep and memory. Shri Krishna also says it in the seventeenth chapter of the *Bhagavad Gītā*, that *tāmo-, rājo-* and *sattva-guṇas* (inertia, activity and luminosity), fill these five types of fluctuations in each individual. Misperception or false knowledge and misconception, or imaginative knowledge are defects of the senses of perception, mind and intelligence. Sleep is the replica of the *tāmasic* nature of the vestments of the Self. Memory is the playground for the other four *vṛtti* of the consciousness. Interestingly, these five *vṛtti* bring five types of pain and five types of pleasure. It is very difficult to trace pleasure that is not mixed with pain.

---

* See table n. 11, p. 172.
** See table n. 6, p. 127.

A non-painful state may become painful and a painful state may become non-painful; for pain is hidden in pleasure and pleasure in pain. These cognisable and non-cognisable felt/unfelt feelings have been explained as *puṇya/apuṇya* and *dṛṣṭa/adṛṣṭa* (right action/wrong action, or virtues/vices and perceivable/invisible). Patañjali puts his thoughts not to make us intellectuals or scholars, but to the practical *sādhaka*. He says that the *ātman* is pure, but on account of coming in contact with objects, he becomes tainted. (*Y.S.*, II.12 – II.20). If a mirror is clean, it reflects clearly; if it is unclean, it does not reflect well. Here the mirror of the *ātman* is the intelligence; and hence intelligence has to be scrubbed from moment to moment to see that it does not function as an unclean mirror or an instrument to taint the *ātman*.

Lord Krishna says beautifully in *Bhagavad Gītā:*

> *"Dhūmenā'vriyate vahnir*
> *yathā'darśo malena ca /*
> *Yatho'lbenā'vṛto garbhas*
> *tathā tene'dam āvṛtam //*

(*B.G.*, III.38)

(As fire is covered by smoke, as a mirror by dust, as an embryo is enveloped by the womb, the *jīvātman* is enticed by mind, intelligence and ego).

THE EFFECT OF THE CONJUNCTION BETWEEN *PRAKṚTI* AND *PURUṢA*

Patañjali's *Yoga Sūtra*, *āyurvedic* texts and *sāṁkhya* philosophy state that the conjunction of the seer *(puruṣa)* with the seen *(prakṛti)* is the cause of pain. He advises to 'snap that thread' and says that "liberation *(mokṣa)* follows immediately with this dissociation". (*Y.S.*, II.17).

Having realised that it is not possible for all to snap the thread of conjunction of the *puruṣa* with *prakṛti*, he comes down to our mental level and makes us understand the *bhūtendriya*.* He wants us to use them in a right direction, through self-discipline and self-study so that they serve not only the seer, but move closer to the seer also.

The moment the *ātman* is evolved by the right usage of nature's vehicles, they recede from the seer. However, nature's vehicles will not easily leave ordinary persons. Patañjali says that chances are there even for the cultured *citta* to develop fissures or holes and his advice is to continue the *sādhanā* to retain the consciousness without fissures. As the *vijñānamaya kośa* has

---

* *Bhūtendriya* (*bhūta* = elements, *indriya* = eleven senses: mind, five senses of perception and five organs of action). See the author's *Light on the Yoga Sūtras of Patañjali*, especially under II.18, III.17 and III.44, and also pp. 124 -125, 213, 292.

the power to fascinate the self causing it to oscillate and fluctuate, the *sādhaka* has to use the potency of intelligence to keep the self away from the influences. I request you all to reflect very carefully on the meaning of the following aphorism.

Sattva puruṣayoḥ śuddhi sāmye kaivalyam iti (*Y.S.*, III.56).

When the exalted intelligence is as pure as the seer, perfect aloofness, unmingled with nature comes into his being. This is *kaivalya* or an indivisible state of existence.

HOW YOGA UTILISES THE CONJUNCTION BETWEEN *PRAKṚTI* AND *PURUṢA* FOR EVOLUTION

Having explained how the *bhūtendriya* are essential for human growth, Patañjali offers the eight petals of yoga to use the *bhūtendriya* through yogic *sādhanā* till the realisation of the Self.

The principle of *yama* is connected to discapline the *karmeñdriya* and the *niyama* to educate the *jñāneñdriya* in a right direction. The effect of each facet of *yama* is in *niyama*, and the effect of each facet of *niyama* is in *yama*. By following the principles of *ahiṁsā*, *śauca* (cleanliness) sets in. By following *satya*, *santoṣa* (contentment) sets in. *Brahmacarya* leads to *svādhyāya*. See how the five facets of *yama* are beautifully aligned with the five facets or five principles of *niyama* and vice versa (see Table n. 14). Whatever we possess, it is the gift or grace of God, and it has to be maintained by surrendering to Him. The moment we surrender, selfish motives are removed and the motive itself becomes different.

When we act with lust, greed and anger, they create various afflictions *(kleśa)* and fluctuations *(vṛtti)*, while with the practice of *āsana* and *prāṇāyāma*, the mind's afflictions and fluctuations are minimised or brought under control, as these cleanse and purify the five *kośa*.

When you are doing *Sālamba Śīrṣāsana* or *Halāsana*, do you study the state of your consciousness and how it moves. Similarly, do you observe the state of consciousness in other *āsanas?* That is why I said that the intelligence is connected to air *(vāyu)*, and its *tānmatra*, *sparṣa* or touch, and to consciousness *ākāśa*, sound *(śabda)*. Have you studied in each *āsana* where this power of touch and space are? The flow of intelligence and consciousness vary in each *āsana*. Thus, *āsana* and *prāṇāyāma* teach us to feel the movements of consciousness and show ways of making them unite as a single flow.

Table n. 14 - Interconnection of *yama* and *niyama*

Yama (moral injunctions)	*Niyama* (fixed observances)
Ahiṁsā (harmlessness)	*Śauca* (cleanliness)
Satya (truthfulness)	*Santoṣa* (contentment)
Asteya (non-stealing)	*Tapas* (religious zeal)
Brahmacarya (continence)	*Svādhyāya* (study which leads to the knowledge of the Self)
Aparigraha (non-greediness)	*Īśvara praṇidhāna* (surrender to God)

In the first chapter, Patañjali speaks of *prāṇāyāma*: *"Pracchardana vidhāraṇābhyāṁ vā prāṇasya"*, (Y.S., I.34); to experience calmness and quietness during a passive retention of the breath after soft and steady exhalation. In the second chapter, he shows the ways of controlling the *indriyas* and how they can be freed from the contact of their object. In the first chapter he explains *pratyāhāra* as *"Viṣayavatī vā pravṛttiḥ utpannā manasaḥ sthiti nibandhanī"*. (Y.S., I.35): "The consciousness becomes favourably disposed, serene and benevolent, by contemplating on an object that is perceived by the mind". This means that when one gets completely engrossed in a thought, the mind is controlled and silenced. If this is not *pratyāhāra*, then what is it? Further, he advises us to contemplate on enlightened sages who are free from desires and attachments. (Y.S., I.37). This is the technique through which the conquest of *manōmaya kośa* is achieved *Dhāraṇā* is meant for *jñānamaya kośa* and *dhyāna* for *ākāśamaya kośa* (the inner space) till it traces the *cidākāśa* – the seer.

According to Patañjali:

- *Deśa bandhaḥ cittasya dhāraṇā*. (Y.S., III.1): Attention on a point or region within the body or outside of it is *dhāraṇā*. It is the control of *vijñānamaya kośa*.
- *Tatra pratyaya ekatānāta dhyānam*. (Y.S., III.2): *Dhyāna* is an uninterrupted flow of attentive awareness from one end to the other. It is the control of *ākāśamaya kośa*.
- *Svapna nidrā jñāna ālambanaṁ vā*. (Y.S., I.38): To study, recollect and compare the states of mind during the wakeful state, the dream-filled and the dreamless sleepy states in order to experience a steady state of consciousness.

- *Viśokā vā jyotiṣmatī.* (*Y.S.,* I.36): To contemplate on the sorrowless luminous effulgent light, which is nothing but the intelligence of the heart, to achieve calmness.

See how systematically Patañjali offers the method to keep a single thought in the states of sleep, dream and attentiveness, and to study the light that never fades. All contemplation leads to mature steady intelligence, *"Ṛtambharā tatra prajñā".* (*Y.S.,* I.48): When consciousness dwells in wisdom, a truth bearing state of direct spiritual perception dawns.

The conquest of the eight petals of yoga comes when the *triguṇa* (the three *guṇas)* are used in the right direction in words, thoughts and deeds. When this happens the gate of the Self opens *(ātma sākṣātkāra).* This is the abode of the *ātman* where all oscillations culminate. In this unoscillating state, you become free only from *kleśa karma.* (*Y.S.,* IV.30).

Aṣṭadaḷa yoga is the code of conduct followed as reverential practice, in the form of self-discipline, self-study and surrender of oneself to God. They are the progressive foundations for one to become perfect. Then, one becomes free from *prakṛti* and the *guṇas* and hence, free from ambitions and aims in life. Thus, the pursuit of yoga ends when one dwells in the glory of the seer.

Patañjali begins with the call of yoga and ends where the rest is beyond words or explanations.

May God bless you all in your yogic practices.

YOGĀÑJALI *
YOGA – AN OFFERING TO MANKIND

Epitome of the four chapters of Patañjali's *YOGA SŪTRA*

SAMĀDHI PĀDA

Patañjali's *Yoga Sūtra* expound the art and science of disciplining the conduct of man in order to enable him to experience the supreme goal of life, so that he drinks the spiritual ambrosia of poise and peace under all circumstances. Actually, this is the summum bonum of Indian philosophy.

KNOWING THE MIND

Before dealing with the discipline of yoga, Patañjali analyses the consciousness or *citta* through his rational and scientific method. The mind is like mercury, very difficult to grasp because it easily slips away. Patañjali concludes that when the *citta* is stilled, it rests in its source, the seer. If the *citta* is not subdued, it gets absorbed by the objects heard, seen, smelt, felt or tasted and through these creates for itself sorrow, misery and unhappiness.

There are five senses of perception for the consciousness to wander in, amassing various imprints. These imprints are painful, nonpainful and pleasing. The *citta* gathers these imprints through direct and valid perception, false thoughts and behaviour, imagination, sleep and memory. The *citta* or consciousness travels in these fields.

Direct perception is dependent upon one's experience and inference and upon the perusal of sacred books or utterances by authoritative masters. Perverse thinking leads to false conceptions and actions. Imagination may remain on a verbal or visual level without facts. Sleep is a state of forgetfulness of oneself, while memory is an assortment of accumulated experiences.

---

* From *70 Glorious Years of Yogacharya B.K.S. Iyengar*, p. 147. published by *The Light on Yoga Research Trust*

All these contribute to the formation of various moods and modes of the thinking mind, which may make or mar his cultural development. They form the base upon which civilisation is developed or destroyed.

EDUCATION OF THE MIND

After discussing the causes for the moods and modes in thinking, Patañjali shows ways of controlling them. The methods prescribed are practice and renunciation. A bird cannot fly with one wing. Practice and renunciation are the two wings with which man ascends to the height of the spiritual world.

Practice involves methodology and when that methodical practice is maintained uninterruptedly for a long time, with attention and poise, it controls one's moods and builds up stability and poise in body and mind, leading one towards a good foundation.

Things that disturb the path of practice and hinder progress are to be renounced. When practice and renunciation are followed with intensity, the goal of silencing the consciousness is attainable. Then there is stillness and clarity. This leads us to explore further to know what is beyond consciousness. Temptations do not daunt the practitioner and he becomes one within himself along with the vestures or sheaths he wears. He begins to consider seriously, think ably and reason with clarity. From here, he moves towards elation that touches the self *(asmitā).* He gets engrossed in this state and reaches a state of quietude, which is an alert passive state. This alert passive state is a crossroads in the spiritual path. It becomes a spiritual desert as he does not know which road to take. He may become stuck there forever. In this state, the brain is not only silenced but becomes an inactive object. This state of quietude is *manōlaya.* This *manōlaya* state can be experienced while practising inverted *āsanas* such as *Śīrṣāsana*, *Setu Bandha Sarvāṅgāsana*, *Viparīta Karaṇi*, *Halāsana*, or *Uttānāsana* when done in a modified way so as to rest and bring stillness and silence in all the organs of action and perception. One is able to feel that sense of alert passivity and experience a state of witnessing. Here, the observer and the observed lose their identities. As long as this state of quietude remains in the intelligence of head and heart, the hidden tendencies also remain inactive and subdued, but they rise up as soon as that passive state disappears and the mind becomes active to the world.

If this state is mistaken as the highest goal of yoga, then one's life would be like that of King Triśanku. He was sent to heaven by Sage Viśvāmitra, but Indra (the King of Gods) refused him and pushed him back. Burning with rage, Viśvāmitra ordered the king to remain where he was and created a new heaven for him. Thus, the king could neither reach heaven nor was he allowed to return to the earth. The same is the state of a yogi at this juncture. No doubt, this state of achievement is a great success in the yogic *sādhanā*. If the *sādhaka* is stuck in that state, he loses the feel of his body. Though nature does not disturb such a *sādhaka*, he still gets caught between the void and the non-void.

If he is prudent with this success, he intensifies his *sādhanā* from the state of *manōlaya* and to go towards *amanaskatva* aloneness, freedom and beatitude.

If the intensity of practice is strong, the *sādhaka* reaches that goal fast. If he slackens his efforts, the goal recedes further and further.

WAYS OF ACHIEVING THE STATE OF ALONENESS

There are many ways of achieving the state of aloneness or *amanaskatva*. Patañjali gives various means, he speaks first on the surrender of oneself to God. He speaks of God, by defining God as the "Supreme Being", totally free from afflictions and fruits of actions. In HIM abides the matchless seed of all knowledge. HE is the FIRST and FOREMOST amongst all masters and teachers.

HE is symbolically known by the word *āuṁ*. This word is divine as it stands in praise of the DIVINE'S FULFILMENT. No word can be uttered without the alphabet *ā*, *u* and *ṁ*. As *ā, u, ṁ* are the seeds of all words it becomes a divine syllable. These three sounds represent the word of contact to communicate and commune with one another as well as the Universal Soul. That is why God is worshipped in India by the word *āuṁ*, known as *praṇava*. It is repeated, to get the feel of its true meaning, in order to eradicate the hindrances that come in the path of health, spiritual success and freedom.

THE HINDRANCES TO SELF REALISATION

The hindrances to spiritual health are ailments, mental lethargy, disbelief, carelessness, physical lethargy, sensual gratification, living in the world of illusions, missing the point and inability to maintain steadiness in practice. They are further aggravated through sorrow, fickle-mindedness, tremor of the body and heavy breathing.

WAYS OF COUNTERING THE IMPEDIMENTS

The ways of countering the impediments to minimise or eradicate them are many. They are checked by either adherence to a single-minded effort in *sādhanā* or by friendliness, compassion and goodwill towards all. Developing the will to be indifferent towards pleasure and pain, virtue and vice helps to build up equipoise in the mind, both within and without. Patañjali also explains several methods to be easily adopted by the *sādhaka* that diffuse the forces of consciousness, according to their mental frame. These are: (a) holding the breath after each exhalation, (b) getting involved in an interesting topic conducive to the principles of yoga, (c) contemplation of the luminous, effulgent, sorrowless light (the Self), (d) following the methods adopted by noble personalities, (e) maintaining a single state of awareness in the wakeful, sleep and dream states, and lastly (f) contemplation on an all-absorbing and conducive thought or object that enables the mind to spread evenly in its abode, the body.

When these methods are judiciously and meticulously practised, the *sādhaka* gets control over his mind. He begins to see the objects clearly whether they be near or far, infinitely big or infinitesimally small, and he develops a highly sensitive mind to remain choiceless, stainless and pure. When this state is felt, then he realises that the self, the seeker and the instrument used to see or seek is none other than himself, the seer. From then on his words, their meanings and feelings are so well blended that it is as if a new light of wisdom has dawned upon him. This new light of wisdom, being intuitive, is independent of anything heard, read or learnt, makes the *sādhaka* intensify his *sādhanā* further to gain illumined unalloyed wisdom, bliss and poise which is beyond the reach of the mind or consciousness. This is the *amanaskatva* state. From here the core of the being shines brilliantly on its own. This Patañjali calls *nirbīja samādhi* or the seedless state of *samādhi*.

SĀDHANĀ PĀDA

As the consciousness *(citta)*, is close to the self, Patañjali compiled the *Yoga Sūtra* beginning with the spiritual quest, as the intellectual calibre of that time was very high. For our own standard of intelligence this quest becomes *antaraṅga sādhanā* or the inner quest. Now, the culturing of consciousness appears next to impossible without first cultivating the senses of perception and the mind.

After taking the intellectuals of those days towards the pinnacle of yoga, Patañjali, realising that the intellectual stature may not be the same, next gives the basics of yoga to build up within us an extra-ordinary, sensitive intelligence from our average intelligence through his expositions in the *Sādhanā Pāda*. He begins with the visible components – the body and senses – so that even the average intelligent man may find a point of access to undertake yogic *sādhanā*. Here, he unfolds the path involving the training of the external gross body (the visible soul of man). From training the body, he proceeds towards the mind, intelligence and consciousness to explore the true being that is within man.

He begins this chapter by introducing *kriyā yoga* or yoga of action. These actions or *kriyā* are: enthusiastic and diligent practice *(tapas)*, study of spiritual scriptures to become familiar with morals and ethics and comprehend one's own being from the body to the self *(svādhyāya)*, and finally the surrender of oneself to God *(Īśvara praṇidhāna)*. He coins these actions as *kriyā* in order to reach the goal of self-realisation.

ORIGIN OF SORROW

Patañjali explains the five types of causes which inflict sorrow and suffering. These sorrows appear or enter man's mind on account of want of correct understanding *(avidyā)*, pride *(asmitā)*, attachment *(rāga)*, aversion *(dveṣa)* and fear of death *(abhiniveśa)*. The causes of sorrow may remain latent, hidden, attenuated or highly active. *Asmitā* is like two sides of a coin. If one side represents pride, the other side represents the cultured individual self. If pride dominates, the self gets submerged. If the self dominates, then pride fades out.

Mistaking or taking for granted the transient as everlasting, the impure as pure, pain as pleasure, worldly pleasure as spiritual joy, and pride or ego as the Self is lack of knowledge *(avidyā)* or perverse knowledge *(viparyaya jñāna)*. This lack of understanding becomes the breeding ground of sorrows.

Desire leads to attachment and non-fulfilment in desire leads to hatred *(dveṣa)*. Clinging to the preservation of one's life's is *abhineveśa*.

Past actions mould the present and future life. Good actions attract less misery, while bad deeds harvest sorrow. Past actions affect the present life and lives to come. They shape birth and the span of life to experience their effects in this life. So a wise man notices the tinge of sorrow even in the highest of pleasures and likes to remain aloof from those, whereas ordinary souls get enmeshed in the mixed joys and sorrows.

Sorrow originates on account of lack of understanding of the conjunction between the seer *(puruṣa)* and the seen *(prakṛti)*. The external world lures and suffocates the individual desire and its non-fulfilment. Nature and her beauties are there for enjoyment, or for freedom. Only prudent, judicious use of them is needed to experience the bliss that is free from mixed pleasure and pain. Here, Patañjali explains through the eight-pettalled yoga how to keep pleasure and sorrow in abeyance and postponement.

Pain may be self-inflicted *(ādhyātmika)*, hereditary *(ādhidaivika)*, or through imbalance of the elements in one's constitution *(ādhibhautika)*. Lust, anger and greed precipitate one to participate in these by direct indulgence *(kṛta)*, or by provocation *(kārita)*, or by countenancing *(anumodita)*, resulting in mild *(mṛdu)*, moderate *(madhyama)* or intense *(adhimātra)* sorrow.

By a minute analysis of the causes of lust, anger and greed, one may directly counter or subdue them through the cultivation of their opposites.

NATURE'S MAP

In order to know the relationship between nature and *puruṣa*, let me stretch the map of nature and the way it functions.

Nature has five elements: earth, water, fire, air and ether. These five elements have subtle manifestations: odour, taste, sight, touch and sound or vibration. Odour is connected to earth, taste to water, sight to fire, touch to air and sound to ether. Nature has its first principle in *mahat* or cosmic intelligence. This cosmic intelligence *(mahat)* is transformed in human beings as consciousness or *citta*, composed of mind, intelligence and pride or ego. Then there are five senses of perception (eyes, ears, nose, tongue, skin) and five organs of action (arms, legs, mouth, generative and excretory organs). In addition to these nature has been bestowed with three qualities, *(guṇa)* namely; illumination *(sattva)*, action and motion *(rajas)* and inertia *(tamas)*. All functions of nature's manifestations are permeated by these three qualities. *Puruṣa* uses nature's manifestations either for enjoyment *(bhoga)*, or for emancipation.

NATURE *(PRAKṚTI)*

Prakṛti or nature is divided into specified or defined *(viśeṣa)*, unspecified or undefined *(aviśeṣa)*, phenomenal *(liñga)* and noumenal *(aliñga)*.

The elements, intelligence (both cosmic and individual), mind, senses of perception and organs of action are definable and distinguishable. Ego or pride *(ahaṁkāra)* and the subtle manifestations of the elements (odour, taste, sight, touch and sound) are indefinable and are entities in themselves. All these have the power to merge into the root of nature *(mūlā prakṛti)*, after enabling the seer to realise his own nature.

ĀTMĀ (PURUṢA)

Puruṣa, the seer or the Self *(ātman)*, is pure. Its knowledge and its existence is eternal and unchanging, whereas nature's characteristic is to change. *Puruṣa* is the knower of everything. It is nature's intelligence that ensnares him and sullies his purity. Like a mirror covered with dust, the seer is coerced with its mirror the intelligence. If this intelligence follows the path of yoga, it gets cleansed and becomes equal to the seer. Then the seer reflects himself like a clean mirror that reflects images accurately.

SAPTA PRĀNTABHŪMI PRAJÑĀ: SEVEN STATES OF KNOWLEDGE

Practice of yoga brings about sevenfold wisdom, or *prajñā*. These are: (1) what has to be known is known, (2) what has to be discarded is discarded, (3) what has to be attained is attained, (4) what has to be done is done, (5) the peace which has to be acquired is acquired, (6) the consciousness which has to be freed, is freed and (7) the Self – the seer is sighted.*

THE EIGHT PETALS OF YOGA

After explaining the wisdom that accrues from yoga, let us move to know the eight fold petals of yoga. They are *yama* (restraint), *niyama* (discipline), *āsana* (posture), *prāṇāyāma* (breath control), *pratyāhāra* (mind-control), *dhāraṇā* (attention), *dhyāna* (meditation) and *samādhi* (total absorption).

Yama and *niyama* are tradition-bound. *Āsana*, *prāṇāyāma* and *pratyāhāra* are progressive *sādhanā* as they help to explore the inner being of the *sādhaka*. *Dhāraṇā*, *dhyāna* and *samādhi* are the natural terminations of yoga *(yoga svarūpa)*, as *vibhūti*. All these eight fold petals woven together are called *aṣṭāṅga* yoga.

YAMA AND *NIYAMA*

The five parts of *yama* are *ahiṁsā* (non-violence), *satya* (truthfulness), *asteya* (non-stealing), *brahmacarya* (celibacy) and *aparigraha* (non-covetousness).

Honest and faithful, wishing no evil in word, thought and deed; rejecting gifts as they lead to greed, and disciplined living are the *yamas*.

Ahiṁsā disarms hostility in others. *Satya* carries power with words. *Asteya* brings the gems of treasures. *Brahmacarya* leads to spiritual knowledge. *Aparigraha* trains one to live fearlessly.

Niyama has five disciplines. They are *śauca* (cleanliness), *santoṣa* (contentment), *tapas* (religious fervour), *svādhyāya* (study of the self) and *Īśvara praṇidhāna* (surrender of the self to the Supreme).

---

* For further details, see the author's *Light on the Yoga Sūtras of Patañjali*, pp. 130-132. Harper Collins, London.

Śauca cleanses the body for its divine occupant. *Santoṣa* cultivates cheerfulness and benevolence. *Tapas* purges and purifies the body, senses and mind. *Svādhyāya* inculcates knowledge of the inner divinity. *Īśvara praṇidhāna* is the surrender to the Creator, the Supreme God.

Hence, these two aspects build up a noble character in the practitioner.

ĀSANA

Āsana means a posture. Posture is the positioning of the body as a whole, with the involvement of mind and Self. It has 'pose' and 'repose'. 'Pose' is the artistic assumption of a certain position with total awareness and 'repose' is to retain and maintain evenly the physical, mental, vital, *prāṇic* and spiritual metabolism, with unity, calmness and composure.

Āsana becomes perfect when proficiency has been acquired and the effort of the mind and consciousness becomes effortless and natural. *Āsana* helps to transform one by taking one away from the awareness of the body towards awareness of the Self. In the perfection of *āsana*, the polarities between body and mind, mind and Self, disappear.

PRĀṆĀYĀMA

Patañjali categorically states that *prāṇāyāma* should be undertaken only after proficiency in all the *āsanas* and not in one *āsana* alone, as is often suggested.

Normal breathing flows irregularly according to one's physical and emotional state. So one has to deliberately regulate this zigzag flow of breath with attention. When this attention is brought in the flow of the inbreath and outbreath know that *prāṇāyāma* has begun.

Prāṇāyāma consists of inhalation *(pūraka)*, exhalation *(recaka)* and retention *(kuṁbhaka)*. Elongation and prolongation of *pūraka* and *recaka* is time *(kāla)*. The inhalation-retention and exhalation-retention is done by the torso *(deśa)*, while precision of movement *(saṁkhya)* is maintained through the rhythmic, smooth flow of breath. Please know that in *pūraka* the causal body *(kāraṇa śarīra)* moves from the inner depth towards the vastness of the body, covering the entire place of the gross part of the torso *(deśa)* with space *(ākāśa)*. Retention *(antara kuṁbhaka)* is to hold on to that created space as long as possible without shrinking the place. In *antara kuṁbhaka* the causal, the subtle and the gross bodies are merged into a single unit. In *recaka* the gross body *(deśa)* moves closer to merge with the inner most body via the inner body without shrinking in place but receding the space. In *bāhya kuṁbhaka* there is the feel of that state of oneness where the gross and subtle bodies unite with the causal body. This is *prāṇāyāma*.

From the deliberate *prāṇāyāma*, (*Y.S.*, II. 49 & 50) Patañjali adds one more *prāṇāyāma* that transcends the deliberately modulated method; namely, inhalation *(pūraka)*, exhalation *(recaka)* and retention *(kuṁbhaka)*. Here, the breathing is done by the breath itself, in an unpremeditated way.

Practice of *prāṇāyāma* not only removes the veil of haziness covering the light of intelligence, but makes the mind a fit instrument for meditation.*

PRATYĀHĀRA

As the mind is cleared from haziness by *prāṇāyāma*, *pratyāhāra* practice enables the mind directly to refrain itself and fall away from its entanglement and involvement in the senses of perception and organs of action, whereas in the earlier petals of yoga, the mind was made to come under control with the help of the senses of perception and the organs of action in an indirect way.

Table n. 15 – The *yogāṅga* and their corresponding *nirodha*

Aṅga or petal	*Nirodha* or the fluctuations restrained	
Yama	***Karmeñdriyavṛtti nirodha*** (cessation of movements of the organs of action)	***Guṇavṛtti nirodha*** (cessation of the movements of the elements and their qualities by the practice of *yama* and *niyama*)
Niyama	***Jñāneñdriyavṛtti nirodha*** (cessation of movements of the senses of perception)	
Āsana	***Snāyuvṛtti nirodha*** (cessation of movements of all constituents of the body - whether nerves, tendons, muscles, veins, etc... and their faculties)	
Prāṇāyāma	***Prāṇavṛtti nirodha*** (cessation of movements of *prāṇa*)	

* For details, see author's *Light on Yoga* and *Light on Prāṇāyāma* – Harper Collins, London.

Pratyāhāra	***Manōvṛtti nirodha*** (cessation of movements of mind)
Dhāraṇā	***Buddhivṛtti nirodha*** (cessation of movements of intelligence)
Dhyāna	***Ahaṁkāravṛtti nirodha*** (cessation of movements of ego)
Samādhi	***Cittavṛtti nirodha*** (cessation of the movements of consciousness)

When the mind becomes ripe for meditation the senses rest quietly in their places and cease importuning the mind for their gratification.

From here on, the mind that acted as a bridge between the senses and the consciousness, turns inwards towards the intelligence and consciousness to explore its spiritual wealth – the Soul *(ātman)*.

VIBHŪTI PĀDA

In the previous chapter, Patañjali gave the reasons for sorrow that affects the intelligence and showed practical ways to unveil the dust that covers it so that the *sādhaka* develops a clear head and an untainted mind. When clarity in head and cleanliness in mind are established, then he says that the intelligence and the consciousness become ripe instruments to do meditation on the real Self.

This chapter shows ways of stabilising the subtlest parts of nature, namely, intelligence, ego (the feeling of the 'I' or 'me') and consciousness. In order to sublimate these three finer sheaths of the seer, concentration *(dhāraṇā)*, meditation *(dhyāna)* and abscrption *(samādhi)*, are introduced in this *pāda*.

Dhāraṇā is *buddhivṛtti nirodha*, for developing steady and enlightened, matured intelligence. *Dhyāna* is *ahaṁkāravṛtti nirodha* or the sublimation of *ahaṁkāra*, the 'I', and the expansion and diffusion of the consciousness *(citta parikarma)*. *Samādhi* is to move from this state of consciousness *(citta prasādana)*, towards the gracefulness of the seer *(ātma prasādana)*.

SAṀYAMA

After explaining *dhāraṇā, dhyāna* and *samādhi* Patañjali says that the blending together of these three petals is *saṁyama.*

From this integration the *sādhaka* realises that the contemplator, the instrument used for contemplation and the objects on which he contemplated are nothing but the 'seer' in him. Thus, he realises that the subject, the object and the instrument used are one and the same.

A GUIDE TO THE REFINED *SĀDHAKA*

Patañjali guides the refined *sādhaka* trace the movements of each action and each thought, which spring forth in a definite order or sequence. By retracing his steps, the *sādhaka* co-ordinates his actions and thoughts without creating space between thought and action. This brings in him extraordinary powers – *vibhūti.*

Patañjali describes thirty-eight properties of yoga. Out of these, even if one of them is felt then the *sādhaka* should note that he is on the right path in his practice of yoga* and that the methods followed are appropriate. With this he warns the *sādhaka* not to mistake them as the ultimate goals of yoga, but to continue the *sādhanā* so that the gate of everlasting bliss opens to experience the indivisible, absolute state of existence.

KĀLA OR TIME

Patañjali explains that time has three movements. These are past, present and future. Moment without movement is the present and the present is the eternal now. Moment is changeless and real. When it slips into movement, it becomes time creating changes. As it rolls into movement, the past and future appear and the moment disappears. Forward movement of moments is the future and movements prior to the moment is the past. Because of this movement of moments, perception of objects may vary at different times, though the objects remain as their own entities. Hence, action and fulfilment differ according to the movement of time. If the mind and intelligence are kept aware of moments without being caught in the movement of moments, then a feeling of no time is experienced. Then the *sādhaka* becomes a *vivekaja jñāni* or *tāraka jñāni* with exalted intelligence which gradually leads him towards *vivekakhyāti,* the crown of wisdom.

This exalted intelligence is pure, untainted and uncontaminated and remains as clear as the Self. Then, his body, cells, senses, mind, intelligence, consciousness and conscience ring the bell of the Self. This is *kaivalya* – an indivisible absolute state of aloneness.

---

* See *Light on the Yoga Sūtras of Patañjali,* III.16-50, 52, 54-55. Harper Collins, London.

KAIVALYA PĀDA

This chapter is very exhaustive but difficult to understand. Here the theme is the content of consciousness that is untarnished and unsullied by white *(sāttvic)*, grey *(rājasic)* or black *(tāmasic)* actions, (*Y.S.*, IV. 7), and remains pure, absolute and divine.

This refinement of consciousness is precipitated by propitious birth, use of herbs, incantations, spiritual fervour or meditation. In the *sādhaka*, nature's energy flows in abundance and accelerates the process of evolution, enabling them to gain spiritual insight.

HOW THE MASTERS SERVE THE WORLD

Patañjali shows how these realised souls should serve the world usefully without tainting their intelligence or their inner peace by defining the actions that they have to follow.

Actions are of four types, black, white, grey and without any taint in them. This last type of action is pure, sorrowless and outside the laws of cause and effect. The realised yogi performs his actions free of desire, pride and motivation.

Cause and effect are nothing but the reactions of actions. Memory links together the chain of cause and effect, even across many lives, whether in human form or otherwise, because they are encoded in our deep memory and turn the spokes of the *kārmic* wheel to experience it. By yoga we can keep them in postponement or in abeyance or make them leave no impressions or excite no reactions.

VĀSANA (IMPRESSION) IS ETERNAL AS LONG AS IGNORANCE PERSISTS

Impressions *(vāsanā)* and desires *(āśā)* exist from the beginning of time and are stored in the memory. Hence, memory connects impressions of past actions as if the present life is just a continuation of the past. In a perfect yogi's life, desires and impressions have an end; when the mechanism of cause and effect is disconnected by pure, motiveless action, desire and attachment wither and fall away as the yogi transcends beyond actions and reactions.

As I pointed out earlier, though nature is eternal, the qualities are ever changing. This blending of the qualities of nature creates diversity in the mind. So it often perceives objects at different times, in different ways. As the untrained mind has many qualities of mood and behaviour, they cause the mind to be moulded and remoulded due to the functioning of the *guṇa* throughout one's life. As the *guṇa* move in rhythmic unity, intellectual development differs qualitatively in each person and everyone sees objects differently though the essence of the objects does not change. For example, a lover finds pleasure in a woman while the same woman is an object of pain to a rival and an object of no interest to an ascetic.

The yogi studies in depth this rhythmic mutation of the *guṇa* and keeps aloof from it. He rests in his own true Self and keeps the essence aloof from the essence of himself and of the object seen. Hence, he is free from bias and free from the reaction of *karma.*

PURUṢA AND *CITTA*

The seer is ever present, changeless, constant, ever-luminous. He is aware of all mutations taking place in his consciousness.

If Self is the seed, the conscience is its seedling. When the seedling opens out with a stem, this is consciousness. This branches off as 'I', intelligence and mind. They grow as trunk and branch out as leaves as *vṛtti* or thought-waves and become the objects of the Self. As the branches of the tree have no existence of their own without the root, similarly, the consciousness has no existence of its own, but is dependent upon the Self. It borrows light from the Self and hence *citta* cannot be subject and object at the same time. As the objects of the world are knowable to the *citta, citta* is a knowable object to the Self. Only intelligence acts as a bridge to merge the *citta* with *puruṣa* or the *ātman.*

There is a good analogy in the *Muṇḍaka Upaniṣad,* which explains the two facets of consciousness. This will enlighten us to know the difference between the *citi* (Self) and *citta* (consciousness).

It is said that two birds were resting on the same tree and became good companions. One of them remained steady, observant and free of involvements. The other one moved restlessly from branch to branch and came closer to the first bird. The moment it came close, it too became silent and restful like the first bird. The first bird here represents the Self while the second bird represents consciousness which plays a dual role of creating strife, or uniting with the Self.

The *citi* (seer, Self) is a passive omniscient witness, whereas the *citta* (created or 'sprouted' consciousness) is active and impressionable involving itself in direct relationship with the outside world. When this involvement of *citta* is brought to a stillness, then it gravitates towards the *citi* or *puruṣa.*

Yet Patañjali cautions that even evolved yogis are not beyond the danger of relapse. Inattention or pride creates fissures in the *sādhaka.* Then old thoughts and habits may resurge and disturb the harmony that was cultivated by yogic *sādhanā.*

If the yogi's unwavering, indivisible state is sustained then virtue pours from his heart like torrential rain *(dharmamegha samādhi). Dharma* means duty and *megha* means cloud. The religion of clouds is to pour rain. The moment it has rained the clouds disappear and the sun's rays shine forth. Similarly, the consciousness gets transformed through yogic discipline, with the crown of wisdom. Here ends yoga.

PEARLS OF YOGIC WISDOM

Yogena cittasya padena vācām
Malaṁ śarīrasya ca vaidyakena
Yopākarottaṁ pravaraṁ munīnāṁ
Patañjaliṁ prāñjalirānato'smi

Ābāhu puruṣākāraṁ
Śaṅkha cakrāsi dhāriṇam
Sahasra śirasaṁ śvetaṁ
Praṇamāmi Patañjalim

(To the noblest of sages, Patañjali,
Who gave yoga for serenity of mind,
Grammar for purity of speech,
And medicine for the health of the body, I bow.

I prostrate before Patañjali,
Whose upper body has a human form,
Whose arms hold a conch and disc,
Who is crowned by a thousand-headed cobra,
O incarnation of Ādiśeṣa, my salutations to Thee).

Friends, to speak on Patañjali's *Yoga Sūtra* is not easy. As you all know, it is a concise and concentrated book. It is difficult to penetrate the feelings of Patañjali's words without his blessings. Today is an auspicious day to learn about this great work. May the blessings of Lord Patañjali be on us, may his wisdom dawn on us, so that the glimpse of his understanding may flash on us.

I request all of you to recite the invocation on Patañjali when you start your classes. If you cannot recite it in *Sanskṛt*, you may recite the translation. In this way, we may invoke his presence at the time of our practices. We recite this invocation for the simple reason that we consider him as our *guru* in yoga. This great sage gave us grammar for right speech, medicine for health and yoga for mind culture. When we are in our *yoga sādhanā*, we should think of him and pay our reverential respects to him so that our minds may be tuned to the good thoughts of his works.

Patañjali finished first his works on grammar and medicine, but he must have been very unhappy within himself feeling that something was missing. He thought, "I have given the grammar for the use of right words and I have shown various ways to develop health, but I have not said anything about the cultivation of the mind". Some commentators say this is the reason for which the first *sūtra** begins with the word *atha* which means 'now'. Some people translate this *sūtra* as "Now, the exposition of yoga", interpreting the 'now' to explain that the science of yoga didn't exist before Patañjali. But Patañjali did not create yoga. He only gave a format to what had been said in the past. The term 'now' does not indicate a new idea. It is like in our classes. We say, "Now, come on, do *Trikoṇāsana*," or "Now, do *Pārśvakoṇāsana!"* Don't we say that? This use of the word 'now' is to bring the hearer's attention to the present situation. So Patañjali was bringing the attention of his readers to a past tradition which had been evaded or neglected. Also, *anuśāsanam* does not mean exposition (as it is usually translated in English). I refer to the oral tradition of the sages (sayings passed down). *Śāsana* means 'code of law to oneself', like the law codes of this world. However this book is a code for the spiritual development of mankind and contains direct instructions in the code of right living. Hence the *sūtra* begins with 'Now', and explains what the code of conduct for right living is.

Patañjali thought, "I have dealt with health and with the usage of words," and said, "Now let me speak about the mind." His words refer to the co-ordination of various texts, *Vedas* and *Upaniṣads*, which were scattered, regarding the theory and practices of yoga. He systematised and presented them as a subject comprehensible to the truly interested students. When the composition of the text was over, he disappeared from this world. As the story goes, he joined his Master, Lord Vishnu, to please Him with his dance. The text *Pātañjala Yoga Sūtra* has survived till today. As I said, there are still discussions going on about the exact date of its composition, but as students of yoga we are more concerned about what Patañjali said than about his time or place of birth.

THE *YOGA SŪTRA*

The *Yoga Sūtra* is the seed for the total growth of a human being. In the first three *sūtra*, Patañjali sums up the essence of the whole work.

---

* *Atha yogānuśāsanam* (*Y.S.*, I.1) (Now begins, auspiciously, the discipline of yoga for self enlightenment).

Atha yogānuśāsanam (*Y.S.,* I.1).

Now begins, auspiciously, the discipline of yoga for self-enlightenment.

Yogaḥ cittavṛtti nirodhaḥ (*Y.S.,* I.2).

Yoga is the cessation of the movements within the consciousness.

Tadā draṣṭuḥ svarūpe avasthānam (*Y.S.,* I.3).

When the consciousness is silent, the seer *(ātmā)* radiates in his own grandeur.

Anuśāsanam is a code, a discipline. What do you develop through this discipline? You are able to restrain the consciousness (*Y.S.,* I.2). But how can the consciousness *(citta)* be restrained *(nirodhaḥ)?* As thoughts are uncontrollable, so too is *citta.* Before we begin to control the consciousness, we must first understand its functions. This understanding will come as we discover the profound meaning of the terms that Patañjali uses in his very first *sūtra.*

Patañjali concludes this summary by saying that as soon as the consciousness is restrained, the core of the being surfaces and rests in its abode (*Y.S.,* I.3). The self is like the cobra, the cobra does not raise its hood unless it is provoked. Usually the consciousness prevents the hood of the self from surfacing. And that is why the consciousness must be restrained because only then can the Self *(draṣṭuḥ)* be woken up and brought to the surface. The moment the *citta* is successfully restrained, you enter a state of beatitude and freedom. You feel this beatitude, because the mind gets dissolved in the seat of the Self, and then the Self acts directly.

If the first three *sūtras* cover the whole subject of yoga, then why the hundred and ninety three extra *sūtras?* The ancient texts of India always begin with the conclusion and then move on to details. Today, books are quite different; the authors begin at the base and move towards the summit. In ancient books the initial summary was there to attract the intellectuals and allow them the freedom to ponder its meaning and then to draw them into the main text.

Anuśāsanam is intimately related to *yama* and *niyama.* Ethical disciplines are deeply involved in character building. We are made up of three *guṇa.* The mind is sometimes dull, sometimes vibrant and sometimes serene. You have experienced these states at one time or the other. They come in a flash and disappear in a flash. Through the science of yoga we learn to free our mind from the states of inertia and vibration and keep it everlastingly in a state of serenity. In order to reach that serenity and to retain it, Patañjali arranged various methods and techniques of yoga in the four chapters, *Samādhi Pāda, Sādhanā Pāda, Vibhūti Pāda* and *Kaivalya Pāda.*

SAMĀDHI PĀDA

(Chapter on Total Absorption)

Samādhi contains two words. *Sama* means 'alike', 'similar', 'auspiciousness', 'goodness' and 'virtue'; *ādhi* means 'origin' and 'over and above'. Hence, *samādhi* means, "to be at one with the *ātman* which is over and above everything". In *sūtra* I.3, Patañjali says that the *ātman,* the core of the being, should be awakened with virtuous *sādhanā*. Then the core is to be diffused throughout the body to illuminate the fibres, blood cells, nerve cells, the senses of perception, the organs of action, mind, intelligence and consciousness. This is the true meaning of *samādhi*. *Samādhi* is not just 'trance'. *Ādhi* refers to the core of our being, the root of our existence, and when the goodness of this core fills the entire human system, it is *samādhi*. The first chapter is named *Samādhi Pāda*, as it deals with the internal practices *(antaraṅga sādhanā)* for restraining as well as silencing the consciousness. It is very difficult for people of average intelligence to understand the internal practices.

CITTA (CONSCIOUSNESS)

Why does Patañjali choose to talk about the most difficult subject first? He wants to know the root that causes afflictions and sufferings and begins by defining the first fundamental term, *citta;* then he explains its constitution and its functions. I feel it is especially important for students of yoga to distinguish that mind is not *citta* but a part of *citta*. *Citta* includes three different aspects of the human being: *manas*, *buddhi* and *ahaṁkāra*.

Suppose the *manas* dominates the entire region of the *citta*, then the *buddhi* and the *ahaṁkāra* get compressed and the *manas* appears to be the whole *citta*. Suppose you are given some deep subject to think about, then the *buddhi* swamps the *citta* whilst the *manas* and the *ahaṁkāra* are compressed. If the *ahaṁkāra* dominates, the *buddhi* and the *manas* gets overshadowed. If you are totally absorbed in something without the functioning of the *manas* or the *buddhi* or the *ahaṁkāra*, then it is the *citta* that appears like a ray of light.

This is where one fails to distinguish between the various compartments of the *citta* or consciousness. The Indian sages have precisely described the mind as the outer cover of the intelligence, the intelligence as the outer cover of the 'I', 'I' as the outer cover of the consciousness, and the whole of consciousness as the outer cover of the Self.

CITTA VṚTTI: THE FLUCTUATIONS IN CONSCIOUSNESS

The three layers that form the consciousness have their origin in the Self; they 'sprout' from the Self. These different aspects of *citta* create *vṛtti*, translated as 'thought-waves'. It is the presence of these thought-waves that creates a 'disturbed state of mind' or 'stressful mind'. Patañjali analyses these thought-waves and divides them into five types (I.5-I.11). Sometimes you experience thought-waves by direct contact with objects, or through the perception of ideas. This is the first type. The second type is when the senses of perception misperceive or deceive us. The example often given is of the observer who claims that the rabbit has horns. In the same way a jaundiced personality cannot see colours correctly. The senses are not well trained and wrong perceptions arise in the form of various thought-waves. The third type is misconception. Here, the senses of perception work, but the mind cannot conceive correctly and thought-waves are produced according to the misconceptions. The fourth is sleep. In sleep everything is silent. If there is no silence, you will not sleep. When you wake up after good sleep, then you remember your existence and say, "Oh, I slept well". However, that 'seer' as the witness remained awake throughout and expressed after that "I slept well". The *yogi* says that you must search that which witnessed your sleep. In this way, a thought-wave can be a guide to understanding the *citta*. Sleep should not be confused with dream. Patañjali uses the word *abhāva* (non-existence, or the feeling of non-being). *Bhāva* means existence, *abhāva* is the negative side of existence or the non-feeling of existence. It is only emptiness: Patañjali refers to this emptiness in deep sleep. For the ordinary person, the part of their experience that is nearest to the state of *samādhi* is sleep. In sleep there is no pain. Even a cancer patient sleeps. During sleep he or she is not aware that he or she has cancer. It is only when he or she wakes up that the impressions return, "I am a cancer patient!". So sleep is the highest state that an ordinary individual encounters. If we can retain the mind free of fluctuations in our waking state, or achieve that state of consciousness as in sleep, then we are in *samādhi!*

The last type of fluctuation is memory. According to Patañjali, memory is both a friend and an enemy, a hindrance and a help. Later on he talks on the profound level of memory, (*Y.S.*, I.20 and I.43), but here he is referring to the superficial functioning of memory. He explains that this memory consists of the imprints, which come from the other four types: direct perception, misperception, misconception and the non-feeling of the consciousness. Through memory we bring the past experiences of these states to the surface. Can one use the memory to recollect these experiences and use them to bring illumination? This does not mean that one stays in those experiences. It means that one uses them as a springboard to move on from those previous experiences. This is the transformation of thought-waves that takes place through memory. So memory must be understood in connection with the other four *vṛtti*.

VṚTTI AND THEIR ASSOCIATED *KLEŚA*

As there are five kinds of *vṛtti*, there are five kinds of pain or five kinds of pleasure associated with them. The *vṛtti* can be painful *(kliṣṭa)* or pleasurable *(akliṣṭa* – literally means 'non-painful'). It is very difficult to grasp this non-painful state, since a pleasurable thought-wave sometimes results in pain or a painful one in pleasure. We must then ask ourselves: "What are these five pains and pleasures?" The five pains are explained in *Sādhanā Pāda*. There he defines the five *kleśa* (*Y.S.*, II.3). *Kleśa* is derived from the same root as *kliṣṭa* and although it is usually translated as 'affliction', it has essentially the same meaning.

The first affliction, *avidyā* (ignorance), means the lack of right understanding and want of spiritual knowledge. *Asmitā* refers to the attitude of pride, ego or 'I know'. If someone is telling somebody something, before the speaker finishes, the 'I' of the other person says, "Oh, there is nothing new in that, I knew that!". This is *asmitā*. The next two are *rāga* and *dveṣa* – 'attachment' and 'aversion'. Joys and pleasures lead to attachment and attachment leads to hatred and pain. Patañjali describes the process of attachment and malice and advises the *sādhaka* to avoid attachment by developing equipoise in mind. Otherwise one develops psychosomatic and psychological diseases.

We run to the psychoanalysts for help. Yoga says we must be our own psychoanalysts and study and grip the problems of *avidyā*, *asmitā*, *rāga* and *dveṣa* within ourselves. This is what Patañjali wants us to study.

The last *kleśa* is *abhiniveśa* (attachment to life). We know that sometimes the instincts rise to the surface. The practice of yoga transforms instincts into intuition. This intuition is a knowledge that is tutored from within as the inner voice. This is directly communicated from the core of the being (Self) towards the individual self, intelligence, mind, cells, fibres, tendons and so forth. By this process, emotional upheavals come to an end and fearlessness sets in. When this intuition takes the lead through *yogic sādhanā*, then all *kleśa karma* come to an end. (*Y.S.*, IV.30).

ABHYĀSA–VAIRĀGYA: PRACTICE AND RENUNCIATION

In *sūtra* I.12 and I.16 Patañjali says that we can accomplish this intuitive power by practice and renunciation. But why does the idea of renunciation appear so soon? Surely this doesn't look easy to understand. How can the uncontrolled mind be renounced? How can we renounce it? Patañjali has given the answer in the fourth *sūtra*.

Vṛtti sārūpyam itaratra (*Y.S.*, I.4).

At other times the consciousness involves the seer and drags him in its fluctuations and wanderings.

Consciousness is close to the seer as well as to the mind, senses of perception, organs of action and body. Due to this closeness of consciousness with the seer and the body, it involves the seer with the body and the body with the seer.

By restraining the consciousness you reach that exalted state in which you feel the Self, but you cannot maintain this state for long. The consciousness likes to be supreme and prefers to have control over all. The consciousness reasserts itself and the Self recedes. Like a powerful magnet that draws the iron ore, the consciousness drags the Self towards its thoughts. Patañjali says, "you must renounce that". As soon as you renounce this pulling of the Self towards the thought-waves, then the consciousness moves towards the seer. Then the seer is at a distance from the thought-waves. If the seer goes with the consciousness, you are trapped; but if the same moves towards the seer, you are freed from thought-waves.

This process is known as *abhyāsa-vairāgya* (practice and renunciation). These two aspects cannot be separated. You have to go on practising. What must you practise? He has not described any practice, but he refers to *anuśāsanam* of the first aphorism as a code of conduct to be practised to restrain the *guṇa* and to get control over the fluctuations of the consciousness. This practice corresponds to the eight petals of yoga as described in the second and third chapters. By conquering our habitual patterns of behaviour, our character changes and we stabilise the mind and consciousness. By character building, the consciousness is stabilised. Patañjali wants us to understand this connection of the consciousness between the body and the seer.

What is the practice?

Often people ask, "How long do I have to do yoga to experience the fruits of its practice? When will I be able to realise the Self?" Patañjali answers these questions in *Y.S.*, I.14:

Sa tu dīrghakāla nairantarya satkārāsevitaḥ dṛḍhabhūmiḥ.

As long as the effort is continued for a long period, with devotion and without interruption the foundation gets firmly established in practice.

He does not speak of the final goal. He talks about the foundation. What is that foundation? He means that the consciousness, which is the origin of all disturbances, becomes stable. He does not speak of *samādhi* but of stability. When that stability comes, the consciousness comes under *vaśīkāra*, which means subjugation.

Dṛṣṭa ānuśravika viṣaya vitṛṣṇasya vaśīkārasaṁjñā vairāgyam (*Y.S.*, I.15): Renunciation is the practice of detachment from desires. That is: bringing the consciousness to a state of *vaśīkāra vairāgya*. *Abhyāsa* and *vairāgya* are like *yama* and *niyama*, 'what not to do' and 'what to do'. *Vairāgya* is such a practice to be free from attachment. In the second chapter he describes how happiness leads to *rāga* or attachment: *Sukha anuśayī rāgaḥ* (*Y.S.*, II.7): Pleasure leads to desire and emotional attachment. To stay free from this *rāga* is *vairāgya*. Thus, *abhyāsa* and *vairāgya* are the methods of practice to keep the consciousness away from the body and closer to the seer.

TYPES OF PRACTITIONER

Patañjali says that there are four types of practitioners *(sādhaka)*, *mṛdu, madhya, adhimātra* and *tīvra* (*Y.S.*, I.21-22): Feeble, average, keen and supremely enthusiastic. *Haṭha yoga* texts also describe four types of practitioners. Many commentators on Patañjali count only the first three and forget *tīvrasamvegin*. *Tīvrasamvegin* is a supremely enthusiastic *sādhaka* who has already restrained his consciousness and for whom freedom is in his hands. For him freedom is not bound by time whereas for the other practitioners, it is time-bound.

Many say that those who have succeeded in renunciation, freedom is quick and realisation easy. But can an individual like you and I renounce so fast? Only when one reaches the highest level of a genius is renunciation quick and freedom at once attainable. Know that they are geniuses as a result of their previous efforts. They have been practising in the way described by Patañjali in their early lives and the imprints of those lives have moulded their geniusness. We may say that we do not believe in *karma* (past lives) or rebirth. Are we not refining our actions every day? The process of refining has to continue; the quality of consciousness that we develop in this life is the seed of our future life. This is continuity.

All say 'train yourself!', even amidst failure. We must encourage all those who say, "Oh, I practise once a week," those who say, "I do it twice a week," "three times a week," and so on. They are *mṛdu* and *madhyama* practitioners. One who says, "I am practising five hours a day with total involvement," is an *adhimātra sādhaka*. Remember that *adhimātra sādhanā* does not mean the inclusion of the hours of teaching as practice. Teaching is not practising, it is not *abhyāsa*. The student who devotes five or six hours a day and practises meaningfully, attentively and devotionally is considered a keen student. Intensity of practice can similarly be graduated. If your practice is at a lower ebb, that is *mṛdu;* average intensity is *madhya* (or *madhyama)*, and high intensity is *adhimātra*. Whatever be the hours spent in *sādhanā* or the intensity of the practice, let us encourage them all to continue regular practice though it takes time to attain stability in the consciousness and the realisation of the Self.

THE FOUR ASPECTS OF THE BRAIN

Uninterrupted practice cultures the uncontrolled consciousness. The vacillations between *pramāṇa* (direct knowledge), *viparyaya* (misperception), *vikalpa* (misconception), *nidrā* (sleep), and *smṛti* (memory) disappear. *Vitarka* (analysis) becomes auspicious *savitarkā* and *vicāra* (reasoning) becomes judicious synthesis or *savicārā*. *Savitarkā* and *savicārā* transform *asmitā* (the power of 'I') into *sāsmitā* (auspicious self), whilst *ānanda* becomes auspicious *sānanda*.

These aspects cover the four parts of the brain; the front brain as the analytical part, the back brain is the reasoning part. The bottom brain is the emotional brain where pleasure and pain are experienced. The top brain is considered the seat of the individual self. Patañjali analyses and mirrors the functional and structural divisions of the brain like modern psychology. If the analytical brain thinks rightly and the reasoning brain decides the thinking process judiciously, then the emotional brain attains auspicious joy, establishing the stability of the self in the top brain.

Out of these four aspects, namely, *vitarka*, *vicāra*, *ānanda* and *asmitā*, the last is the most difficult to explain. In the second chapter, *asmitā* is said to be ego or the pride, while in the fourth chapter, it conveys a different meaning: *Nirmāṇacittāni asmitāmātrāt* (*Y.S.*, IV.4). Here, he describes *asmitā* as cultured consciousness. This cultured consciousness takes one closer to the individual self. When consciousness gains stability through yogic discipline its identity changes into seasoned wisdom *(ṛtaṁbharā prajñā)* (*Y.S.*, I.48).

VIRĀMA PRATYAYA: THE STATE OF SILENCE

When the four functions of the brain are inter-woven, one experiences a state of silence. Patañjali calls it *virāma pratyaya* (*Y.S.*, I.18). There is a pause in the brain as well as in the consciousness. Then one becomes a *prakṛtilayan*, undisturbed by the five elements and their infrastructures *(tanmātra)*, or lives in a bodiless state.

For example, we all experience a bodiless state in sleep. Then does that state become *samādhi?* Certainly not. That is why one is called *nidrā* and the other *sāsmita prajñā*. It is a state called *virāma pratyaya* – a state between *sabīja* and *nirbīja samādhi*.

Coming to the point, Patañjali's concern is on the understanding and progress of the yoga *sādhaka*. He warns the *sādhaka* not to be caught in this bodiless state or *prakṛtilaya* state and guides them to come out from this state and pursue *abhyāsa* with intensity:

> *Śraddhā vīrya smṛti samādhiprajñā pūrvakaḥ itareṣām* (*Y.S.*, I.20).
>
> Continue practice with faith, vigour, memory, complete absorption and total awareness.

After educating the *sādhaka* up to this *virāma pratyaya* state, he introduces here the notion of faith, because he does not want anyone to start by simply believing, but to have one's own experiences, which develop faith. Subjective truth surfaces and so one gains faith. Faith comes after experience. From this experience of faith one gains vigour *(vīrya)*. These two come through discipline.

He is telling us not to stop after such experiences as the state of void or the freedom from the body but to pursue the *sādhanā*. It may appear like resting in space. But he says that is not the end. This is a flash of the divinity that comes in the *sādhaka* to continue the *sādhanā* in order to proceed towards the *nirbīja samādhi* state.

YOGA AND GOD

Patañjali introduces the idea of God, and expresses Him in a syllable and not in a symbol. Patañjali was the first to introduce the characteristics of God. The other five orthodox schools of Indian philosophy, *sāṁkhya, nyāya, vaiśeṣika, mīmāṁsa* and *vedānta*, are highly dependent on the authority of the *Vedas*, though they accept God; whereas the two heterodox systems, Buddhism and Jainism, do not believe in God. Patañjali introduces the belief in God as an alternative method for quietening the mind and defines God as "He who is free from the reaction of actions". (*Y.S.*, I.24). God has neither pain nor pleasure. He advises us to concentrate and meditate on the syllable *āuṁ*, (*Y.S.*, I.28), *Śabdha Brahman*. In order to communicate, one opens first the mouth with *ā*. For continuance, one rolls and moves the tongue with *u*. And at the time of finishing, one closes the mouth with *ṁ*. Thus the base of *Śabdha Brahman* is dependent on *āuṁ*. That is why it is considered as the seed or the *bīja mantra* in our prayers. According to our philosophy, surrendering oneself to *bīja mantra* is surrendering oneself to God or *Brahman*.

MEDITATION

The moment the word 'meditation' is introduced, the present generation thinks that this is an easy method. When you ask them what they are doing, they all say, "I am meditating." Patañjali gives a variety of methods because he knows that meditation is not possible for all. The *citta vṛtti* keeps wandering here and there. And even if the practitioner has controlled the senses and the mind, he does not know at what time he may fall back. So he says, continue *sādhanā* from the *yama* to *dhāraṇā* as a right method, so that meditation comes naturally. First of all, do we have the capacity to accept our weaknesses and find out whether it is easy to become free from pain, sorrow and affliction, through meditation?

Have you heard of Ramakṛishna Paramahamsa? When he was suffering from terminal cancer, all his followers pleaded with him: "As you have totally surrendered to *Śakti*, why do you not ask Her to expel your suffering from cancer?" You know what his answer was. "Have I done meditation all these years just to ask for this disease to be taken away?" Do we (you and I) have that kind of mentality? You have heard of Ramana Maharshi – he also had cancer and the cancer had spread to such an extent that the doctors said that they would prefer to amputate his arm under anaesthesia. He immediately said, "You want my arm, don't you? Then, why must I go under anaesthesia? Cut it off!" Do you have that courage? Please understand Patañjali from this angle when he speaks of meditation as a method: He speaks first to the *sādhaka* of supreme intensity *(tīvra saṁvegin)* about the ways of meditation as they are close to the seer to achieve the goal. As *dhyāna* is very subtle and hard for the *sādhaka* who is keen *(adhimātran)*, average *(madhyama)* and mild *(mṛdu)*, he shows various alternative methods for them to follow. From this know how difficult meditation is for those who have not reached ripeness in their intelligence *(buddhi-paripakvatā)*.

ALTERNATIVE TO MEDITATION

Patañjali offers various methods for those who cannot meditate on God and begins with:

a) *Maitrī karuṇā muditā upekṣāṇāṁ sukha duḥkha puṇya apuṇya viṣayāṇāṁ bhāvanātaḥ cittaprasādanam* (*Y.S.*, I.33): If these above guidelines, of friendliness, compassion and joy are built up in a *sādhaka*, towards his fellow beings and if he cultivates indifference in himself, towards his pleasure and pain, good and bad, then his consciousness gets favourably disposed to live in serenity. As a yoga practitioner, I have learnt how one has to behave with people and how one has to handle oneself when one is confounded by the hindrances of body, mind and consciousness that come in the way of spiritual evolution. He wants each one of us to study the hindrances judiciously, so that one knows when to observe friendliness and compassion, feel gladness in progress and to show indifference to the things which disturb one's *sādhanā*.

b) *Pracchardana vidhāraṇābhyām vā prāṇasya* (*Y.S.*, I.34).
Another alternative way is by maintaining the pensive state felt at the time of soft and steady exhalation and during passive retention of the breath after exhalation.

From the exalted state of meditation *(dhyāna)*, Patañjali comes down to *prāṇāyāma*. Can you see the significance? One who suffers from a disease has only two choices, to accept his illness and surrender to God, or to challenge the disease and to fight it out with positive thoughts. Both acceptance and surrender are a form of meditation. However, as meditation is not possible to all, he wants us to watch the outgoing breath and to hold it passively. In this process the consciousness moves into a passive state and deepens into a quiet state before inhalation. This state of quietude is *prasānta citta* or tranquil state as the thought waves are made to fade at least during and after exhalation.

c) Then, he says, "go wholeheartedly into whatever subject that attracts one". (*Y.S.*, I.35). (I follow this guidance and get fully and totally absorbed in the *āsanas* and *prāṇāyāma*. By this statement of Patañjali one cannot call the *āsanas* physical exercises). Any ideal thought that attracts one totally to get absorbed in it, moves naturally towards the higher plane of consciousness. For twenty-four hours a day, great scientists' minds and bodies are fixed with dedication on one subject. By this total involvement, focus and absorption on their subject, they may be considered as yogis.

As I told you, this is the way I practise the *āsana* and *prāṇāyāma*. My critics are suffering from *vikalpa* or misconception; the terminology that they use to describe my practice is based on their misconception. Consequently they do not approach this subject as it should be tackled. With an open mind, one has to practise in depth to totally interpenetrate the art. One must be open to learning. The scientists want to break down the particles to understand the inner structure and mechanism of matter. I am interested in breaking down the molecules of my body into atoms to discover the internal processes of my being. I have to continue exploring the quality of movement and the quality of effort. If I say, "My head aches and head-balance brings relief," is that the end of it? No! What more can *Sālamba Śīrṣāsana* give? How I make my consciousness be in *Sālamba Śīrṣāsana* while keeping the body alert? How I can draw my mind away from the body, to bring alertness? This way I do and I have shown you the process. But this can only be understood when the student is ready. Then there will be total absorption.

d) Now, he shows another alternative: *Viśokā vā jyotiṣmatī* (*Y.S.*, I.36).
Contemplation on the serene and luminous light of the spiritual heart.

This sorrowless light is the *ātman*. But can we directly reach the *ātman?* Can you imagine how difficult it is?

e) So, he guides in the next *sūtra*, "Take those who have experienced and transcended sorrows, as objects of your concentration." (*Y.S.*, I.37). He says, "Take ideal persons such as Ramana Maharshi, Ramakṛishna Paramahamsa, Christ, Buddha or any other. Take them as examples. Develop character by studying their ways of behaviour and see that they help to quieten the consciousness".

f) He suggests we study, recollect and compare the states of consciousness during the wakeful state, the dream-filled and dreamless sleepy states, in order to live and experience steadiness throughout (*Y.S.,* I.38).

g) At the end, he says to contemplate on a pleasing object, conducive to the steadiness of the consciousness, for serenity (*Y.S.,* I.39).

CITTA PRASĀDANAM: THE DIFFUSION OF THE CONSCIOUSNESS

These various means help the consciousness to diffuse itself evenly throughout the body at each and every level. It is like water that is spilt and spreads evenly over the floor. It diffuses through the system and finds its resting level. This is *citta prasādanam* or *citta parikarma,* (*Y.S.,* I.33), where consciousness equates itself with each part, each cell, each molecule and each atom of the body, then experiences the whole body as nothing but consciousness. In this state, memory loses its power to restrict and block the control of consciousness.

Smṛtipariśuddhau svarūpaśūnya iva arthamātranirbhāsā nirvitarkā (*Y.S.,* I.43).

When memory is purified *(smṛti pariśuddhau),* memory, mind and consciousness cease to exist. Then it shines purely without reflection as non-analytical *samādhi.*

As a fruit which has fully ripened falls to the ground, memory falls from its previously held position. Since mind, consciousness and memory are inextricably linked, they ripen together and fall together. When that happens, a new light, a new knowledge dawns. Consciousness cuts off from the contact with the outer world and comes in contact with the inner world. This inner world is the seer or the Self. From then on, one gains intuitive wisdom as *ṛtambharā prajñā,* the truth bearing state of awareness which never wavers (*Y.S.,* I.46).

In this unwavering state, do not allow memory to hanker after, "I want to repeat such and such an experience", or "Oh, today I had a wonderful experience". In such moments the memory takes charge and one is caught again in thought waves. Then consciousness withers and one moves back to the intelligence of the head. So be very careful not to fall into the trap of memories. So keep away from memorising past experiences, but think afresh and do afresh.

Nirvicāra vaiśāradhye adhyātmaprasādaḥ (*Y.S.,* I.47).

With the attainment of purity in non-deliberate contemplation, there flows a profound and serene spiritual light.

At this moment, instead of the *citta* covering its frontier, the Self engulfs it. The self occupies the body everywhere, without any support, form, *mantra*, concentration on exhalation or on an ideal human being. You and I become a sorrowless light.

Here culminates the *Samādhi Pāda* of the *Yoga Sūtra* with this supreme state of *nirbīja samādhi* and then begins the *Sādhanā Pāda* with basic instructions for unevolved souls like us, or for those who have fallen from yogic grace.

Patañjali wants those who might have reached this state to continue practice, because sorrows may come at any time and disturb the equilibrium of the consciousness, the life force and the seer.

Heyaṁ duḥkham anāgatam (*Y.S.*, II.16).
The pains that are to come are to be avoided.

One does not know what pitfalls lie ahead. There are nine types of 'diseases'. They are physical, mental and spiritual discomforts and distractions. They are described in *sūtra* I.30. The last of these is *anavasthitattva* or the failure to maintain that exhalted state of *ṛtaṁbharā prajñā*. Hence, one must recognise the possibility of falling from that state. You may lose the power that has been gained. This loss of vision makes you become once more a beginner.

We have the examples of Godmen who have reached the spiritual heights and then think that they have everything. They forget their *sādhanā* and fall from their height. They not only do not accept the downfall, but are not willing to re-start their *sādhanā* and later end up in a state of failure and disappointment. We have read, seen or heard of such evolved souls who have fallen from spiritual heights. They may be born geniuses but they did not keep on educating and cultivating their consciousness to reach towards the supreme state of *nirbīja samādhi* (seedless state of *samādhi*). Therefore, I feel that *Sādhanā Pāda* is essential even for God-men and geniuses to maintain intellectual vigilance throughout their lives.

SĀDHANĀ PĀDA
(Chapter on Practice)

The *Sādhanā Pāda* begins with the background of the philosophy of affliction *(kleśa)* that man inherits in life. Patañjali explains what *kleśa* is and then shows the ways to overcome it.

KLEŚA

Sādhanā Pāda begins with the background of the causes of *kleśa* –affliction or pain, and the ways of eradicating them.

Avidyā asmitā rāga dveṣa abhiniveśaḥ kleśāḥ. (*Y.S.,* II.3).

Lack of right knowledge, pride or egoism, desire and joy, sorrow and hatred and fear of death are the afflictions.

Draṣṭṛdṛśyayoḥ saṁyogaḥ heyahetuḥ. (*Y.S.,* II.17).

The cause of pain is the conjunction of the seer with the seen.

Patañjali says, "Do not allow the core of being to come in contact with the world, but keep away from its contact in order to be free from pains and sorrows, whether they are physical, mental or spiritual". But he does not stop there. He goes on further and shows the origins of attachment and how both good and bad actions of past lives continue reacting in the present life. He draws our attention to *sāṁkhya* philosophy, which also states that "the contact of the seer with the seen is the origin of pain and the impressions of present actions determine a man's future". Both yoga and *sāṁkhya* systems state that man is entirely responsible for his future, since his life is moulded by the impressions of past actions. He must correct and develop himself, so that he is not trapped by these past impressions. He guides through yoga to mould a good future, by sowing a seed for a favourable *karma.*

He says that the instruments of the seer are all there to help the seer to come to an understanding of himself with the ingredients or the principles of nature. Nature is there for the evolution of the seer. These vestments, namely, the body, organs of action, senses of perception, mind, intelligence, ego and consciousness are meant for him to use to evolve towards transcendence. These vestments are to be treated as aids and not as hindrances in the progress of evolution, says Patañjali.

Though the consciousness continually drags the seer towards external objects, it is also there to serve the seer. Unfortunately, they take it the other way round, as if they are the lords of the seer. This is exactly what is happening in the world, hence Patañjali wants us to have command over these vestments through yogic discipline, so that the afflictions or *kleśa* are minimised or eradicated once and for all.

CONTROLLING THE SENSES

Just as the *prāṇāyāma* texts advise you to tame the breath as one would tame a tiger, Patañjali says to tame the organs of action by harmlessness, honesty, non-misappropriation, chastity and freedom from greed and unnecessary possessions. Suppose your mind tells you, "I want to hit this man, I want to kill this man," but your hands and legs refuse to act, can you kill that man? Similarly, if you want to tell a lie, but you keep your mouth shut, can you tell a lie? From this angle, Patañjali begins the subject with the peripheral body, especially the organs of action *(karmeñdriya),* for feeble and average practitioners.

Niyama is concerned with the inner body. They are hidden in *āsana*. *Āsanas* are practised because they give an internal bath through circulation; they purify the inner cells of the body. You may take a bath and clean the skin, but what about the inside body? We are all fighting against pollution in the atmosphere, but what about the pollution of the internal body? How do we discharge these impurities? Cleanliness, one of the components of *niyama,* means purification of both the internal and external body, as a congenial vehicle for a happy life. This cleanliness and happiness certainly leads one to culture the body, mind and conscience to unite with the Self through the thread of purity, as consciousness is the link between the external body and the internal body. Cultivation of *niyama* is self-discipline.

Psychedelic drugs trigger the senses of perception and the brain reacts. The yogi tries to learn to get this feeling in a natural way. Cleanliness controls senses of perception and organs of action. Contentment brings a sense of calmness in the nervous system and the consciousness; whereas zealousness, i.e., *tapas* and *svādhyāya,* develops discriminative discernment *(viveka khyāti).* This way Patañjali takes one from physical happiness and mental poise to spiritual delight, where the neurological and psychological systems are completely pacified. This is possible only to a person who has achieved complete restraint of the consciousness and has control over the central nervous system that is involuntary. That is how *yogis* are able to stop the heart and brain functions.

ĀSANA AND THE CELLULAR SYSTEM

If the *karmendriya* is tamed by *yama*, the *jñāneñdriya* is tamed by *niyama*. But the cellular system must be attended to, because the physiological body is the medium linking the skeletal body and the mental body. Unless we discover these links by ourselves within ourselves, we cannot study yoga properly. Changes in the personality take place when one gains control over the organs of action and the senses of perception. Here, a 'jump forward' takes place in the human system. If the cellular system is unhealthy, illness follows. So, the cells must be made healthy. Hence, the practice of *āsana* is given as the third petal of yoga.

Let me illustrate the intricacies involved by referring to a few of the *āsanas*. When you do *Utthita Trikoṇāsana* you stretch both the legs downward towards the feet. Then you suck the energy of the feet upwards, connecting the joints of the legs in order to re-adjust the torso to feel oneness and concord between body, mind and self. When you do *Utthita Pārśvakoṇāsana*, while bending one knee, you feel the cellular system encircling upwards from the lower legs.

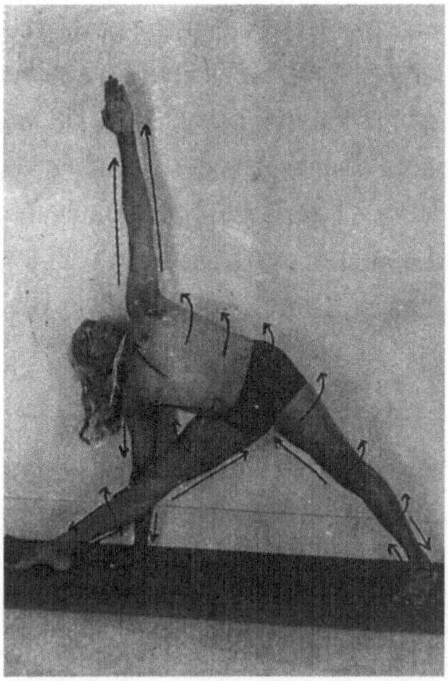

Plate n. 16 – *Utthita Trikoṇāsana*

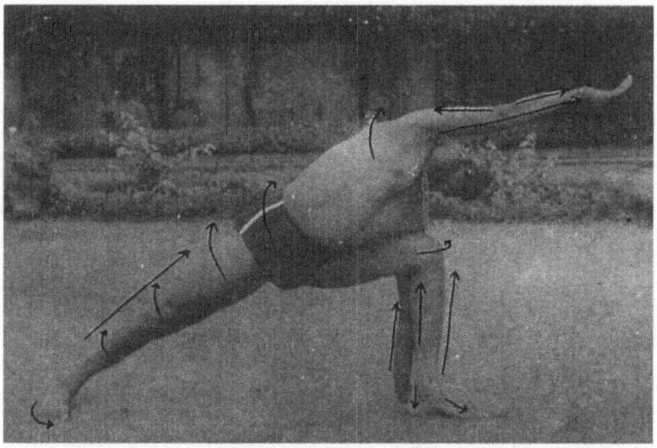

Plate n. 17 – *Utthita Pārśvakoṇāsana*

Plate n. 19 – *Vīrābhadrāsana* I

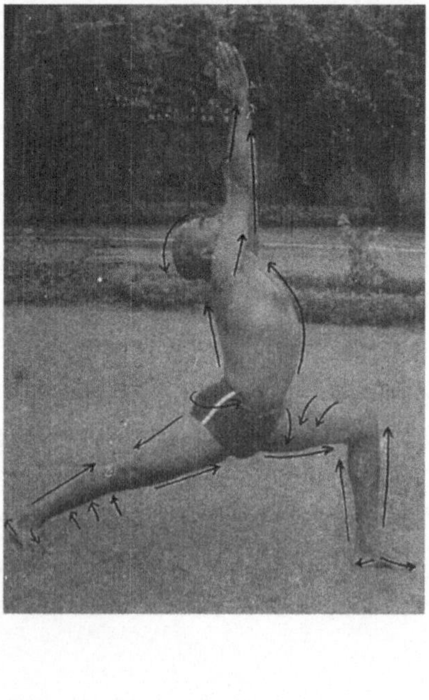

Plate n. 18 – *Vīrābhadrāsana* II

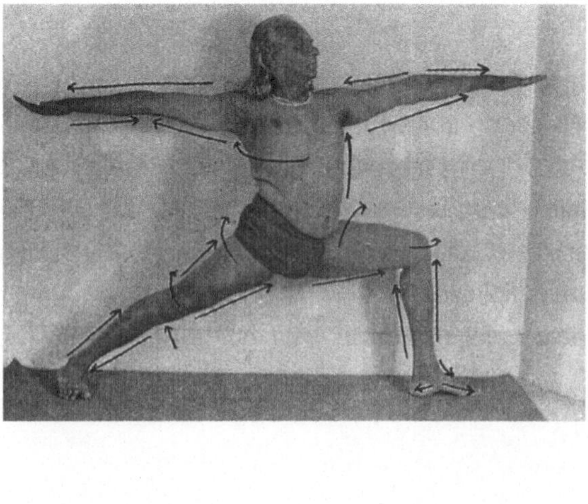

Here the energy and circulation moves upwards, whereas in *Utthita Trikoṇāsana* you direct the energy to be firm on the feet. In *Utthita Pārśvakoṇāsana* you observe that the blood is flowing towards the knee from the bottom foot. Have you ever felt it?

Observe *Vīrabhadrāsana* I. Here the blood circulates from the bottom of the knee towards the pelvis. In *Utthita Pārśvakoṇāsana*, you feel the blood flowing upwards from the lower leg and backwards from the knee to the hip of the front leg. The moment you change to *Vīrabhadrāsana* II, you feel the blood flowing on the back portion of the leg. By correct performance with the range of *āsanas* this way, the circulation of blood and the flow of energy in various directions in the leg increase and the entire leg gets cleansed. In order to do precisely, first you have to find out how to move the blood and energy in different areas by feeling the warmth generated by energy and circulation. In *Utthita Pārśvakoṇāsana*, if you feel warmth in the outer leg but not in the inner leg, then the circulation is taking place only on the outside and not inside. When the circulation is balanced inside as well as outside, it means you are doing a healthy pose. This is cleanliness *(śauca)*, which is implicit in *āsanas*. Otherwise the blood does not reach from the flesh to the marrow; the inner leg cells do not receive nutrients and they die; only the outer cells get a supply and are kept healthy.

With your conscious effort and attentiveness, the blood and the energy are supplied evenly throughout the body, and the cells are kept healthy. *Varāha Upaniṣad* speaks of *ratna pūrita dhātu* (the blood filled with jewels), a special constituent and essential ingredient of the blood in the body. This *Upaniṣad* uses the word jewel *(ratna)* for the healthy particles of blood *(rakta)*. It conveys that the quality of the blood should be brought to the level of a jewel. That is the effect of the *āsanas*, which build up the cellular system as jewels so that the body can take care of itself and the consciousness can attend to the higher aspects of life.

Take the example of AIDS. Scientific research has shown that the cellular system possesses its own intelligence and its own memory. It does not work with the dictates of the brain. It follows that yogic science works directly on the cells without the use of the brain. This is only possible if a thorough practice of *āsanas* is maintained, continuously for the cells to look after themselves. That is another reason why Patañjali advises not to discontinue practice. Even if one has experienced *samādhi*, one may fall from that state of illumination*. The cellular system, which occupies the entire body, needs discipline, toning, purification and sanctification through the practice of the eight-petalled yoga. The modern yogis who can barely stand, let alone walk, and have nothing to teach, say, "Oh, I have experienced such and such things, hence this practice is no longer required". The fact is that they have neglected their practice and lost their

* See *Vyāsabhaśya*, I.30.

power and hence use such words. This is escape from the truth. As ardent students of yoga do not listen to such words, but carry on the *sādhanā* disengaging from such advice.

PRĀṆĀYĀMA

When the cellular system has been cleansed and the nervous system purified, then the life force can pass through the tubes *(nāḍī)* without obstruction. That is why Patañjali says,

Tasmin sati śvāsa praśvāsayoḥ gativicchedaḥ prāṇāyāmaḥ. (*Y.S.,* II.49).

Tasmin sati means, "after this is accomplished"; i.e. when perfection is achieved in *āsanas*, he advises the *sādhaka* to begin *prāṇāyāma*. It is the art of regulating inhalation, exhalation and retention. This is the only instance where Patañjali shows space between two successive petals of *aṣṭāṅga yoga*. He does not say that you have to practise *yama*, then *niyama* and then *āsana*. Absolutely not. But for the real practice of *prāṇāyāma*, a restriction is brought in that it should be done only after the mastery of *āsanas*.

Unless the body is clean, the life force cannot move freely. Hence, *prāṇāyāma* practice is suggested after the mastery of *āsanas*. Mastery comes when the effort ceases and the dualities between body and consciousness and consciousness and Self disappear. (*Y.S.,* II.47)*.

Many underestimate the meaning of the *sūtra* II.46 *(Sthira sukham āsanam)* and translate it as "any comfortable pose is sufficient to go ahead in *prāṇāyāma* and *dhyāna*". But *sūtra* II.47 clearly mentions, *"Prayatna śaithilyānantasamāpattibhyām*", meaning that when the effort ceases, the consciousness becomes one with the *āsana* and the seer. For him, *āsana* is the seer and the seer is the *āsana*. You must experience this state in any *āsana* to understand its meaning. When the effort becomes effortless, then only the *sādhaka* experiences *sthirata*** (stability) and *sukhata**** (delightfulness). This applies to all the *āsanas*.

People do not study Patañjali thoroughly. They may sit in one pose comfortably for five minutes; when it becomes uncomfortable they change their position. Does this way of changing bring the effect of the *āsana*? I doubt it. The significance of *sthiram* and *sukham* is further elaborated in *Y.S.* III.47, by Patañjali, where he mentions that stability and pleasantness must be accompanied by adamantine willpower, strength, grace and beauty. When all these are accomplished, then the meaning of *āsanānuśāsana* (the code of conduct to be observed in *āsana*) is well understood. Remaining stale in an *āsana* and sagging the body and mind is not the meaning of the *āsana*.

---

* See *Vyāsabhaśya,* I.49.

** *Sthiratata* is the stability of mind

*** *Sukhata* is the delight of the body

Each *āsana*, like a sharp arrow, has to sharpen the intelligence, sensitise the consciousness and 'electrify' the doer. These are the fruits gained through uninterrupted practice and mastery of the *āsanas*. If you just sit in any comfortable pose, is there any beauty, grace or strength in it? In Patañjali's name todays yogis speak otherwise; this pains me.

After having achieved perfection in *āsana*, begin with the practice of *prāṇāyāma*, which is regulation of inhalation, exhalation and retention.

Many commentators say that Patañjali explains very little about *prāṇāyāma* and that it is in the *Haṭhayoga Pradīpikā* that it is described. But let us examine what Patañjali says. First he describes the aspects that we all know – *pūraka* (inhalation), *recaka* (exhalation), *pūraka-kumbhaka* (inhalation retention) and *recaka-kumbhaka* (exhalation retention). *Kumbhaka* is the connecting link between *pūraka* and *recaka*. Patañjali condenses language. However, he deals with various phases of *prāṇāyāma* in one *sūtra: Bāhya abhyantara stambha vṛttiḥ deśa kāla saṁkhyābhiḥ paridṛṣṭaḥ dīrgha sūkṣmaḥ.* (*Y.S.*, II.50): Here he explains the deliberate movements of *prāṇāyāma*. They are: regulated inhalation, regulated exhalation and regulated retention. One has to learn to regulate, spacing the breath in its place, by making full use of the space in the torso. Then he proceeds by suggesting the maintenance of depth and measured precise flow of the breath. This measured flow of movement and cessation of breath is to be prolonged and refined according to one's capacity. This is how he introduces the various facets in the art and science of *prāṇāyāma*. In II.51: *"bāhyābhyantara viṣayākṣepi caturthaḥ"*, he deals with the fourth movement of *prāṇāyāma* that transcends the first three movements and becomes non-volitional and non-deliberate. The brevity of these two aphorisms make it difficult for us to penetrate their meaning. In the above *sūtras* he gives us the full and precise technique of *prānāyāma*, guiding us how to place the breath accurately in the body, with measured time and precision, whether in gross or subtle levels.

TWO TYPES OF *KUMBHAKA*

The first is the deliberate retention of breath *sahita kumbhaka*, which I have explained in depth in my work *Light on Prāṇāyāma*.

The second is non-deliberate retention of breath. Here the consciousness gets absorbed. *Haṭha yoga* texts name this non-deliberate retention as *kevala kumbhaka*. In this type of *prāṇāyāma* you are not aware of the movement or the retention of the breath. It is like when we are absorbed in the vision of the beauty of the setting sun, we are not aware whether we inhale or exhale or retain the breath. Patañjali classifies this unintended *kumbhaka* as the fourth type of *prāṇāyāma* (*Y.S.*, II.51).

THE EFFECT OF *PRĀṆĀYĀMA*

Then Patañjali continues, saying that when the first four aspects of *prāṇāyāma* are mastered, the clouds which cover the mind and brain – the doubts and confusions that we all are aware of are dissolved (*Y.S.,* II.52). At that time the mind and consciousness get cultured to become a fit instrument for concentration *(dhāraṇā).*

Dhāraṇāsu ca yogyatā manasaḥ. (*Y.S.,* II.53). The mind and consciousness have now acquired the competence to move on towards the gateway of concentration for the realisation of the seer.

THE TWIN BROTHERS: *PRĀṆA* AND *CITTA*

When *āsana* and *prāṇāyāma* control the cells and life force, then stability in bio-energetical force *(prāṇa śakti)* takes place. *Prāṇa* is close to the individual self. According to the *Upaniṣads, prāṇa* and *citta* move together. Consider the consciousness and its parts as a tree. The seed is the seer. The part of seedling, which gives birth to the bud, is *citta* or consciousness. From the *citta* only one single bud shoots out. You see the bud and you say, "Here is a plant". That is the sprout or *asmitā,* the ego. First the seed did not show any form. Then the bud forms into a stem, which branches into two parts as intelligence *(buddhi)* and mind *(manas).* Then various branches and subsidiary branches grow out of them. These are the organs of action and the senses of perception. The leaves move and breathe sending energy to the base. This process is the involutionary method of yoga, by which the energy is drawn from the leaves and sent back to the base, whereas in the first process, the energy is drawn from the root and then is supplied to the top end of the tree as an evolutionary method.

Similarly, in our yogic system, we distribute energy through *prāṇāyāma,* by channelling it into the nervous system, which acts as a bridge between consciousness and Self. One often says, "I don't have enough energy"; it is because the energy cannot find clear avenues to pass through. As the course of the river changes when the banks change, similarly the energy avenues change according to our own occupation and modes of living. When we question, "Why is this part of me wearing out?" it is because the course of the energy channels have changed. Often we express that this part is alive but such and such part is dead. By the practice of *prāṇāyāma,* the vital energy is made to touch those areas with needed energy to revitalise those insensetive parts of the body.

The *Praśna Upaniṣad* says that breath and consciousness are twin brothers. These twins always move together. If the movements of the consciousness go wrong, then *prāṇa* loses its direction and if the *prāṇa* moves wrong, then consciousness gets disturbed. Hence, the theme of the *Praśna Upaniṣad* is that these twins must act in unison with each other as they are inextricably linked. When one is controlled, the other follows.

PRATYĀHĀRA

Patañjali defines *pratyāhāra* in the last *sūtra* of this chapter. *Pratyāhāra* is freeing the organs of action and senses of perception through the cultured mind and consciousness. Here begins the ethic of the mind and consciousness (*Y.S.*, II.54). Now you can see the gap that exists in understanding of yoga today. Patañjali, the organiser of the yoga system, declares that when the mind becomes ready for *dhāraṇā* (single pointed attention), it means that *pratyāhāra* is a table land which has built up stability in the mind for a long time at a stretch. Having learnt the control of the organs of action and the senses of perception through *yama* and *niyama*, and having silenced the cognisable pains by the practice of *āsana* and *prāṇāyāma*, now the mind, the cause of volition, has to be kept silenced by *pratyāhāra* so that it detaches completely from the *jñāneñdriya* and *karmeñdriya*. The mind is considered as the inner sense *(antareñdriya)*. The *sādhanā*, from *yama* to *prāṇāyāma*, is the evolutionary method from the self towards the periphery; while *pratyāhāra* is a transitory state, a plateau, for stabilising the earned evolutionary growth. The other three *(dhāraṇā, dhyāna* and *samādhi)* are the involutionary methods from the intelligent 'I', the imposter of the true Self and consciousness, towards the Self. (This involutionary journey in a way is also an evolutionary journey).

The first *sūtra* on *pratyāhāra*, (*Y.S.*, II.54), speaks of the effort to restrain the individual's wavering conduct by *yama* and *niyama*, while *āsanas* control the cellular system, which is non-cognisable to our eyes, yet keep it healthy.

As cancer or AIDS cannot be diagnosed quickly, they remain as unfelt *(adṛṣṭa)* diseases and the affected person feels fine and appears happy because the sickness is hidden and has not surfaced. Hence, it is a non-cognisable and non-painful sickness. The moment it surfaces, it becomes painful. That is why practice of *āsana* is required, so that non-cognisable diseases may be controlled through the culture of the cells. From *pratyāhāra* onwards, the *sādhanā* begins to work on the non-painful states of consciousness. (*Y.S.*, II.55).

ŚAKTI OF FIVE ELEMENTS

What is the *śakti* (power) that the cosmic breath carries? The explanation is very simple. We all talk about *kuṇḍalini*. Patañjali also talks about this, but the readers miss the point because he refers to it as *prakṛti śakti*. Later texts talk of *kuṇḍalini śakti*. A river has life; running water has life, but can it produce electricity? It cannot, unless water is channelled to move into the turbines in the hydroelectric power stations. Similarly, our normal breathing has life, but it cannot produce as much energy as required by the human system. In thermo-nuclear power stations, the water is heated to high temperatures and kept under high pressure. It is this super-heated water that rolls the turbines and generates electrical power.

The chemical composition of water is H_2O; hydrogen and oxygen, representing the elements of *āp* and *tej*, present in the water. By adding more heat *(tej* element) to the water, a new energy gets created. This is *prāṇa śakti*. We are made of five elements: earth, water, fire, air and ether. In human relations, one person introduces another person to a third one and they become three members. The same is true in the case of elements. The three co-operating elements are earth, air and ether, whereas water and fire are the antagonistic elements. If a house is on fire, what do you do? You call the fire brigade and they pour water on the fire to get it extinguished. Though water and fire are antagonistic elements, they also have the capacity for a kind of fusion, which produces a very powerful energy. The process of yogic discipline increases the potency of the energy within the human system through the interaction of these two elements. Then this *śakti* is stored in the *cakras* of the body and gets distributed by the element of ether, which works through the nervous system maintaining harmony, balance and concord between body, mind and self.

VIBHŪTI PĀDA
(Chapter on Attainments)

Here, Patañjali takes us from mind towards the subtle senses, namely, intelligence, 'I' or *ahaṁkāra* and consciousness. He shows the way of integrating these subtle senses to reach the seer. He describes the fruits *(vibhūti)* of yoga, that accrue before reaching the seer. These do not mean supernatural powers as it is so often translated, but it refers to the fruits of action. *Sādhanā* being the action, *vibhūti* refers to the fruits of actions. The *Samādhi Pāda* describes *antarātma sādhanā* (innermost practice), whilst the *Sādhanā Pāda* focuses on *bahiraṅga sādhanā* (external practice) and touches the transition from *bahiraṅga* to *antaraṅga sādhanā* (internal practice). *Samādhi Pāda* describes the practice at its most refined level, while *Sādhanā Pāda* gives a more basic and practical approach for non-initiates, novices and also for those who have fallen away from spiritual grace. This *pāda* explains *antaraṅga sādhanā* in depth and how the transition takes place from *antaraṅga* to *antarātma sādhanā*.

POINTS OF CONCENTRATION

Patañjali describes the ways of concentration to be practised on several different points from within the body or from outside the body. Many people now stress the use of external objects such as candlelight or flowers. If one advocates external objects, why not concentrate within oneself, like looking into one's throat, looking at one's heart, looking between the eyebrows, etc.? Can't one see the light of the intelligence, which is burning inside, although one is unaware of it?

Vyāsa, in his commentary, offers points for external as well as internal concentration. When someone suggests that you look at a beautiful rose, why not look at the beautiful balancing actions in your body. Are they not both acts of concentration? If you gaze at a candle, you are working with an organ of perception; if you work with the skin in controlling an *āsana*, that is another organ of perception. Do you see how false this distinction of the physical and the mental is? So do not get caught in such confused terms, always try to find out the truth yourselves.

For example, in *Setu Bandha Sarvāṅgāsana*, you concentrate on the heart. Where should you exactly concentrate when you do *Viparīta Daṇḍāsana?* Is it on the legs, arms or chest, or to integrate all these three as the focus of concentration? As you cannot concentrate wholly for a long time, you give up and say, "Oh, Mr. Iyengar, this is nothing but physical yoga!" But, you have no patience to stay longer in the pose, until the mind is ready to concentrate on the *āsana*.

Take for example *Sālamba Śīrṣāsana*. In *Sālamba Śīrṣāsana*, if you do not keep the shoulders parallel to each other, you have pain and you lose your balance. Do you not concentrate continuously in order to maintain the balance by raising your shoulders and keeping them parallel? Think about this and you will realise that you are doing something which is more than physical. You are working for the mind and body to unite as a single unit, by igniting the light of the Self. When we do not study the depth of each *āsana*, then we say, "Oh, I'm doing this for my health". By saying this you close the door to the possibility of other fruits which may come to you through that *āsana*. If you say, "Yes, I am doing this for my health, but let me also observe what other things come along with health", then you may receive more inner light. If you block your mind, your mind will never go beyond that block; this cannot be considered as concentration or meditation.

Please know that the objects of the world are the vestments of the Universal Soul: it is possible to concentrate on the outer objects, but they do not take you to the inner world; whereas yogic practices take you deep into the core of the body. The inner body consists of mind, intelligence, consciousness and Self. *Āsana* and *prāṇāyāma* help the body to connect the mind, intelligence and consciousness, for them to keep focus on the seer.

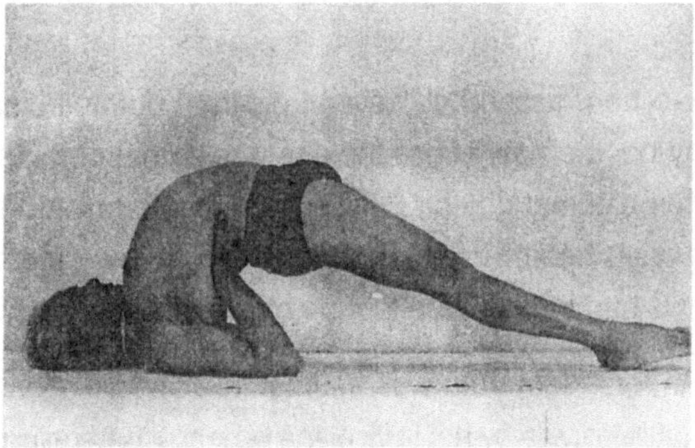

Plate n. 20 – *Setu Bandha Sarvāṅgāsana*

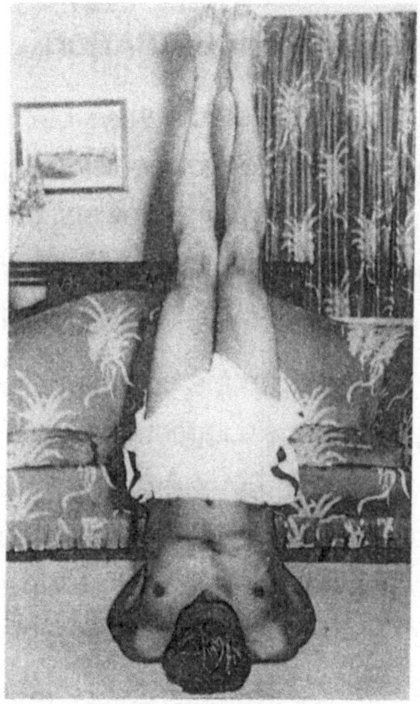

Plate n. 21 – *Sālamba Sarvāṅgāsana*

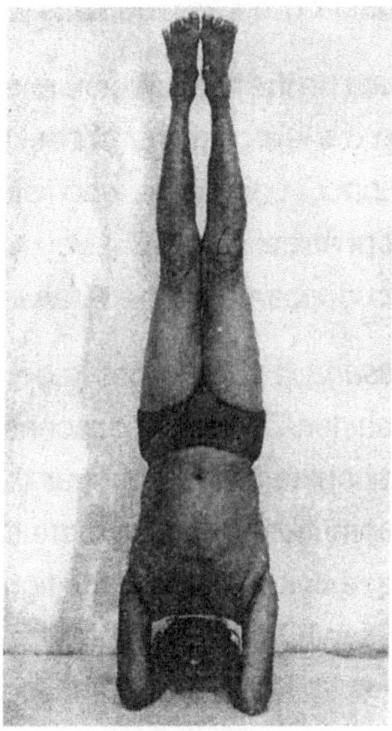

Plate n. 22 – *Sālamba Śīrṣāsana*

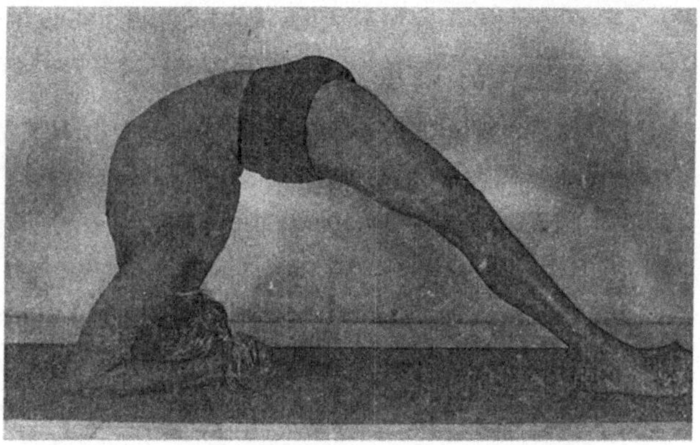

Plate n. 23 – *Dwi Pāda Viparīta Daṇḍāsana*

DHYĀNA (MEDITATION) IS AN UNINTERRUPTED FLOW OF ENERGY AND CONSCIOUSNESS

Yoga refers, however, to different kinds of blocks. These blocks are like the *bandha* (lock). In *Sālamba Sarvāṅgāsana*, when the chest is brought to touch the chin, it is called chinlock or *jālandhara bandha*. *Bandha* are used to consciously prevent the mind and the consciousness from going beyond certain points. With these restraints, we must try to extend the period of concentration a little longer in order to realise the oneness between the centripetal and the centrifugal movements. Patañjali says:

Tatra pratyaya ekatānatā dhyānam (*Y.S.*, III.2)

When attention is maintained on a single thread or a point without interruption from the beginning to the end, it is *dhyāna* or meditation.

Dhyāna happens automatically when concentration on an object, or on the self, or on an *āsana* or on movement of breath, does not fluctuate. If one maintains a single flow of energy with a single flow of consciousness, then that is *dhyāna*.

In *prāṇāyāma* sometimes you observe the breath; it begins to come well, then your attention fades and suddenly the breathing becomes rough. That is broken meditation. It is not *dhyāna*. You must control these tendencies and see that there is no break in the measured inflow or the outflow of breath. In the same way in *āsana* too: you must overcome all the blocks and brakes in the joints and muscles of the body, which interrupt the flow of movement and concentration. If you practise *āsana* in such a way, then the flow of movement and consciousness remains uninterrupted. When you achieve this state, prolong it. You are in meditation.

SAMĀDHI

In *Samādhi Pāda*, Patañjali explains the restraint of the fluctuating mind like shock treatment, "I restrain you and stop all your fluctuations". In *Vibhūti Pāda*, he says that the inner consciousness does not want to fluctuate and has a spontaneous tendency to restrain the mind. Between the moment of fluctuation and the moment of restraint of that fluctuation there is a pause, a space.

Vyutthāna nirodha saṁskārayoḥ abhibhava prādurbhāvau nirodhakṣaṇa cittānvayaḥ nirodhapariṇāmaḥ (*Y.S.*, III.9).

Study of the silent moments between rising and surfacing impressions *(vyutthāna saṁskāra)* and restraint of these impressions *(nirodha saṁskāra)* is the transformation of consciousness towards restraint *(nirodha pariṇāma)*.

Patañjali wants you to discover this silent space. You have to watch this space and learn to prolong this silent moment of pause. Only then do you draw near to *samādhi*. In this pause you have a glimpse of tranquillity. Instead of concentrating on restraint, concentrate on this silent moment. Develop this in your practice of *āsana* and *prāṇāyāma*. Cultivate your brain to get the sensitivity and stability to respond to this change. Learning to become familiar with this pause is *nirodha pariṇāma* (the restraining transformation). When you begin to lengthen this silent moment consciously, then you have achieved *samādhi pariṇāma*, or the transformation to *samādhi* (*Y.S.*, III.11). In *Samādhi Pāda* Patañjali defined *samādhi*; here he shows the process and method to learn.

See how beautifully Patañjali delineates the three transformations:

a) *nirodha pariṇāma*, the phase in which the mind switches between a state of fluctuation and a state of restraint;

b) *samādhi pariṇāma* being where the *sādhaka* begins to lengthen the pause between these two states;

c) *ekāgratā pariṇāma*, which is still a higher state has to be reached. *Ekāgratā* is usually translated as concentration; but if we break this word into *eka* and *agra* we find a subtler sense for this compound, meaning literally, 'one base' or 'one foundation'.

In *samādhi pariṇāma* there is a feeling of tranquillity. In this prolonged 'quiet space', there is no feeling of the self. In *ekāgratā pariṇāma* you penetrate deeper, the mind and consciousness rest in the abode of the *ātman*, the Self. Then there is no division; you are the Self in body, mind, intelligence, consciousness.

THE FRUITS OF PRACTICE

In the following part of *Vibhūti Pāda*, Patañjali has given a list of thirty-five experiences out of which one or a few may come to you as a result of your right practice. From mind reading to the ability to distinguish externally indistinguishable objects, are the fruits of practice. As human beings are all different, so are the fruits of their practice. If you persevere in your practice, one or the other of these powers surely will be felt. Patañjali says that such yogic fruits should be taken merely as a sign of right practice. He wants you to show indifference to these fruits and carry on with your *sādhanā*. Some who have tasted such fruits have been caught up in the net. They say, "Oh! See what I have attained!", they will be instantly caught up with the new type of *kleśa* or pain; whereas they have already fought to get rid of the *kleśa*. Patañjali's message throughout the *Yoga Sūtra*, is to be beware of oneself and to persevere with one's practice only and not to be carried away with attainments.

THE SEER AND THE SEEN

The last *sūtra* of the *Vibhūti Pāda* describes the state of *kaivalya*, which finally comes if one persists in one's practice.

Sattva puruṣayoḥ śuddhi sāmye kaivalyam iti (*Y.S.*, III.56).

When the exalted intelligence is as pure as the seer, the yogi has reached *kaivalya*, the perfect independence of the seer.

The seer is freed from the seen the moment the intelligence of nature becomes equal to the intelligence of *puruṣa* (the seer). *Kaivalya*, according to Patañjali, occurs the moment the intelligence of the seer and the intelligence of the seen become one. This is the highest state in which there is perfect freedom. It is a divine marriage of the Self with nature.

KAIVALYA PĀDA
(Chapter on Absolute Liberation)

Patañjali defines *kaivalya* (absolute state of aloneness or absolute emancipation) and shows how a yogi has to lead his life from this state of absolute emancipation. How the yogi who has achieved *kaivalya* should continue to live in the world is the essence of this *pāda*. At this state, all the yogi's desires for external things have vanished and his desires are now transformed towards the seer. At the very beginning of this *pāda*, he defines five types of yogis with divine powers who take birth:

Janma auṣadhi mantra tapaḥ samādhijāḥ siddhayaḥ (*Y.S.*, IV.1).

The divine powers come by birth, herbs, incantations and scrupulousness in practice and meditation.

Patañjali says that some are gifted by birth, some gain power through *mantra* and some through *auṣadhi* (medicine or herbs). In this context, he does not refer to the use of psychedelic drugs, with which we are so familiar in this century. Some attain powers through earnest practice and some through meditation. But only the last two types are capable of reaching *kaivalya*.

THE ENERGY OF NATURE

The energy of nature is *kuṇḍalini*. In the early traditions it was called *prakṛti śakti*. The later texts speak of it as *kuṇḍalini śakti*. In the *Haṭhayoga Pradīpikā*, *puruṣa* is called Śiva and *prakṛti* is called *śakti*. Patañjali refers always to *puruṣa* and *prakṛti*. He uses the word *prakṛti* to describe how the energy of nature flows abundantly in these yogis. This does not happen for you or me. It happens when one reaches that purified stage. You have all been misinformed on this point that *kuṇḍalini* can be awakened without *tapas* and I am trying to correct that misunderstanding. Patañjali says:

Jātyantara pariṇāmaḥ prakṛtyāpūrāt (*Y.S.*, IV.2).

In evolved souls the potential energies of nature flow in abundance to transform their consciousness dynamically.

So what should we do when this tremendous energy begins to flow? You have heard how many saints have become sinners and sinners have become saints. Though they experienced *samādhi*, they became victims of this extraordinary energy that is released from their genius. Patañjali gives a beautiful example of a farmer, to illustrate how the yogi should deal with this energy.

He says the farmer builds embankments to regulate the flow of water to his fields, whereas the yogi channels this abundant flow of nature's potential energies for the development of spiritual illumination and frees himself from the clutches of nature. *Nimittaṁ aprayojakaṁ prakṛtīnāṁ varaṇabhedaḥ tu tataḥ kśetrikavat* (*Y.S.*, IV.3). Later, he transforms the same potencies of nature into divine energy to flow in his mind and heart. Hence, one who is advanced in yoga must build banks in his body so that the energy is controlled, conserved and directed.

FREEDOM IN ACTION

When one has gained such a control over this abundant energy, then one is capable of understanding the true nature of *karma*. It is said in the *Bhagavad Gītā*, "Yoga is skill in action": *Yogaḥ karmasu kauśalam*. (*B.G.*, II.50). This is the common translation of the stanza, but it makes no sense to the common man. He thinks that the skill is to do actions without any expectation. But Patañjali explains this skill as a control. Let us see what Patañjali says about *karmasu kauśalam*.

Karma aśukla akṛṣṇam yoginaḥ trividham itareṣām. (*Y.S.*, IV.7).

Actions *(karma)* are of three types for average people. They are: white, black or a mixture of these two. The yogi's actions are neither white nor black, nor mixed. They constitute a fourth type: the pure action.

We of average intellect are susceptible to good actions, bad actions and mixed actions. A mixed action, for example, is when we want to offer help to someone or give something to somebody and then keep changing our minds about whether to help or not. These are the actions which you can define in these three categories. We are full of such things, but the yogi does not oscillate in thoughts. He has no mixed ideas or thoughts and feelings in his actions. He is free from these kinds of actions. When he gains that freedom, his actions become skilful. He is free from motivations and as His actions are free from motivations. He studies his actions and their effects dispassionately and gains the foreknowledge of both the short-term and the long-term effects of all his actions. (*Y.S.*, III.23).

FREEDOM FROM TIME

Patañjali goes on to show the connection between action and time. He does not discard the reality of past, present and future and as far as I understand, he is the only person who explained the relationship of past, present and future and also between time and timelessness. He says that action is dependent on time, as well as on timelessness.

A moment is timeless. The movement of moments is time. If the movement of moments goes back, it is the past. When the movement of moments moves forward, it is the future. Do not allow the moment to move into movement, observe it as moments only, without allowing yourself to get gripped in the thought of movement. It is like the spokes of a moving wheel; if you can see the spokes, you see the movement; if you do not see the spokes, then you cannot tell where the movement begins or where it ends. When your action is free, you are also free from time.

A moment is virtuous but the movement of moments is non-virtuous and that creates oscillation. If you can learn to observe the moment and live in it, you can avoid being caught in the movement of moments and remain stable in the moment. You are now beyond motivity. You have conquered action. That is the true skilfulness. If you reach this state, then you have conquered time. Here, the consciousness loses its identity. It is inexorably drawn, due to the spiritual force of gravity, towards the seer. Now the seer is freed from time and action.

PERSEVERANCE IN PRACTICE: THE ULTIMATE *SAMĀDHI*

Breaks may still occur in this new state of consciousness as a result of impressions from previous experiences: *Tat cchidreṣu pratyayāntarāṇi saṁskārebhyaḥ.* (*Y.S.,* IV.27): With all this progress, the force of subliminal impressions may still surface, often creating a fissure in the consciousness *(citta)* disturbing its unity with the seer and creating a divisible state between the consciousness and the seer. When the fissures appear and the *citta* begins to fluctuate and move away from the seer, then the *sādhaka* must intensify his *sādhanā.* See how Patañjali is consistent in his instruction, that practice is essential throughout. Only when the fissures stop appearing and all the subliminal impressions are exhausted, then the search of the *sādhaka* comes to an end. There is no need to search further because the *ātman* exists within and without. The seeker discovers that the object of seeking and instrument of seeing is himself, the seer. This ends the spiritual quest as the seeker becomes the Soul and goal.

In the *Yoga Sūtra* two terms are used to describe this ultimate state: in *Samādhi Pāda,* Patañjali calls it *nirbīja samādhi (samādhi* without seed) and in *Kaivalya Pāda* he calls it *dharmamegha samādhi,* (*Y.S.,* IV.29), literally *"dharma-pouring samādhi".* These two terms are like the two sides of a coin; they are two ways of viewing the same phenomenon. How can we explain the *"Dharma*-pouring *samādhi"?* Sometimes the sky is covered by clouds for days and days. You see neither the sun nor the rain and you become gloomy. Is this not true? You ask, "Why does it not rain? Why can we not see the sun?". It is the divine duty, the *dharma* of clouds, to pour down rain, but still they do not pour. Such weather is like our brains. The clouds are formed in our intelligence and stay for days together, obscuring the intelligence *(buddhi),* which is like the rays of the sun within us. Do not let those clouds settle! Keep the light of the intelligence striking the entire frontier of your body, as it has its own rhythms like the moon, which waxes and wanes.

Ātmā, the Self, is the sun in us. It never fades. So when the *citta*, this fluctuating part of us, rests in the sun – the Self – the clouds pour down their rain and finally disappear. When these clouds disappear, the light of the intelligence of the seer shines everywhere in the body with perfect clarity. This means that one has conquered the *guṇa* – the qualities of nature, and has sighted the *puruṣa*. Thus ends yoga.

This is what everybody is seeking and everyone wants to experience. If not today, then tomorrow, if not tomorrow, then next week, next month, next year or even next life. Even if it takes several lives, have patience and continue *sādhanā* until the seer is sighted.

We are all involved in this process of progression. As I have said before, casual practice brings casual results, temperamental practice brings temperamental results and total practice brings total results.

So my friends, this is the way to light the lamp of intelligence. Begin with the body because the body is the cover of the seer. Just as you open all the doors and windows of a closed house for the stale air to go out and for the fresh air to enter, maintain your practice in a way that your body, mind, consciousness and self do not become polluted and obscured, creating darkness within and without. Throw away the pollution and cast off all the coverings of the skeletal, physiological, mental, intellectual and conscious sheaths or layers, one by one, till you become the seer within and without. This is the indivisible state of existence! *"Tadā draṣṭuḥ svarūpe avasthānam!"** (*Y.S.*, 1.3).

PREPARING FOR THE LIGHT

I hope you have grasped the points. The study and exposition of the *Yoga Sūtra* of Patañjali is an extremely difficult subject, but an extremely important one for self-progression. If you do not

* Then the seer dwells in his own true splendour (*Y.S.*, I.3).

provide the necessary preparation, what will happen to you when the light of the Self comes? You will fall spiritually sick! Remember when Arjuna asked Lord Krishna, "I want to see if you are really the Lord of the Universe; show me your true form and your pure original nature and not the pictures of imagination you have used till now". Lord Krishna showed to Arjuna His true form. He became not only nervous but also afraid to see His true manifestation. So he begs Lord Krishna to bless him with divine eyes, so that he could have His *viśvārūpa darśana* (God's manifestation in full form) (*Bhagavad Gītā*, chapter XI,8).

Remember Patañjali's aphorism always: *"Heyaṁ duḥkham anāgatam."** You do not know what pains await you. If you are not strong enough, the joy of the divine light can also be unbearable. Then people say, "It happened to me in my meditation! I am so frightened. I don't know what to do!" They cannot cope and become mentally ill. How many meditators have become schizophrenics? Have you not heard of these cases? So one has to be careful and cautiously tread the path of spiritual practice. Develop the strength to endure this and work to keep that strength. That is why *āsana* and *prāṇāyāma* must be practised regularly, so that the nervous system and the will-power are kept strong enough to bear the divine light when it dawns. Carry on and may God bless you all.

---

* The pain which is yet to come, can and is to be avoided.

THE YOGA SŪTRA CODIFIED ACCORDING TO THE THEMES FOR READY REFERENCE

1. WHY YOGA

I.30 *vyādhistyānasaṁśaya pramādālasyāvirati bhrāntidarśanālabdhabhūmikatvānavasthitatvāni cittavikṣepāste'ntarāyāḥ*
I.31 *duḥkhadaurmanasyāṅgamejayatvaśvāsapraśvāsā vikṣepasahabhuvaḥ*
II.16 *heyaṁ duḥkhamanāgatam*
II.17 *draṣṭṛdṛśyayoḥ saṁyogo heyahetuḥ*
II.23 *svasvāmiśaktyoḥ svarūpopalabdhihetuḥ saṁyogaḥ*
II.26 *vivekakhyātiraviplavā hānopāyaḥ*
II.33 *vitarkabādhane pratipakṣabhāvanam*
II.34 *vitarkā hiṁsādayaḥ kṛtakāritānumoditā lobhakrodhamohapūrvakā mṛdumadhyādhimātrā duḥkhājñānānantaphalā iti pratipakṣabhāvanam*
IV.10 *tāsāmanāditvaṁ cāśiṣo nityatvāt*
IV.11 *hetuphalāśrayālambanaiḥ saṅgṛhītatvādeṣāmabhāve tadabhāvaḥ*
IV.30 *tataḥ kleśa karma nivṛttiḥ*

2. PREVENTION AND CURE

II.16 *heyaṁ duḥkhamanāgatam*
IV.28 *hānameṣāṁ kleśavaduktam*

3. WHAT IS YOGA

I.1 *atha yogānuśāsanam*
I.2 *yogaścittavṛtti nirodhaḥ*
II.1 *tapaḥsvādhyāyeśvarapraṇidhānāni kriyāyogaḥ*
II.4 *avidyā kṣetramuttareṣāṁ prasuptatanuvicchinnodārāṇām*
III.9 *vyutthānanirodhasaṁskārayor abhibhavaprādurbhāvau nirodhakṣaṇacittānvayo nirodhapariṇāmaḥ*
III.10 *tasya praśāntavāhitā saṁskārāt*
III.11 *sarvārthataikāgratayoḥ kṣayodayau cittasya samādhipariṇāmaḥ*

III.12 *tataḥ punaḥ śāntoditau tulyapratyayau cittasyaikāgratāpariṇāmaḥ*
III.14 *śāntoditāvyapadeśyadharmānupātī dharmī*
III.19 *pratyayasya paracittajñānam*
III.20 *na ca tatsālambanaṁ tasyāviṣayībhūtatvāt*
III.51 *tadvairāgyādapi doṣabījakṣaye kaivalyam*
IV.18 *sadā jñātāścittavṛttayastatprabhoḥ puruṣasyāpariṇāmitvāt*
IV.25 *viśeṣadarśina ātmabhāvabhāvanānivṛttiḥ*
IV.26 *tadā vivekanimnaṁ kaivalyaprāgbhāraṁ cittam*
IV.29 *prasaṁkhyāne'pyakusīdasya sarvathā vivekakhyāterdharmameghaḥ samādhiḥ*

4. *AṢṬĀÑGA YOGA* AND ITS EFFECTS (EIGHT PETALS OF YOGA)

I.3 *tadā draṣṭuḥ svarūpe'vasthānam*
II.18 *prakāśakriyāsthitiśīlaṁ bhūtendriyātmakaṁ bhogāpavargārthaṁ dṛśyam*
II.20 *draṣṭā dṛśimātraḥ śuddho'pi pratyayānupaśyaḥ*
II.25 *tadabhāvāt saṁyogābhāvo hānaṁ taddṛśeḥ kaivalyam*
II.28 *yogāñgānuṣṭhānādaśuddhikṣaye jñānadīptirāvivekakhyateḥ*
II.29 *yamaniyamāsanaprāṇāyāmapratyāhāradhāraṇādhyāna-samādhayo'ṣṭāvañgāni*
III.34 *prātibhādvā sarvam*
III.35 *hṛdaye cittasaṁvit*
III.36 *sattvapuruṣayoratyantāsaṁkīrṇayoḥ pratyayāviśeṣo bhogaḥ parārthatvāt svārthasaṁyamāt puruṣajñānam*
III.37 *tataḥ prātibhaśrāvaṇavedanādarśāsvādavārta jāyante*
III.39 *bandhakāraṇaśaithilyāt pracārasaṁvedanācca cittasya paraśarīrāveśaḥ*
III.43 *kāyākāśayoḥ saṁbandhasaṁyamāllaghutūlasamāpatteścā'kāśagamanam*
III.46 *tato'ṇimādiprādurbhāvaḥ kāyasaṁpat taddharmānabhighātaśca*
aṣṭasiddhi (aṇimā, mahimā, laghimā, garimā, prāptī, prākāmya, īśatva and vaśitva)
III.47 *rūpalāvaṇyabalavajrasaṁhananatvāni kāyasaṁpat*
III.48 *grahaṇasvarūpāsmitānvayārthavattvasaṁyamādindriyajayaḥ*
III.49 *tato manōjavitvaṁ vikaraṇabhāvaḥ pradhānajayaśca*
III.50 *sattvapuruṣānyatākhyātimātrasya sarvabhāvādhiṣṭhātṛtvaṁ sarvajñātṛtvaṁ ca*
III.51 *tadvairāgyādapi doṣabījakṣaye kaivalyam*
III.55 *tārakaṁ sarvaviṣayaṁ sarvathāviṣayamakramaṁ ceti vivekajaṁ jñānam*
III.56 *sattvapuruṣayoḥ śuddhisāmye kaivalyamiti*
IV.3 *nimittamaprayojakaṁ prakṛtīnāṁ varaṇabhedastu tataḥ kṣetrikavat*
IV.22 *citerapratisaṁkramāyāstadākārāpattau svabuddhisaṁvedanam*
IV.25 *viśeṣadarśina ātmabhāvabhāvanānivṛttiḥ*

IV.26 *tadā vivekanimnaṁ kaivalyaprāgbhāraṁ cittam*
IV.29 *prasaṁkhyāne'pyakusīdasya sarvathā vivekakhyāterdharmameghaḥ samādhiḥ*
IV.30 *tataḥ kleśa karma nivṛttiḥ*
IV.31 *tadā sarvāvaraṇamalāpetasya jñānasyānantyāt jñeyamalpam*
IV.32 *tataḥ kṛtārthānāṁ pariṇāmakramasamāpattirguṇānām*
IV.33 *kṣaṇapratiyogī pariṇāmāparāntanirgrāhyaḥ kramaḥ*
IV.34 *puruṣārthaśūnyānāṁ guṇānāṁ pratiprasavaḥ kaivalyaṁ svarūpapratiṣṭhā vā citiśaktiriti*

YAMA

II.30 *ahiṁsāsatyāsteyabrahmacāryāparigrahā yamāḥ*
II.35 *ahiṁsāpratiṣṭhāyām tatsannidhau vairatyāgaḥ*
II.36 *satyapratiṣṭhāyāṁ kriyāphalāśrayatvam*
II.37 *asteyapratiṣṭhāyām sarvaratnopasthānam*
II.38 *brahmacaryapratiṣṭhāyāṁ vīryalābhaḥ*
II.39 *aparigrahasthairye janmakathaṁtāsaṁbodhaḥ*
III.24 *maitryādiṣu balāni*
III.25 *baleṣu hastibalādīni*

***YAMA* FOR ALL**

II.31 *jātideśakālasamayānavacchinnāḥ sārvabhaumā mahāvratam*

NIYAMA

II.32 *śaucasantoṣatapaḥsvādhyāyeśvarapraṇidhānāni niyamāḥ*
II.40 *śaucāt svāñgajugupsā parairasaṁsargaḥ*
II.41 *sattvaśuddhisaumanasyaikāgryendriyajayātmadarśana-yogyatvānica*
II.42 *santoṣādanuttamaḥ sukhalābhaḥ*
II.43 *kāyendriyasiddhiraśuddhikṣayāttapasaḥ*
II.44 *svādhyāyādiṣṭadevatāsaṁprayogaḥ*
II.45 *samādhisiddhirīśvarapraṇidhānāt*

ĀSANA

I.33 *maitrīkaruṇāmuditopekṣāṇāṁ sukhaduḥkhapuṇyāpuṇya viṣayāṇāṁ bhāvanātaścittaprasādanam*
II.46 *sthirasukhamāsanam*
II.47 *prayatnaśaithilyānantasamāpattibhyām*
II.48 *tato dvandvānabhighātaḥ*
III.47 *rūpalāvaṇyabalavajrasaṁhananatvāni kāyasaṁpat*

PRAṆĀYĀMA

I.34	*pracchardanavidhāraṇābhyāṁ vā prāṇasya*
II.49	*tasminsati śvāsapraśvāsayorgativicchedaḥ prāṇāyāmaḥ*
II.50	*bāhyābhyañtarastambhavṛttirdeśakālasaṁkhyābhiḥ paridṛṣṭo dīrghasūkṣmaḥ*
II.51	*bāhyābhyañtaraviṣayākṣepī caturthaḥ*
II.52	*tataḥ kṣīyate prakāśāvaraṇam*
II.53	*dhāraṇāsu ca yogyatā manasaḥ*
III.40	*udānajayājjalapaṅkakaṇṭakādiṣvasaṅga utkrāntiśca*
III.41	*samānajayājjvalanam*
III.42	*śrotrākāśayoḥ saṁbandhasaṁyamāddivyaṁ śrotram*
III.43	*kāyākāśayoḥ saṁbandhasaṁyamāllaghutūlasamāpatteścā'kāśagamanam*

PRATYĀHĀRA

I.35	*viṣayavatī vā pravṛttirutpannā manasaḥ sthitinibandhanī*
II.54	*svaviṣayāsaṁprayoge cittasya svarūpānukāra ivendriyāṇāṁ pratyāhāraḥ*
II.55	*tataḥ paramāvaśyatendriyāṇām*

DHĀRAṆĀ

I.36	*viśokā vā jyotiṣmatī*
I.37	*vītarāgaviṣayaṁ vā cittam*
II.53	*dhāraṇāsu ca yogyatā manasaḥ*
III.1	*deśabandhaścittasya dhāraṇā*

DHYĀNA

I.29	*tataḥ pratyakcetanādhigamo'pyantarāyābhāvaṣca*
I.38	*svapnanidrājñānālambanaṁ vā*
I.39	*yathābhimatadhyānādvā*
II.11	*dhyānaheyāstadvṛttayaḥ*
III.2	*tatra pratyayaikatānatā dhyānam*
IV.6	*tatra dhyānajamanāśayam*

SAMĀDHI

I.20	*śrāddhāvīryasmṛtisamādhiprajñāpūrvaka itareṣām*
I.46	*tā eva sabījaḥ samādhiḥ*
I.51	*tasyāpi nirodhe sarvanirodhānnirbījaḥ samādhiḥ*
II.2	*samādhibhāvanārthaḥ kleśatanūkaraṇārthaśca*
II.45	*samādhisiddhirīśvarapraṇidhānāt*
III.3	*tadevārthamātranirbhāsaṁ svarūpaśūnyamiva samādhiḥ*

III.11 *sarvārthataikāgratayoḥ kṣayodayau cittasya samādhipariṇāmaḥ*

III.38 *te samādhāvupasargā vyutthāne siddhayaḥ*

IV.1 *janmauṣadhimantratapaḥ samādhijāḥ siddhayaḥ*

IV.29 *prasaṁkhyāne'pyakusīdasya sarvathā vivekakhyāterdharmameghaḥ samādhiḥ*

***SAMĀDHI VIBHĀGA* (types of *samādhi*)**

Samādhi is of two types.

i) *Saṁprajñāta Samādhi* or *Sabīja Samādhi*

ii) *Asaṁprajñāta Samādhi* or *Nirbīja Samādhi*

i) *Saṁprajñāta Samādhi* or *Sabīja Samādhi*

I.17 *vitarkavicārānañdāsmitārūpānugamāt saṁprajñātāḥ*

I.18 *virāmapratyayābhyāsapūrvaḥ saṁskāraśeṣo'nyaḥ*
(a stabilising state)

I.42 *tatra śabdārthajñānavikalpaiḥ saṅkīrṇā savitarkā samāpattiḥ*

I.43 *smṛtipariśuddhau svarūpaśūnyevārthamātranirbhāsā nirvitarkā*

I.44 *etayaiva savicārā nirvicārā ca sūkṣma viṣayā vyākhyātā*

ii) *Asaṁprajñāta Samādhi* or *Nirbīja Samādhi*

I.51 *tasyāpi nirodhe sarvanirodhānnirbījaḥ samādhiḥ*

IV.29 *prasaṁkhyāne'pyakusīdasya sarvathā vivekakhyāterdharmameghaḥ samādhiḥ*

IV.34 *puruṣārthaśūnyānāṁ guṇānāṁ pratiprasavaḥ kaivalyaṁ svarūpapratiṣṭhā vā citiśaktiriti*

5. *SAṀYOGA* (UNION)

II.17 *draṣṭṛdṛśyayoḥ saṁyogo heyahetuḥ*

II.23 *svasvāmiśaktyoḥ svarūpopalabdhihetuḥ saṁyogaḥ*

II.25 *tadabhāvāt saṁyogābhāvo hānaṁ taddṛśeḥ kaivalyam*

6. *ABHYĀSA* (PRACTICE)

I.1 *atha yogānuśāsanam*

I.12 *abhyāsavairāgyābhyām tannirodhaḥ*

I.13 *tatra sthitau yatno'bhyāsaḥ*

I.14 *sa tu dīrghakālanairantaryasatkārāsevito dṛḍhabhūmiḥ*

I.18 *virāmapratyayābhyāsapūrvaḥ saṁskāraśeṣo'nyaḥ*

I.20 *śrāddhāvīryasmṛtisamādhiprajñāpūrvaka itareṣām*

I.32 *tatpratiṣedhārthamekatattvābhyāsaḥ*

I.33 *maitrīkaruṇāmuditopekṣāṇāṁ sukhaduḥkhapuṇyāpuṇya viṣayāṇāṁ bhāvanātaścittaprasādanam*